Introduction to Behavioral Pharmacology

For Jessie, Catherine, and the Dragons

Introduction to Behavioral Pharmacology

Edited by

Alan Poling

Western Michigan University

and

Thomas Byrne

Massachusetts College of Liberal Arts

CONTEXT PRESS

Reno, Nevada

Publisher's Note

This publication is designed to provide accurate and authoritative information in regard to the subject matter covered. It is sold with the understanding that the publisher is not engaged in rendering psychological, financial, legal, or other professional services. If expert assistance or counseling is needed, the services of a competent professional should be sought.

Distributed in Canada by Raincoast Books

© 2000 Context Press

Context Press is an imprint of New Harbinger Publications, Inc.
5674 Shattuck Ave.
Oakland, CA 94609
www.newharbinger.com

Printed in the United States of America

Library of Congress Cataloging-in-Publication Data

Introduction to Behavioral Pharmacology/ edited by Alan Poling and Thomas Byrne.
    p. cm.
    Includes bibliographical references
    ISBN-13: 978-1-878978-36-3
    ISBN-10: 1-878978-36-5
    1. Pharmacology.   2. Behavior Analysis.

    I. Poling, Alan, 1950- II. Byrne, Thomas, 1972-

RM315.I588 2000
615.78—dc21   00-025399   CIP

Preface

On superficial examination, it appears that drugs, like gods, work in mysterious ways. One has only to see a group of people drinking in excess to recognize that not everyone responds in the same way to a given substance. Some drunks are aggressive, others are maudlin. More than a few are depressive or amorous. What makes them different? This is the kind of question than interests behavioral pharmacologists, and it is the purpose of this book to provide a conceptual framework adequate for answering such questions. The reader who masters its contents won't be able to provide a detailed explanation of why S. F. cries and F. S. sings when they are in the hops, but he or she will have a better understanding of how drugs produce their behavioral effects, and of the many variables that influence drug action. Such information is worth having, for we are constantly exposed to, and affected by, drugs.

Introduction to Behavioral Pharmacology comprises 10 chapters. Chapter 1 describes the fundamental features of behavioral pharmacology, which combines procedures and concepts of behavior analysis and pharmacology to explore and explain the behavioral effects of drugs, and summarizes important historical events in the field's development. Chapter 2 introduces behavior analysis and Chapter 3 does the same for pharmacology. Chapter 4 describes how drugs affect the brain and how these actions relate to behavior change. Chapters 5 and 6 summarize procedures commonly used by behavioral pharmacologists to study drug effects in nonhumans and humans, respectively. Chapter 7 describes how drugs affect behavior by acting as functional stimuli in the context of respondent and operant conditioning. Chapter 8 summarizes the variables that may influence the effects of a given drug. Chapter 9 considers how behavioral pharmacology can contribute to the evaluation of psychotropic drugs, which are medications prescribed to deal with behavior disorders, including mental illness. Chapter 10 discusses drug abuse from the perspective of behavioral pharmacology. To aid students, important terms appear in **bold-faced type** throughout the book.

Introduction to Behavioral Pharmacology is written for people with no special training in pharmacology or behavior analysis, although at least passing familiarity with the latter area will make certain sections easier to understand. The book is an edited text, but all chapters were contributed by faculty and students from the Psychology Department at Western Michigan University, and one of us (AP) is a co-author of each chapter. Our aim was to minimize the unevenness characteristic of edited texts, while retaining the breadth of coverage that multiple contributors bring to a work. If we have succeeded in either regard, it is due largely to the good efforts of those who worked with us. We thank them. We also thank Steve Hayes for his patience in allowing us to complete this project years after our promised date of completion. Finally, and most importantly, we thank Catherine, Jessie, Serah, and Kristal for their love and support, which make all efforts worthwhile.

Alan Poling and Thomas Byrne
Spring 2000

Table of Contents

Chapter 1

Introduction

Alan Poling
Western Michigan University

The discipline known as behavioral pharmacology uses methods and concepts from behavior analysis to explore and explain the behavioral effects of drugs. Behavior analysis is a unique natural science approach to the study of behavior popularized by B. F. Skinner (e.g., 1938, 1953, 1974). Because behavior analysis forms the theoretical and methodological foundation of behavioral pharmacology, it deserves careful attention. This chapter summarizes the behavior analytic approach to understanding behavior in general, and considers how this approach is used to analyze drug effects.

The Science of Behavior Analysis

Like several other early psychologists, Skinner argued that the best way to understand human behavior is to study it from the perspective of the natural sciences. The specific perspective that he advocated has been both influential and controversial. Many psychologists and laypeople criticize what they believe to be Skinner's position, but in fact they are objecting to views that he never held. Others, of course, actually understand behavior analysis and are opposed to it, usually on philosophical grounds. Table 1-1 summarizes what behavior analysis as developed by Skinner is and is not; the balance of this section justifies the contents of the table.

When he died in 1990, Skinner was the most well known psychologist ever to live. Shortly before he died, the American Psychological Association (APA) awarded him its lifetime achievement award, the only such award ever given. It is ironic that at the ceremony where Skinner received the APA's Lifetime Achievement Award, he lamented that psychology still had not become a natural science and that many psychologists continued to try to explain behavior by referring to cognitive or mental events, not the real causes of behavior. For Skinner, those causes were genetic, physiological, and environmental variables.

Although Skinner recognized that genetic and physiological variables play a role in controlling how an organism responds in a given situation, his own research and theorizing focused on the relation between environmental events and behavior. He focused on environmental events because:

1. Environmental variables clearly influence behavior.
2. Environmental variables are directly observable and can be studied with the technology available.

Table 1-1. Characteristics of Behavior Analysis

Behavior Analysis Is:

A natural science that emphasizes the effects of environmental variables on behavior.

Concerned with behavior in its own right, not as an indication of events at another level of analysis.

A proven and practical approach to dealing with a wide variety of behavioral problems.

Behavior Analysis Is Not:

Stimulus-Response psychology.

Unconcerned with mental events (thoughts, feelings, etc.), genotype, and physiology.

Simple common sense.

Dead.

---

3. Environmental variables that affect behavior often are subject to direct manipulation; if they are manipulated appropriately, desired behaviors can be fostered.

Prior to Skinner's work, the Russian physiologist Ivan Pavlov (e.g., 1927) had provided clear laboratory evidence of the importance of environmental variables in controlling behavior. Pavlov was interested in digestion, and his early work involved presenting various stimuli (e.g., dilute acid, food) to dogs and measuring the amount of saliva produced in response to them. Some stimuli, food in particular, reliably elicited salivation, so long as the dogs were hungry. Pavlov noticed that salivation was also produced by stimuli that reliably preceded food delivery, such as the sound of his footsteps or the laboratory light being turned on. Initially, Pavlov called salivation controlled by such stimuli psychic reflexes, or psychical secretions, but he soon labeled them as conditioned (or conditional) reflexes. Stimuli that automatically elicited salivation, such as food, were called unconditional stimuli and the salivation that they elicited was called an unconditional response. Conditional stimuli acquired the capacity to elicit salivation by reliably preceding unconditional stimuli in a process variously (and synonymously) termed **respondent, classical**, or **Pavlovian conditioning**. The salivation that they elicited was termed a conditional response. Pavlov spent most of his life exploring classical conditioning. In doing so, he rapidly recognized the futility of trying to explain the process in terms of mentalistic or subjective events occurring in the dogs. He wrote:

[In our first experiments] we conscientiously endeavored to explain our results by imagining the subjective state of the animal. But nothing came of this except sterile controversy and individual views that could not be reconciled. And so we could do nothing but conduct the research on a purely objective basis. (Quoted in Cuny, 1965, p. 65).

Pavlov recognized that speculations about the internal state of subjects were of no value in explaining the changes in behavior produced by conditioning. Of far greater explanatory value were the relations between stimuli that were responsible for the conditioning. Pavlov and his many collaborators explored these relations with great care and discovered the basic principles of respondent conditioning. These principles, outlined in Chapter 2, basically describe how learning can occur through the correlation, or pairing, of neutral stimuli (e.g., the sight or smell of food) with stimuli (e.g., food in the mouth) that reflexively control responding (e.g., salivation). Note that in respondent conditioning events outside the organism - that is, stimulus-stimulus pairings—are responsible for changes in behavior.

Pavlov's studies of respondent conditioning clearly demonstrated that behavior is lawfully related to measurable changes in the environment and can be explained without recourse to unobserved, hypothetical entities. One of his students, Igor Zavadskii, conducted a study that is thought to be the first in the tradition of behavioral pharmacology. In this study, Zavadskii measured the effects of caffeine, cocaine, ethanol, and morphine on the respondently-conditioned salivation of dogs (Laties, 1979). Zavadskii's procedures share much with those favored by many behavioral pharmacologists today: A wide range of doses was studied, within-subject controls were used, and effects were measured under a range of conditions. This line of research apparently held little appeal for the Russians, however, and the emergence of behavioral pharmacology as an organized discipline awaited the birth of behaviorism in America.

John Watson introduced the term "behaviorism" in 1913, and it was he who first put forth a strong natural science view of psychology. According to Watson, the only way to make sense of human behavior is to analyze it scientifically. He wrote, for instance, "It is the business of behavioristic psychology to be able to predict and control human activity. To do this it must gather scientific data by experimental methods" (1930, p. 11). These methods demand directly observable data, and Watson argued for a psychology concerned only with how overt behavior (responding) changes as a function of other observable changes in the environment (stimuli):

The rule, or measuring rod, which the behaviorist puts in front of him always is: Can I describe this bit of behavior I see in terms of "stimulus and response"? By stimulus we mean any object in the general environment or any change in the tissues themselves due to the physiological condition of the animal, such as the changes we get when we keep an animal from sex activity, when we keep it from feeding, when we keep it from building a nest. By response, we mean anything the animal does—such as turning toward or away from a light, jumping at a sound, and more highly organized activities such as building a skyscraper, drawing plans, having babies, and the like. (1930, p. 6)

Watson's psychology was a stimulus-response (S-R) psychology, and he attempted to explain behavior primarily in terms of respondent conditioning, which is impossible.

Like Watson, Skinner assumed that the proper business of psychology is predicting and controlling behavior. Unlike Watson, Skinner did not attempt to explain behavior primarily in terms of respondent conditioning. Instead, Skinner recognized that many important behaviors are strongly influenced by their consequences. This recognition was, of course, not novel. For instance, Thorndike's **law of effect** called attention to the importance of the consequences of behavior in determining whether or not the behavior recurred under similar circumstances:

> Any act which in a given situation produces satisfaction becomes associated with that situation, so that when the situation recurs the act is more likely than before to recur also. Conversely, any act which in a given situation produces discomfort becomes disassociated from that situation, so that when the situation recurs the act is less likely than before to recur. (Thorndike, 1905, p. 203)

Although Skinner was not the first psychologist to recognize the importance of consequences in controlling behavior, he was the first to develop a comprehensive system for studying their effects. His approach to analyzing and explaining behavior is often, but imprecisely, termed behaviorism. It is also called **behavior analysis**, which is the term I prefer. Skinner referred to his preferred tactics and strategies of research as **the experimental analysis of behavior**, and the terms **applied behavior analysis** and **behavior modification** refer to attempts to improve human behavior by using methods consistent with the experimental analysis of behavior.

Radical behaviorism refers to the philosophical position adopted by Skinner; this term is used in contrast to the **methodological behaviorism** of John B. Watson. Methodological behaviorism deals only with publicly observable responses, that is, movements made by organisms, and ignores what are traditionally viewed as mental events (e.g., thoughts, feelings, and beliefs). Radical behaviorism conceptualizes behavior as involving both public and private events; it acknowledges the existence of a "behavioral world within the skin," encompassing what are commonly termed thoughts, feelings, beliefs, attitudes, and related phenomena. But it assigns these private events no special status. They do not cause overt behavior, save as stimuli that function in the same fashion as directly observable stimuli, and are special only in the sense of being especially difficult to study.

Skinner emphasized the importance of relations among antecedent stimuli, responses, and consequences in determining the behavior of humans and other animals. He termed these relations **contingencies**. Contingencies of reinforcement are present when behavior is strengthened by its consequences; contingencies of punishment are present when behavior is weakened by its consequences. Skinner used the term **operant** to refer to behaviors that could be modified by their consequences, and the term **operant conditioning** to refer to the process of modifying some characteristic of behavior (e.g., probability of occurrence) by altering its consequences. Chapter 2 covers the basic principles of operant conditioning.

Although Skinner emphasized that the past consequences of behavior play a crucial role in determining whether such behavior occurs under similar present circumstances, he recognized the role of other variables, such as the organism's motivational state. He also acknowledged that in humans verbal rules concerning the consequences of behavior, even if those consequences had never been directly experienced, could influence whether or not a given kind of responding occurred. That is, as explained in Chapter 2, behavior could be both rule-governed and contingency-controlled. Given the complexity of the contingencies that influence human behavior, and the fact that both rules and contingencies affect it, it is obvious that a simple S-R psychology is impossible.

Skinner did not attempt to develop an S-R psychology, but he did emphasize that behavior is fundamentally orderly, and that it is the task of the experimental psychologist to delineate orderly functional relations between classes of independent and dependent variables. Observed functional relations constitute the raw material of science, and allow for prediction and control of the subject matter.

As noted, Skinner's approach to delineating functional relations is termed the experimental analysis of behavior (EAB). The *Journal of the Experimental Analysis of Behavior (JEAB)* was founded in 1958 and continues as an important outlet for

Table 1-2. Comparison of Research Strategies Characteristic of the Experimental Analysis of Behavior and of Traditional Experimental Psychology

Dimension	Experimental Analysis of Behavior	Traditional Experimental Psychology
Number of subjects	Few	Many
Research design	Within-subject	Between-subjects
Data collection	Direct, repeated measures of behavior	Various methods, often indirect and nonrepeated measures of behavior
Data analysis	Visual	Statistical
Approach to variable data	Consider the variability as imposed; isolate and control the responsible extraneous variables	Consider the variability as intrinsic; use statistics to detect effects of the independent variable despite the variability

behavior analytic research. The book *Tactics of Scientific Research* by Murray Sidman (1960) covered the logic and practice of EAB with admirable clarity and its contents have influenced many researchers.

The essential features of EAB research are outlined in Table 1-2, which contrasts EAB with the approach to research favored by many traditional experimental psychologists. In essence, behavioral pharmacologists use the methods of EAB to understand drug effects. The approach assumes that:

1. **Behavior is important in its own right.** That behavior is important in and of itself may seem obvious, but many psychologists are primarily concerned with behavior as a reflection of some underlying process or condition, such as personality, mental illness, or neurochemical activity. Behavior analysts, in contrast, emphasize that behavior is a rich and fascinating subject matter in and of itself, and is the proper subject matter of psychology.

2. **Intensive study of a few subjects is generally a fruitful research strategy.** Behavior analysts recognize that different organisms have different histories, genotypes, and physiologies, hence, they are likely to differ to some degree in their sensitivity to independent variables. Given this, within-subject experimental designs, in which each subject is exposed to all levels of the independent variable and behavior is compared across levels for individuals, are superior to between-subjects designs, in which different subjects are exposed to different levels of the dependent variable and mean group performances are compared. Within-subject designs require extensive study of each subject, and can yield meaningful information with as few as one subject. In practice, two to six subjects are involved in most studies, in part to allow for detection of individual differences in sensitivity to independent variables.

3. **Visual (graphic) analysis of data is desirable.** Behavior analysts recognize that group means often provide no useful information about the behavior of the individuals whose scores yielded the means. Therefore, mean differences in behavior under different levels of an independent variable are uninteresting, and the inferential statistics used to compare means are unnecessary. All that is required to discover lawful behavior processes that operate at the level of the individual organism is to plot values of the independent variable against values of the dependent variable, and to determine by visual inspection whether the two are related.

4. **Direct and repeated measures of behavior are invaluable.** Because behavior is of interest in its own right, it should be directly measured. Procedures (e.g., questionnaires, checklists) that measure behavior indirectly raise problems of validity and reliability and, in general, should be avoided. Within-subject designs require repeated measures of behavior, and only if measures of behavior are essentially continuous can the fine-grained effects of an independent variable be determined. Skinner believed that the cumulative record was especially valuable because it provided a direct and continuous index of behavior.

5. **Variable data are best dealt with by isolating and controlling the responsible extraneous variables.** Inevitably, psychologists are concerned with variability in

behavior. When they conduct experiments, their task is separating variability in behavior that results from changes in the level of an independent variable from changes in behavior that result from other sources (extraneous variables). This task is made easier if one holds conditions constant until the behavior of interest stabilizes, then repeatedly introduces and withdraws the independent variable, with these probes separated by sufficient exposure to the original conditions for behavior to again stabilize. The steady-state performance that is evident prior to and after probe sessions provides a stable baseline against which the effects of the independent variable can be assessed.

Steady-state experimental arrangements provide sensitive tools for evaluating the behavioral effects of a wide range of independent variables, including drugs (e.g., Poling, Methot, & LeSage, 1995). In some cases, however, excessive variability is evident in the same individual under seemingly constant conditions. In other cases, different individuals differ with respect to their sensitivity to the independent variable, even though it is being assessed under the same conditions. There are basically two strategies for dealing with either form of variability. One is to accept the variability as intrinsic and try to quantify the effects of the independent variable by statistical manipulations (e.g., comparing means across subjects and conditions). The other, recommended by Skinner (and Sidman), is to isolate the variables responsible for the variability and, if possible, to eliminate them. If, for instance, subjects differ in their sensitivity to an independent variable, they do so for reason—that is, they differ in some respect—and it is the scientist's task to determine how they differ.

6. **Study of nonhuman subjects under controlled experimental conditions can be of great value in understanding the variables that control human behavior.** Skinner noted (1953) that several disciplines ultimately concerned with humans, including medicine and physiology, make heavy use of nonhuman research findings. He also provided a good rationale for the use of nonhuman subjects in behavioral research:

> We study the behavior of animals because it is simpler. Basic processes are revealed more easily and can be recorded over longer periods of time. Our observations are not complicated by the social relations between subject and experimenter. Conditions may be better controlled. We may arrange genetic histories to control certain variables and special life histories to control others—for example, if we are interested in how an organism learns to see, we can raise an animal in darkness until the experiment is begun. We are also able to control current circumstances to an extent not easily realized in human behavior—for example, we can vary states of deprivation over wide ranges. These are advantages which should not be dismissed on the a priori contention that human behavior is inevitably set apart as a separate field. (1953, p. 39)

Skinner acknowledged that the processes and laws that account for nonhuman behavior might be inadequate to account fully for human behavior. He argued, however, that whether or not processes demonstrated in nonhumans are applicable to humans might be determined by empirical test, but not by dogmatic assertion.

Most of the early research in behavior analysis involved nonhuman subjects, primarily rats, pigeons, and monkeys. Humans also were involved in several basic research studies (Grossett, Roy, Sharenow, & Poling, 1982). In addition to emphasizing the importance of isolating and describing fundamental principles of behavior, Skinner (e.g., 1953) contended that those principles and the general strategies of EAB could be used to benefit humanity. Following a flurry of studies demonstrating that basic operant principles generally held with humans as well as nonhumans (e.g., Bijou, 1955, 1957; Lindsey, 1956), researchers demonstrated the truth of this contention (e.g., Cooper, Heron, & Heward, 1987; Miltenberger, 1997).

A Brief History of Behavioral Pharmacology

Behavioral pharmacology emerged as a discipline when researchers began applying strategies and tactics characteristic of EAB to the analysis of drug effects. It is unlikely that any five behavioral pharmacologists could reach a consensus as to what events constituted milestones in the field; each would probably opt for her or his own work. Nevertheless, the philosophical underpinnings, methods, and explanatory models of behavioral psychology were initially made public in a small number of books and journal articles. Table 1-3 provides a chronological listing of several publications which appear to have made seminal contributions to the field. Certain other events (e.g., professional meetings) of exceptional importance also are listed. Even though many significant developments in behavioral pharmacology are omitted from the table, anyone familiar with the material presented in the publications listed therein could justifiably claim a sound fundamental understanding of the field.

Perhaps the first analysis of drug effects based directly on EAB methodology was conducted by Skinner and Heron (1937), who investigated the effects of caffeine and amphetamine on the operant behavior of four rats. In the first part of the study, lever-press responses produced food every 4 minutes, an arrangement called a fixed-interval 4-minute schedule of reinforcement. In the second part, lever-presses never produced food, an arrangement termed extinction. Under both conditions, the drugs generally increased rates of responding. Obtained effects with caffeine under conditions where responding produced food are evident in Figure 1-1, which shows mean cumulative responses across 1-hour test periods when drug was and was not given.

In an attempt to explain their findings, Skinner and Heron posited that the drug might increase responding by increasing hunger, and they evaluated this possibility by comparing food consumption and response rate in the presence and absence of drug. As Skinner (1938) explained:

> After the caffeine had been given twice, it occurred to us that the increase in rate might be caused indirectly through an increase in hunger. . . . As a check on this possibility the amount of food eaten by each rat following the experimentation each day was determined by weight. [T]here is a close

Table 1-3. Selected Milestones in the Development of Behavioral Pharmacology	
Year	Event
1937	Skinner and Heron publish a paper in which the methods characteristic of the experimental analysis of behavior are used to examine the effects of caffeine and amphetamine on operant behavior in rats.
1955	Dews publishes an article presenting data indicating that the effects of drugs can be rate-dependent, that is, determined by the rate of occurrence of the response in the absence of drug.
1956	The New York Academy of Sciences sponsors a conference called *Techniques for the Study of the Behavioral Effects of Drugs*. Basic research methods and explanatory principles of behavioral pharmacology are described by participants, who include Dews, Herrnstein, Miller, Morse, Sidman, and Skinner.
1957	The Behavioral Pharmacology Society is founded, the first and only professional association devoted entirely to the field.
1959	Skinner publishes an important chapter arguing that studies using the methods of operant conditioning to study drug effects in nonhumans are of value in understanding the actions of drugs used to treat people with mental illness.
1964	Thompson and Schuster publish a paper showing that monkeys not previously exposed to morphine will self-administer the drug; the study is the first of many in this general area.
1968	Thompson and Schuster publish *Behavioral Pharmacology*, the first text devoted to the subject.
1971	The second behavioral pharmacology textbook appears, Harvey's *Behavioral Analysis of Drug Action*. A book emphasizing that drugs can have functional stimulus properties (Thompson & Pickens) also is published.
1975	A volume edited by Weiss and Laties and devoted entirely to behavioral toxicology appears.
1977	Another major text in the general area of behavioral pharmacology is marketed (Seiden & Dykstra); this book emphasizes both the neurochemical and behavioral effects of drugs.
1978	*Contemporary Research in Behavioral Pharmacology* (Blackman & Sanger), an edited text offering general summaries of research in several significant areas, appears.

correspondence between the variations in the amount of food consumed and the rate of responding for that day. It is apparent that the caffeine does increase the food consumption and that presumably the rat is hungrier when it is in the apparatus [in the presence of drug]. This would account for some of the effect upon behavior but probably not all. (p. 411)

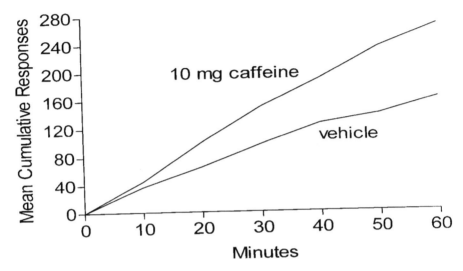

Figure 1-1. *Effects of 10 mg caffeine on cumulative responding by rats exposed to a fixed-interval 4-minute schedule of food delivery during a one-hour experimental session. Data, which are replotted from Skinner and Heron (1937), represent the mean performance of a group of four subjects.*

This study is noteworthy in three regards:
1. Skinner and Heron emphasized the behavioral effects of caffeine, not its chemical or neuropharmacological effects, or their effects on unobservable mental states.
2. Skinner and Heron established stable and repeatable baseline patterns of behavior in the absence of drug and determined drug effects by comparing performance in the presence of drug to characteristic baseline performances. Behavior was measured directly and repeatedly, a within-subject experimental design was used, and data were analyzed by visual inspection.
3. Skinner and Heron explained drug effects by considering how the drug influenced a variable (motivation for food, or hunger) known to influence the behaviors of interest (response rates during reinforcement and extinction conditions) in the absence of food.

4. Skinner and Heron studied drug effects in a nonhuman species, although their ultimate concern was with the effects of caffeine and amphetamine in humans.

The general approach to studying and explaining drug effects that is evident in Skinner and Heron's study was characteristic of much of the early research in behavioral pharmacology. Nonetheless, their study does not appear to have fostered a great deal of interest, and a decade would pass after its appearance before behavioral pharmacology began to emerge as a discipline.

In fact, systematic examinations of the behavioral effects of drugs occurred only sporadically from the turn of the century until its midpoint. In the 1950s, interest in the area skyrocketed; Pickens (1977) reported that between 1917 and 1954 only 28 studies examining drug effects on learned behavior were published in English-language journals, whereas 274 such studies appeared from 1955 to 1963. The factors responsible for this remarkable increase are complex (see Pickens, 1977), but the development of behavior analysis as a recognized approach to psychology was a necessary prerequisite.

By 1955, behavioral psychology had matured into an accepted, if controversial, discipline. In two major books, Skinner (1938, 1953) had expounded the theme that behavior is orderly, therefore subject to scientific analysis, and had developed a technology for this analysis. In 1956, the potential value of this technology for studying drug effects was emphasized at a conference called *Techniques for the Study of the Behavioral Effects of Drugs*, sponsored by the prestigious New York Academy of Sciences and chaired by Skinner and Dews (Annals, 1956). After this conference, and in part because of it, researchers increasingly came to adopt EAB methods for analyzing the behavioral effects of drugs.

Much of the impetus for the development of a science of behavioral pharmacology resulted from the discovery of drugs effective in the treatment of behavioral problems (i.e., psychotropic drugs) and from the widespread public awareness of the ubiquity and seriousness of drug abuse problems. A third, though perhaps weaker, impetus sprang from a growing concern with the effects of chemical contamination of the environment.

Interest in the behavioral effects of drugs was galvanized by the introduction of chlorpromazine (Thorazine) into psychiatric practice in the early 1950s. Chlorpromazine is generally effective in treating psychotic disturbances (i.e., it reduces hallucinations, thought disorders, and delusions in people with schizophrenia), and researchers sought to understand the mechanisms through which it produced beneficial changes in behavior. They also sought to discover other medications with similar effects.

Like scientists from other disciplines, behavioral pharmacologists were quick to examine the effects of chlorpromazine. They primarily examined the drug's effects on learned (i.e., operant) behavior. They also were instrumental in the development of animal models, which are assays that allow the clinical utility of a compound to be predicted on the basis of how it affects nonhuman subjects. Animal models were important to drug companies because they provided a means of discerning new, and profitable, compounds that duplicated or improved upon the actions of legally protected medications.

An early, and well known, animal model used to screen drugs for antipsychotic properties is the pole-climbing (or pole-jump) escape/avoidance procedure (e.g., Cook & Weidley, 1957; Courvoisier, Fournel, Ducrot, Kolsky, & Koetschet, 1953). In this assay, rats are placed in a chamber with a metal grid floor that can be electrified. A wooden pole protrudes upward from the floor. Occasionally, a tone sounds for a brief period, after which a shock is delivered to the grid. The rat can escape from the shock by climbing the pole after the shock starts, or avoid it by climbing during the tone. Neuroleptics interfere with avoidance responding at doses that do not affect escape responding; other drug classes fail to do so. (This is an oversimplification, but aptly captures the rationale of the procedure.)

The success of the escape-avoidance conditioning paradigm for screening neuroleptics initiated a search for assays selectively affected by other drug classes. This search was rather successful, and animal models continue to play an important in drug houses' screening and evaluation of newly synthesized compounds (Porsolt, McArthur, & Lenégre, 1993). For example, drug self-administration procedures involving nonhumans are typically employed in initial evaluations of the abuse potential of drugs being considered for clinical application (see Thompson & Unna, 1977).

Beyond helping to devise drug screening procedures, and in the process gaining much information about the effects of many drugs in a variety of experimental paradigms, behavioral pharmacologists contributed greatly to the development of objective, scientific methods for evaluating the behavioral effects of drugs. Historically, behavioral pharmacologists have favored within-subject experimental designs in the tradition of Sidman (1960) and have insisted that drug-behavior interactions can be adequately assessed only when independent and dependent variables are operationally defined public events, accurately and reliably manipulated and monitored. To date, the approach to drug evaluation advocated by behavioral pharmacologists has not greatly influenced clinical drug assessment, although this appears to be changing as a science of clinical behavioral pharmacology emerges. The applicability of the research methodology of behavioral pharmacology to clinical drug evaluation is addressed in Chapter 9.

As early as 1969, researchers contended that the methods of behavioral pharmacology were appropriate for detecting deleterious effects of relatively low doses of toxins (Weiss & Laties, 1969). This branch of behavioral pharmacology, termed **behavioral toxicology**, grew rapidly (e.g., Evans & Weiss, 1978; Weiss & Laties, 1975), and continues to be viable. Although behavioral toxicologists employ some special techniques, their approach to examining drug effects is equivalent to that of behavioral pharmacologists in general, save that harmful effects are of primary interest to the toxicologists.

Research Areas in Behavioral Pharmacology

Two fundamental principles unite the field of behavioral pharmacology. The first is that the effects of drugs are lawful and thereby subject to scientific analysis. The second is that the behavioral effects of drugs merit attention in and of themselves. Behavioral pharmacologists assume that drugs are environmental events (stimuli), the effects of which, like those of other stimuli, can be understood (i.e., predicted and controlled) without recourse to reductionistic or mentalistic explanations. From this perspective, the study of drug effects should focus upon (1) determination of behavioral loci of drug action, (2) determination of behavioral mechanisms of drug action, and (3) determination of variables that modulate a drug's behavioral effects (Thompson, 1981).

The term **behavioral loci of drug action** refers to the changes in behavior produced by a drug - that is, what the drug actually does at the behavioral level. This determination is made by evaluating the drug's effects under many different assays, which are procedures designed to determine how, and if, a drug influences particular aspects of behavior. For example, evaluating a drug's effect on reaction time constitutes an exploration of a particular locus of action. Behavioral pharmacologists have developed a substantial number of assays for exploring drug effects; many of these assays are discussed in Chapters 5 and 6.

In a general way, **mechanism of action** refer to the processes whereby a drug produces its behavioral effects. In traditional pharmacology, these processes commonly involve events that occur at the biochemical level, for example, changes in neurotransmitter activity (Chapter 4). **Behavioral mechanisms of action**, however, refer to the stimulus functions of the drug, and the effects of the drug on the capacity of other stimuli to control behavior. As Thompson (1981) points out:

Specifying the behavioral mechanism(s) responsible for an observed [drug] effect involves a) identifying the environmental variables which typically regulate the behavior in question, and b) characterizing the manner in which the influence of these variables is altered by the drug. In some instances, the drug assumes the status of a behavioral variable, per se, rather than modulating an existing environmental variable. (p. 3)

The general strategy for determining behavioral mechanisms of action begins with assessment of a drug's functional stimulus properties. In doing this, one evaluates whether the drug serves as an unconditional stimulus, and whether through classical conditioning it can be established as a conditional stimulus. One also assesses whether the drug can be established as a reinforcer and as a discriminative stimulus in the context of operant conditioning.

Once a drug's functional stimulus properties are assessed, the manner in which the drug alters the variables that normally control operant and respondent behaviors is determined. Variables that modulate the drug's effects also can be isolated.

Pharmacology and Behavioral Pharmacology

Although behavioral psychology contributed greatly to the research methods and conceptual principles adopted by behavioral pharmacologists, any attempt to understand drug effects demands knowledge of basic principles of pharmacology. These principles arose from the application of scientific methods to the study of drugs, which began midway through the nineteenth century with the work of Bernard in France, Schmiedeberg in Germany, and Abel in the United States (for histories of pharmacology see Holmstedt & Leljestrand, 1963; Schuster, 1962). These researchers and their successors made it clear, for example, that all drugs have multiple and dose-dependent actions; these are now basic tenets of behavioral pharmacology. In addition, the concepts of tolerance and physical dependence, as well as the receptor model of drug action, come from traditional pharmacology. These concepts form an integral part of the thinking of behavioral pharmacologists (e.g., Thompson & Schuster, 1968). They are covered in Chapters 3 and 4.

Concluding Comments

There is no clear and absolute distinction between psychopharmacology and behavioral pharmacology. In fact, the former term was coined years ago as a descriptor of a then yet to be developed science dealing with the behavioral effects of drugs (Macht & Mora, 1921). Not all attempts to develop such a discipline adopted the research strategies and explanatory principles characteristic of the experimental analysis of behavior; those that did led to the emergence of the discipline herein called behavioral pharmacology. Behavioral pharmacologists have accomplished much over the past 50 years and, as explained in the pages that follow, their procedures and concepts can be used gainfully to analyze the behavioral effects of any drug. Making sense of those procedures and concepts requires some sophistication in behavior analysis, and it is to this area that attention is turned in Chapter 2.

References

Bijou, S. J. (1955). A systematic approach to the experimental analysis of young children. *Child Development, 26,* 161-168.

Bijou, S. W. (1957). Patterns of reinforcement and resistance to extinction in young children. *Child Development, 28,* 47-54.

Blackman, D. E., & Sanger, D. J. (1978). *Contemporary research in behavioral pharmacology.* New York: Plenum Press.

Cook, L., & Weidley, E. (1957). Behavioral effects of some pharmacological agents. *Annals of the New York Academy of Sciences, 66,* 740-756.

Cooper, J. O., Heron, T. E., & Heward, W. L. (1987). *Applied behavior analysis.* Columbus, OH: Merrill.

Courvoisier, S., Fournel, J., Ducrot, R., Kolsky, M., & Koetschet, P. (1953). Propriétés pharmacodynamiques du chlorhydrate de chloro-3(diméthyl-amino-s' propyl)-10 phénothiazine. *Archieves of International Pharmacodynamics and Therapeutics, 92,* 305-361.

Cuny, H. (1965). *Ivan Pavlov: The man and his theories.* New York: Eriksson.

Dews, P. B. (1955). Studies on behavior: I. Differential sensitively to pentobarbital of pecking performance in pigeons depending on the schedule of reward. *Journal of Pharmacology and Experimental Therapeutics, 115,* 343-401.

Evans, H. L., & Weiss, B. (1978). Behavioral toxicology. In D. E. Blackman & D. J. Sanger (Eds.), *Contemporary research in behavioral pharmacology* (pp. 449-488). New York: Plenum Press.

Grossett, D., Roy, S., Sharenow, E., & Poling, A. (1982). Subjects used in *JEAB* research: Is the snark a pigeon? *The Behavior Analyst, 5,* 189-190.

Harvey, J. A. (1971). *Behavioral analysis of drug action.* Glenview, IL: Scott, Foresman.

Holmstedt, B., & Leljestrand, G. (1963). *Readings in pharmacology.* New York: Pergamon Press.

Laties, V. G. (1979). I. V. Zavadskii and the beginnings of behavioral pharmacology: An historical note and translation. *Journal of the Experimental Analysis of Behavior, 32,* 463-472.

Lindsey, O. R. (1956). Operant conditioning methods applied to researching chronic schizophrenia. *Psychiatric Research Reports, 5,* 118-139.

Macht, D. L., & Mora, C. F. (1921). Effects of opium alkaloids on the behavior of rats on the circular maze. *Journal of Pharmacology and Experimental Therapeutics, 16,* 219-235.

Miltenberger, R. (1997). *Behavior modification: Principles and procedures.* Pacific Grove, CA: Brooks/Cole.

Pavlov, I. P. (1927). *Conditioned reflexes.* (G. V. Anrep, Trans.). Oxford, England: Clarendon.

Pickens, R. (1977). Behavioral pharmacology: A brief history. In T. Thompson & P. B. Dews (Eds.), *Advances in behavioral pharmacology* (Vol. 1, pp. 230-261). New York: Academic Press.

Poling, A., LeSage, M., & Methot, L. (1995). *Fundamentals of behavior analytic research.* New York: Plenum Press.

Porsolt, R. D., McArthur, R. A., & LeNégre, A. (1993). Psychotropic screening procedures. In F. van Haaren (Ed.), *Methods in behavioral pharmacology* (pp. 23-51). Elsevier: Amsterdam.

Schuster, L. (1962). *Readings in pharmacology.* New York: Little, Brown.

Seiden, L. S., & Dykstra, L. A. (1977). *Psychopharmacology: A biochemical and behavioral approach.* New York: Van Nostrand Reinhold.

Sidman, M. (1960). *Tactics of scientific research.* New York: Basic Books.

Skinner, B. F. (1938). *The behavior of organisms.* New York: Appleton-Century-Crofts.

Skinner, B. F. (1953). *Science and human behavior.* New York: Macmillan.

Skinner, B. F. (1959). Animal research in the pharmacotherapy of mental disease. In J. O. Cole & R. W. Gerard (Eds.), *Psychopharmacology: Problems in evaluation* (pp. 224-235). Washington, DC: National Academy of Sciences.

Skinner, B. F. (1974). *About behaviorism*. New York: Random House.

Skinner, B. F., & Heron, W. T. (1937). Effects of caffeine and benzedrine upon conditioning and extinction. *Psychological Record, 1*, 340-346.

Thompson, T. (1981). Behavioral mechanisms and loci of drug action: An overview. In T. Thompson & C. Johanson (Eds.), *Behavioral pharmacology of human drug dependence* (pp. 1-10). Washington, DC: U.S. Government Printing Office.

Thompson, T., & Pickens, R. (1971). *Stimulus properties of drugs*. New York: Appleton-Century-Crofts.

Thompson, T., & Schuster, C. R. (1964). Morphine self-administration, food-reinforced, and avoidance behaviors in rhesus monkeys. *Psychopharmacologia, 5*, 97-94.

Thompson, T., & Schuster, C. R. (1968). *Behavioral pharmacology*. Englewood Cliffs, NJ: Prentice-Hall.

Thompson, T., & Unna, K. (1977). *Predicting dependence liability of stimulant and depressant drugs*. Baltimore: University Park Press.

Thorndike, E. L. (1905). *The elements of psychology*. New York: Seiler.

Watson, J. B. (1930). *Behaviorism*. New York: Norton.

Weiss, B., & Laties, V. G. (1969). Behavioral pharmacology and toxicology. *Annual Review of Pharmacology, 9*, 297-326.

Weiss, B., & Laties , V. G. (1975). *Behavioral toxicology*. New York: Plenum Press.

Chapter 2

Principles of Behavior Analysis

Thomas Byrne
and Alan Poling
Massachusetts College of Liberal Arts
and Western Michigan University

As described in Chapter 1, behavioral pharmacologists rely heavily on concepts of respondent and operant conditioning in accounting for the behavioral effects of drugs. The purpose of this chapter is to introduce these concepts.

Respondent Conditioning

All organisms are born with a repertoire that allows them to interact with their environment. Many inborn behaviors occur automatically in response to presentation of particular stimuli. When this is the case, the relation between the stimulus and response is termed an **unconditioned reflex**. Examples of unconditioned reflexes are a bright light causing pupillary constriction, sugar in the mouth causing salivation, and an object approaching the eye causing an eye blink. In each case, no special history is required for the stimulus to cause the person to respond in a given fashion; that is, the relation is **unconditioned**, or unlearned.

Stimuli and Responses

The concepts of stimulus and response are of crucial importance to behavior analysis, and to behavioral pharmacology. In general, a **stimulus** (the plural of stimulus is stimuli) is any object or event. Stimuli are classes of events, and may be defined in terms of their physical characteristics or their behavioral functions. For example, all lights produced by bulbs with an intensity greater than some specified value (e.g., 50 watts) might be described as "bright." Here, the categorization is in terms of a physical dimension (intensity). All lights so categorized might, but need not, produce similar behavioral effects.

It is, for instance, possible that all lights produced by bulbs of 50 or more watts would elicit pupillary constriction when viewed at a distance of 10 feet by a person in a darkened room. If so, each of them could properly be termed an **unconditional stimulus** (US), which is the technical term used to describe stimuli that reflexively control a designated behavior. They are "unconditional" because their ability to affect behavior is not conditional on a particular learning history. The behavior elicited by a US is termed an **unconditional response** (UR). A US is not defined in terms of its physical characteristics alone. Instead, it must have a particular behavioral function, the capacity to elicit a UR.

In essence, a **response** is any defined unit of behavior, usually one that is discrete and recurring. Like stimuli, responses are classes of events. They, too, can be defined in terms of their physical form, and this is characteristically how URs are defined. For example, "eye blinks" are defined by their form, or topography, and comprise a range of specific movements. It is also possible to define responses in terms of their function, that is, the changes they make in the environment. As we shall see, operant responses characteristically are defined in this manner.

Although in a reflex the US elicits a UR, this does not mean that their relation is an invariant one, that is, one in which every US presentation is followed by a response of fixed form and magnitude. Several variables influence unconditioned reflexes, including the intensity of the US and the frequency of its presentation. If, for example, a US is presented continuously or repeatedly over a short period of time, its capacity to elicit a UR declines. This phenomenon is termed **habituation**, which is a rudimentary form of learning.

The Essence of Respondent Conditioning

Of course, not all stimuli elicit a detectable UR. After multiple pairings with a US, however, previously neutral stimuli may come to elicit responses. The process of altering behavior by arranging stimulus-stimulus relations is termed **respondent conditioning** (the terms Pavlovian conditioning and classical conditioning are synonyms), and the best known example of the phenomenon comes from the work of Ivan Pavlov, mentioned in Chapter 1.

As noted there, Pavlov measured in dogs the secretion of saliva (UR) resulting from the oral presentation of meat powder (US). He serendipitously noticed that sounds preceding the presentation of the meat powder (for example, his footsteps) came to elicit salivation before the food was delivered. This observation suggested that stimuli predictive of food came to control a response (salivation) similar to the UR (salivation) controlled by food. Pavlov tested this hypothesis by turning on a metronome just before food presentation. After several pairings of the metronome's sound and food, the sound alone elicited salivation. In technical terms, the metronome sound became a **conditional stimulus**, or CS, which is the name assigned to a stimulus that gains the capacity to control behavior through classical conditioning. Calling the tone a *conditional* stimulus emphasizes that the capacity of the sound to control salivation is conditional on the dog having a history in which the metronome sound was paired with food delivery. The response controlled by a CS is termed a **conditional response**, or CR. CRs frequently resemble URs in form, but they may differ appreciably.

Pavlov used the term **conditioned reflex** to refer to an acquired relation between a CS and a CR. In our example, the relation between food delivery and salivation is an unconditioned reflex, whereas the relation between the sound of the metronome and salivation is a conditioned reflex. Conditioned reflexes involve learning. In general, **learning** occurs when there are enduring changes in relations between behavior and environmental stimuli due to certain types of experience.

For learning to occur in the context of respondent conditioning, the CS must occur shortly before, and be predictive of, the US. That is, the probability of the US occurring must be higher following the CS than at other times, although not every CS presentation need be followed by the US, nor must every US presentation follow the CS. The necessary condition for respondent conditioning is that the CS and US are correlated in time, so that the probability of the US occurring is greatest shortly after the CS occurs. Put differently, the CS must be predictive of the US.

Higher-order Conditioning

After a neutral stimulus has been established as a CS (i.e., acquired eliciting stimulus functions through repeated pairing with a US), it can be paired with other neutral stimuli to make them conditional stimuli. This phenomenon is known as higher-order conditioning. Consider an experiment in which salivation in dogs (CR) is conditioned to the sound of a tone (CS). If a different neutral stimulus, say a light, is paired with the tone, the light alone will eventually elicit salivation. This is second-order conditioning. The process could be extended to third-order conditioning by pairing another neutral stimulus, perhaps a touch on the shoulder, with the light. It too might eventually come to elicit salivation. But it probably would not because third-order conditioning is usually impossible with an appetitive US such as food. Even second-order conditioning is relatively weak, although it can be readily demonstrated (Macintosh, 1974).

Extinction and Spontaneous Recovery

When classical conditioning does occur, the CS continues to elicit the CR only so long as the CS-US pairing is at least occasionally maintained. If the pairing is ended, either by presenting the CS without the US or by presenting the two stimuli independent of each other, the CS-CR relation weakens and eventually ceases to occur. The cessation of responding due to presentation of a CS not paired with a US is termed **respondent extinction**. If, for instance, Pavlov had stopped giving meat to his dogs after sounding the tone, salivating to the sound eventually would have stopped. Like habituation, respondent extinction serves an organism by preventing it from responding needlessly to once significant but now unimportant stimuli. If, however, a considerable period of time (e.g., a day) passes without CS presentation, the effects of respondent extinction wane and the CS again elicits the CR. This phenomenon is known as **spontaneous recovery**.

Stimulus Generalization

Whenever some characteristic of a response (e.g., its rate, magnitude, or probability of occurrence) differs in the presence and absence of a particular stimulus, the response is said to be **stimulus controlled**. In most cases, when a given stimulus controls a particular kind of behavior, other stimuli that are physically similar do likewise. This phenomenon is termed **stimulus generalization**. Envision a two-year-old child who has been stung by a hornet. The sting is a US; it is painful and elicits crying and a general activation response (UR). The physical characteristics of the hornet (its shape, color, size, and sound) preceded the US; therefore, they come to serve as a compound CS (a CS with multiple elements). When another hornet approaches, it elicits crying and general arousal in the child (CR). Similar responses are also likely to be elicited by other hornet-like insects, such as wasps. The likelihood that a given insect, or other stimulus, will elicit such responses depends on their similarity to the hornet. In general, the greater the similarity between a novel stimulus and a CS, the greater the likelihood that the novel stimulus will elicit a response similar to the CR. For example, in our example, a house fly will likely elicit a weaker response than will a bee or a wasp.

Operant Conditioning

In respondent conditioning, behavior is controlled by antecedent stimuli, that is, by events that precede the response of interest. Although antecedent stimuli also play an important role in operant conditioning, events that occur after the behavior of interest are especially important. Specifically, in **operant conditioning**, the consequences of an organism's actions in the past determine, in large part, whether such actions will occur under similar conditions in the future.

Stimuli produced by a response (i.e., its consequences) can have two general effects: The future likelihood of occurrence of the response under similar circumstances can increase, or it can decrease. We use the term reinforcement to refer to the former relation, whereas punishment is used to describe the latter. **Reinforcement** is evident when a response is followed by a change in the environment (reinforcer) and is thereby strengthened. The response-strengthening effects of reinforcement typically involve an increase in the future rate (number of responses per unit time) of the response, although other changes in behavior (e.g., a decrease in response latency) may also be indicative of a reinforcement effect. It is important to recognize that reinforcement always strengthens the behavior that is reinforced, although this process may weaken, strengthen, or have no effect on other behaviors.

A good example of reinforcement is giving a dog a treat after it performs a trick, perhaps barking on command. When this is done, the dog is more likely to perform the trick again in the future. The consequence of the dog's barking was access to a treat, and it is this consequence that affected its behavior. That is, barking was reinforced. (Incidentally, the dog was not—responses, not organisms, are reinforced or punished.)

Reinforcement often is the process responsible for the learning of new behaviors. Assume, for example, that a hungry raccoon is attracted by the smell of food contained in a garbage can. Following the scent trail, it rears alongside the can, lifting its lid and gaining access to the contents. Because of this outcome, the future probability of lid-lifting increases. Therefore, reinforcement has occurred.

Traditionally, psychologists have classified reinforcers according to whether they involve adding something to the environment (e.g., presenting food), or subtracting something from it (e.g., turning off a loud noise). When a stimulus strengthens behavior by virtue of being presented (or increased in intensity) following the occurrence of such behavior, the stimulus is called a positive reinforcer and the procedure is termed **positive reinforcement**.

Negative reinforcement also strengthens behavior, but it does so through the termination or postponement of a stimulus (the negative reinforcer), or by a reduction in its intensity. For example, a driver may find his vision impaired by a dirty windshield. The driver turns on the windshield wipers, which removes the dust and insect remains. Removal of the dust and insect parts negatively reinforces the behavior of turning on the wipers, that is, this outcome increases the likelihood of turning on the wipers when the windshield becomes dirty in the future.

As illustrated in Figure 2-1, the distinction between positive and negative reinforcement is simple logically, but in practice it can be hard to tell the two apart. As a case in point, does a person adjust the tuning on a blurry television because doing so in the past has produced a clear image (positive reinforcement), or because doing so historically has removed a blurry image (negative reinforcement)? Because of such difficulties, and the possibility of confusing negative reinforcement with punishment, there is justification for not differentiating positive and negative reinforcement (Michael, 1975), although the practice remains common.

STIMULUS

		ADDED	SUBTRACTED
STRENGTHENED		Positve Reinforcement	Negative Reinforcement
BEHAVIOR			
WEAKENED		Positive Punishment	Negative Punishment

Figure 2-1. *Reinforcement always strengthens behavior, whereas punishment always weakens it. Positive and negative reinforcement (and punishment) are distinguished on the basis of whether a stimulus is added to, or subtracted from, the environment of the organism whose behavior is reinforced (or punished).*

As discussed in Chapter 10, reinforcement plays a critical role in drug use and abuse. Whenever a person behaves so as to introduce a drug into her or his body (e.g., swallows a pill, inhales on a cigarette) and the frequency of such behavior therefore increases, the drug has functioned as a positive reinforcer. For example, if a person self-administers heroin, a stimulus has been added to that person's environment. If there is a resultant increase in the frequency of heroin injections, then the heroin has functioned as a positive reinforcer.

It is sometimes erroneously argued that heroin functions as a negative reinforcer for a person undergoing withdrawal from the drug, because injecting the drug "removes aversive withdrawal symptoms." This makes no more sense than saying that food is a negative reinforcer because it "removes aversive hunger," or that sexual activity is a negative reinforcer because it "removes aversive horniness." Stimuli are classified as positive or negative reinforcers on the basis of whether adding them to or removing them from the organism's environment strengthens behavior, not on the basis of their subjective effects. Like food and sexual stimulation, heroin strengthens behavior by being added to the organism's environment. Therefore, it is a positive, not a negative, reinforcer. This does not mean, of course, that the withdrawal symptoms are of no importance. They are, insofar as their occurrence is likely to increase the probability of drug-seeking and drug-taking. This effect is, however, best construed as a motivational (or establishing) operation, as discussed later in this chapter.

A variety of environmental changes (i.e., stimuli) can serve as reinforcers. **Unconditioned** (or primary) **reinforcers** strengthen behavior in organisms without any particular history, which is to say in most "normal" members of a particular species. Many primary reinforcers are of direct biological significance. Air, food, sexual contact, and water are examples of positive reinforcers that fit into this category. Primary negative reinforcers, which organisms will escape (respond to terminate) or avoid (respond to postpone), include high-intensity stimulation in most modalities.

In contrast to primary reinforcers, **conditioned** (or secondary) **reinforcers** gain their ability to strengthen behavior through learning. Conditioned reinforcers can be established through respondent conditioning, that is, by being paired with (i.e., immediately preceding the delivery of) primary reinforcers or other established conditioned reinforcers. As discussed later, they also can be established through verbal mediation. Money is a good example of a conditioned reinforcer.

In some cases, the opportunity to behave in certain ways is reinforcing. The **Premack principle** states that the opportunity to engage in a higher-probability behavior will reinforce a lower-probability behavior. In this context, probability refers to the relative amount of time that an organism will engage in the behaviors if unconstrained. If an organism is given a choice between emitting Behavior A or Behavior B and spends more time engaging in Behavior A, then Behavior A is the higher-probability activity. For example, if given a choice between scrubbing a floor or flying a kite, most children spend far more time in the latter activity. If this is true, then according to the Premack principle the opportunity to fly a kite (the higher-probability behavior) will be an effective reinforcer for floor scrubbing (the lower-probability behavior). A parent might well use this relation to increase the time that their child spent cleaning: In order to fly a kite, the child must first scrub the floor. This is the Premack principle in action.

Environmental events may reinforce (or punish) responses that precede them even if the response does not actually produce the reinforcer. For instance, a crap shooter who, for unknown reasons, says "Be there, baby," while rolling the dice is apt to repeat the phrase under similar conditions in the future if the roll is a winning seven, even though there is no plausible mechanism whereby the verbal response could control the dice. Reinforcement of this type has been termed **superstitious**,

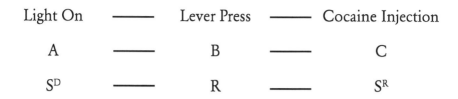

Figure 2-2. *Shorthand descriptions of relations among an antecedent stimulus (light on), a response (lever press by a monkey), and a consequence of that response (intravenous injection of cocaine). The letters A, B, and C refer to the antecedent stimulus, behavior, and consequence, respectively. If this arrangement strengthened lever pressing, it could be described as a reinforcement contingency, where in the presence of a discriminative stimulus (S^D) a given response (R) consistently produces an unconditioned reinforcer (S^R).*

adventitious, or **fortuitous** and probably controls some behaviors that appear counterintuitive. It should be noted, however, that explaining a behavior as being superstitiously reinforced is begging the question of how the behavior is actually controlled, unless the nature of the superstitious reinforcement is apparent.

Operant Extinction

As long as a behavior produces an effective reinforcer, that behavior will recur. But when responding no longer produces the reinforcer that once maintained it, the behavior eventually ceases. This process is **operant extinction.** As an example of extinction, consider again the garbage-raiding raccoon. By now, each night for a month the raccoon's lid-lifting behavior has been reinforced by access to food. Then the family that owns the garbage can has gone away on an extended vacation. This puts an end to the garbage refills. The raccoon will likely open the can nightly for a while, but eventually will cease to do so because the behavior is no longer reinforced.

Responses that have a protracted history of reinforcement are likely to persist for a substantial period despite failing to produce a reinforcer. In fact, when extinction is first implemented, the organism may respond at higher rates than usual. This is known as **extinction-induced bursting.** Emotional responding and increases in the variability of behavior also commonly occur during extinction.

As another example of extinction, consider what happens when a person puts a dollar in a vending machine, pushes a button in a manner that historically has produced a favored candy, and gets nothing. She or he is likely to curse, pound the machine, and push other buttons. Eventually, however, machine-related behavior ceases.

The overall persistence of responding when reinforcement is no longer available is called **resistance to extinction** and is one measure of response strength. Even when responding falls to near-zero levels during extinction, the behavior remains in the organism's repertoire, and may return quickly to previous levels if reinforcement once again becomes available. Interestingly, when motivation relevant to a particular kind of reinforcer is high and responses that recently have produced that reinforcer are unavailable or ineffective, previously-extinguished responses often occur. This phenomenon is termed **resurgence**.

Punishment

Punishment occurs when the future probability of behavior decreases because of the consequences of the behavior. This can be illustrated with an example involving the aversive qualities of ethanol for a novice drinker. Assume that a young child finds a glass of gin and tonic left over from a cocktail party her parents had the night before. The child, who frequently drinks from glasses, takes a sip and immediately spits out the bitter concoction. Being rather careless but active socialites, her parents leave out mixed drinks on many occasions over the next couple of years. But the child does not attempt to drink the mixtures again. In fact, the child refuses to drink out of cocktail glasses altogether. The behavior of drinking from a cocktail glass has been punished, and the gin and tonic has functioned as a punisher.

In the example of the gin and tonic, no special history was required for the stimulus to function as a punisher. Such a stimulus is an **unconditioned punisher**. Other examples of such punishers include extreme heat or cold, loud noise, and strong electric shock. In general, stimuli that immediately and adversely affect the health of an organism will function as primary punishers. But there are exceptions. A stimulus can not function as a punisher if it is not detectable by an organism. For example, humans cannot directly detect the presence of carbon monoxide gas. Therefore, although carbon monoxide can be deadly, it will not function as a punisher.

The same processes that establish stimuli as conditioned reinforcers are also effective in establishing neutral stimuli as conditioned punishers. A common example of a conditioned punisher is the word "no." Without any prior training, a toddler will not have any specific reaction to "no." But early in the life of most English-speaking people, the word is paired with unconditioned punishers, and is thereby established as a conditioned punisher. For example, a young child may reach toward a hot stove in the presence of his parents. A quick, forceful grab of the child's arm (unconditioned punisher), accompanied by a stern "No," will likely decrease the probability of the child reaching for the stove in the future. It will also be an initial step toward establishing "no" as an effective punisher. Of course, several pairings with another punisher may required before the word alone has a response-reducing function.

Discriminative Stimuli

Operant behavior is determined in large part by its historical consequences under particular conditions. Therefore, the momentary probability that such behavior will occur depends, in part, on 1) the nature of the consequences (punishing or reinforcing), and 2) the extent to which current conditions resemble the historical conditions under which the consequences occurred. Consider again one of our examples of reinforcement, giving a dog a treat after it barks on command. When this is done, we noted, the dog is more likely to perform the trick again in the future if the treat is indeed a reinforcer. But what we failed to emphasize was that the barking would be stimulus-controlled. That is, it would occur reliably following the command ("Speak, Sam"), but not at other times. Here, as is often the case, the historical consequences of a particular kind of behavior imbue stimuli that were uniquely present when those consequences occurred with the capacity to evoke that kind of behavior.

To emphasize the importance of events that occur before, as well as after, the response of interest, behavior analysts often depict operant conditioning in terms of relations among antecedent stimuli, responses, and consequences, as in Figure 2-2. This figure depicts an A-B-C analysis, with A being an antecedent stimulus, B a particular behavior, and C the consequence of that behavior. In technical terms, the antecedent stimulus is called **a discriminative stimulus** (S^D) which is a stimulus that a) given the momentary effectiveness of some form of reinforcement, b) increases the frequency of occurrence of a particular behavior because, c) historically, that kind of behavior was reinforced in the presence of that stimulus.

Stimuli present when a particular type of behavior is not successful (i.e., is extinguished) can also influence responding. The term S^{delta} is used to designate such stimuli. An S^{delta} is a stimulus that reduces the frequency of occurrence of a particular type of behavior because in the past, that type of behavior was extinguished in its presence, but was reinforced in its absence. Note that both the S^D and the $S^{deltadelta}$ are defined functionally. That is, both exercise control over behavior, although the control is excitatory in the case of the S^D (i.e., responding increases in its presence) and inhibitory in the case of the $S^{deltadelta}$ (i.e., responding decreases in its presence).

As an example of behavior controlled by a discriminative stimulus, consider a crack addict, R. S., who has not taken cocaine since the previous evening. The noon hour is approaching; R. S. is undergoing withdrawal, and crack would serve as a positive reinforcer. But he is out of money and is unable to buy the drug. Through a history of positive reinforcement, he has acquired the response of asking street dealers to give him a rock of crack on credit. On this occasion two dealers, Mary and John, are both seated in a bar near R. S., in separate booths. Mary never supplies drugs on credit has repeatedly turned down R. S.'s requests. John, in contrast, is more trusting and has consistently given R. S. crack on credit. Hence, with respect to R. S. asking "Give me a rock, I'll pay tomorrow" (or something to that effect), Mary is an S^{delta} and John is an S^D, insofar as the request historically has been reinforced in the presence of the latter and extinguished in the presence of the former. Because of this, R. S. is likely to ask John for credit, but not to ask Mary. This must, of course, be the case if John actually is serving as an S^D.

As this example illustrates, the development and maintenance of stimulus control over operant behavior requires differential reinforcement, wherein a response is reinforced in the presence of one stimulus and extinguished in the presence of one or more other stimuli. These conditions are arranged specifically in operant discrimination training, which is a major part of education. Consider how children are taught to label colors. What we call "color" is determined by the wavelength of reflected light, and we teach young people to name colors by reinforcing their voicing of a particular name in the present of objects that reflect certain wavelengths, but not in the presence of objects that reflect other wavelengths. Humans can detect wavelengths of approximately 350 to 750 nanometers (nm), and we might teach a child to voice the terms red, green, yellow, and blue when presented with objects that reflect wavelengths of 700, 600, 500, and 400 nm, respectively.

What would happen when a child trained in this way was presented with objects that reflected some other wavelength, perhaps 350 nm? In all likelihood, he or she would say that the object was blue. As mentioned in our discussion of the stimulus control of respondent behavior, when stimuli that differ along a given dimension (e.g., wavelength) control the same response (e.g., saying "blue"), stimulus generalization is evident. When two or more stimuli control the same behavior, whether through stimulus generalization or for some other reason, they are said to be **functionally equivalent**.

Obviously, many discriminations are based on multiple stimulus dimensions. You recognize your mother not on the basis of any single physical dimension (e.g., size, color, form), but on the basis of multiple characteristics. Discriminations also can be conditional. In a **conditional discrimination**, whether a response is reinforced (and therefore subsequently recurs) in the presence of one stimulus depends on the presence of one or more other stimuli. For instance, you're sitting in one room, studying, and a friend is in the adjoining room. One room, yours, has a digital clock, the other does not. The numbers 10:32 appear on the clock face, but they exercise no control over your behavior until your friend asks "What time is it?" You respond "It's ten thirty-two." Here a sequence of two stimuli, the auditory one provided by your friend and the visual one supplied by the clock, controlled your behavior.

Establishing Operations

The capacity of a given stimulus to serve as a reinforcer (or punisher) is not fixed, and may vary dramatically across persons, or across situations for the same person. In fact, the same stimulus may serve as a positive reinforcer in one situation and as a negative reinforcer in another situation. For instance, consider a human who has just run five miles on a hot and humid afternoon. At the completion of the run, the opportunity to submerge in a pool of cool water would likely be a powerful positive reinforcer. But if the person had just completed a five-mile walk through an unexpected snowstorm, the opportunity to submerge in the same pool of cool water would likely be avoided - that is, it would serve as a powerful negative reinforcer. The difference between the two scenarios is a change in the motivating variables, which behavior analysts often term establishing operations. The concept of establishing operations (EOs) was formulated by Michael (1982), who defines them as follows:

> An **establishing operation** is an environmental event, operation, or stimulus condition that affects an organism by momentarily altering (a) the reinforcing effectiveness of other events, and (b) the frequency of occur-

rence of the type of behavior that had been consequated by those other events. (p. 58, boldface added)

It is important to realize that establishing operations can have bi-directional effects, that is, they can either increase or decrease the reinforcing (or punishing) effectiveness of a given stimulus, and thereby increase or decrease the likelihood of behavior that historically has produced the stimulus.

Unconditioned establishing operations (UEOs) produce their effects in the absence of any particular learning history. Conditioned establishing operations (CEOs), in contrast, alter the reinforcing (or punishing) effectiveness of other events only as a result of the individual's history. That is, their ability to affect behavior is acquired through learning, or conditioning. In the example above, ambient temperature acted as a UEO to modulate the reinforcing effects of cool water. An example of a CEO is the host of a TV game show saying "I'll give $1,000 for every broken fountain pen you audience members can show me." Following that statement, but not prior to it, broken fountain pens would have substantial reinforcing value.

Some establishing operations are rather complex. Consider the reinforcing effects of ethanol (beverage alcohol). Under what circumstances does the drug function as a positive reinforcer for the typical college student? The answer is "in a social setting." Not just any social setting, of course, but in the kind that is characteristic of bars. Relatively few people drink alcohol when they're alone, having breakfast, even if it's readily available. But many of the same people have a few drinks at evening get-togethers with friends. Here, the social milieu serves as a CEO, and determines whether or not alcohol is reinforcing.

It is important to emphasize that establishing operations affect the likelihood of occurrence of all forms of behavior that historically have produced a particular type of reinforcer. If, for example, a dog historically has received food after nosing its food bowl, scratching at bags of dog food, and exploring the kitchen floor, all of those behaviors will increase in frequency as food deprivation increases. Regardless of their form, responses that produce the same outcome constitute an **operant response class**, and characteristically are affected in similar fashion by environmental variables.

Schedules of Reinforcement

Reinforcers need not follow every occurrence of a behavior to determine the rate and pattern of its occurrence; intermittently occurring reinforcers can strengthen behavior. Specific relations among responses, environmental events, and the passage of time constitute **schedules of reinforcement**. Schedules of reinforcement are important for four reasons:

1. *Schedules of reinforcement are ubiquitous.* They operate throughout the natural environment of humans and other animals, even though it is often difficult to ascertain what schedule is in effect at a given time for a particular response.

2. Schedules of reinforcement determine the rate and temporal pattern of behavior. Some schedules generate high and consistent response rates, others generate very different rates and patterns. As discussed later in this book, rates of responding in the absence of drug often strongly influence drug effects.

3. Schedules of reinforcement affect resistance to extinction. Responding always approaches near-zero levels if extinction is arranged for a sufficient period, but the rapidity with which behavior weakens depends on the schedule in effect prior to extinction.

4. Schedules of reinforcement determine choice. The time and effort allocated to one particular kind of behavior relative to another (i.e., choice) is determined, in part, by the schedules in effect for the alternative behaviors.

Dozens of different schedules have been described and used at least occasionally in animal research; only a few of the most commonly-used schedules will be discussed here. Fixed-ratio (FR) and variable-ratio (VR) schedules are response-based. In the former, a reinforcer follows every *n*th response, for example, every fifth response under an FR 5 schedule. So-called continuous reinforcement is an FR 1 schedule; all other schedules (except extinction) arrange intermittent consequences. Under a VR schedule, on average every *n*th response is followed by the reinforcer, although the number of responses required for reinforcement varies irregularly. Both of these schedules typically engender high rates of responding with protracted exposure. Substantial post-reinforcement (or pre-ratio) pausing, the cessation of behavior following a reinforcer, is characteristic of performance under FR, but not VR, schedules.

In contrast to FR and VR schedules, fixed-interval (FI) and variable-interval (VI) schedules are time-based, although they do require emission of a specified response for reinforcement. The FI schedule specifies that the first response emitted after a given period has elapsed (e.g., 10 minutes under an FI 10-min schedule) will be reinforced. This interval usually is timed from the delivery of the previous reinforcer or the onset of some other stimulus. Relatively low overall response rates are typical under FI schedules; most responses are emitted toward the end of the interval, a pattern known as "scalloping." Variable-interval schedules specify that the first response emitted after some average period of time has elapsed will be reinforced; this interval varies irregularly around the mean value. These schedules generally evoke moderately high and very steady rates of responding.

Progressive-ratio (PR) schedules require an organism to emit an increasing number of responses to earn reinforcement. For instance, under a PR 5 schedule of cocaine delivery for a rat, the number of lever-press responses required to earn cocaine in a given test session begins at 5 and is incremented by 5 every time cocaine is earned. That is, the response requirement for the first five cocaine deliveries are, in order, 5, 10, 15, 20, and 25. The ratio requirement eventually becomes so long that the subject ceases to respond for a specified period, usually 5 to 15 minutes, at which point the session ends. The largest ratio completed before responding ceases is termed the breaking point, and is used as a measure of the efficacy of the scheduled reinforcer, or of response strength.

Under differentiation schedules, reinforcers are presented when responding displays a specified property. The most commonly studied differentiation schedules are those which: (1) deliver the reinforcer only if the time between two successive responses (i.e., the interresponse time, or IRT) exceeds a specified value; (2) deliver the reinforcer only if the IRT is less than a specified value; or (3) deliver the reinforcer only if a certain response fails to occur during a specified period. These schedules are commonly referred to as interresponse-time-greater-than-t (IRT > t), interresponse-time-less-than-t (IRT < t) and differential-reinforcement-of-pauses-greater-than-t (DRP > t), respectively. Other descriptors for the schedules are differential-reinforce-ment-of-low-rates (DRL), differential-reinforcement-of-high-rates (DRH), and dif-ferential-reinforcement-of-other-behavior (DRO). The designations DRL, DRH, and DRO are based on prediction of the patterns of behavior likely, but not certain, to occur under each condition (Lattal & Poling, 1981; Zeiler, 1977).

The patterns of responding that occur under differentiation schedules depend crucially on temporal parameters. In general, under IRT > t schedules most responses occur with an interresponse time approximately equal to t, although response "bursting" soon after a reinforcer is delivered is common. High and consistent rates of responding frequently appear under IRT < t schedules, whereas DRP > t schedules of reinforcement typically result in a rate of responding lower than that which occurred in their absence. This last result may appear paradoxical; how can a schedule of reinforcement result in a lowered rate of responding? The answer is that, under the DRP > t schedule (also referred to as the differential-reinforcement-of-not-responding-greater-than-t) schedule, the response that is reinforced is a period in which a particular bit of behavior fails to occur (i.e., a pause). This response actually increases in frequency under the DRP > t schedule (Poling & Ryan, 1982). Alternatively, the schedule can be construed as involving punishment by the prevention of delivery of a reinforcer (Malott, Whaley, & Malott, 1997).

Simple schedules can be combined to form complex schedules. Concurrent and multiple schedules are examples of complex schedules. **Concurrent schedules** arrange reinforcement simultaneously for two or more response classes. For ex-ample, under a concurrent VI 1-min FR 5-min schedule, left-key responses by a pigeon would be reinforced under the VI component, whereas right-key responses would be reinforced under the FR component. Concurrent schedules are especially useful for studying choice (de Villiers, 1977). They are also commonly used in the quantitative analysis of behavior, which involves developing equations that relate environmental inputs (e.g., reinforcement rates) to behavioral outputs (e.g., re-sponse rates).

Unlike concurrent schedules, **multiple schedules** successively arrange two or more component schedules, each associated with a specific discriminative stimulus. Mixed schedules are like multiple schedules, except that no discriminative stimuli are correlated with the component schedules.

Schedules of reinforcement have proven invaluable for examining the impor-tance of stimulus control and non-drug response rate as determinants of drug action, and for analyzing the stimulus properties of drugs.

Acquiring New Behavior

Novel behavior can be generated in several ways. In humans, verbal descriptions, modeling, or physical prompting often is sufficient to engender new forms of responding. The reinforcement of successive approproximations, or more succinctly **shaping**, is another procedure used to produce novel actions. For instance, shaping characteristically is used to produce lever pressing by rats and key pecking by pigeons.

In shaping, the desired final response is first defined and the closest approximation to that response that is now occurring is ascertained. Thus, a rat's lever press response might be defined as a downward movement of the lever with a force sufficient to operate a microswitch, and the closest observed approximation thereto might be approaching the lever. Initially, a reinforcer is delivered when the closest approximation to the desired response occurs. For example, food might be delivered when the rat came within an inch of the lever. Over time, the requirement for reinforcement is gradually changed until the final response appears. Each time the criterion for reinforcement is changed, extinction is arranged for the previously-reinforced response. As noted previously, extinction increases the variability of behavior, which makes it more probable that behavior will meet the new criterion for reinforcement. When it does, the criterion is again changed. This process continues until the final response form reliably occurs. At that time, the response has been acquired.

To adapt to the incredibly complex world in which they live, humans must constantly acquire new behavior, and new forms of stimulus control over established behavior. Put differently, they must learn. Given the incredibly importance of learning, it should come as no surprise that drug-induced learning impairment has garnered much attention from behavioral pharmacologists.

Verbal Behavior

Humans are unique with respect to the importance that language plays in their activities. Many behavior analysts use the term verbal behavior to refer to the kinds of activities that laypeople would term language use. According to Skinner (1957), **verbal behavior** is behavior that indirectly affects the environment through the behavior of another person. This indirect mode of action is what distinguishes verbal behavior from all other behavior. A smoker may obtain a cigarette through the direct physical act of taking a cigarette out of a pack, or that person may ask a friend for a cigarette. The consequence in each case is the acquisition of a cigarette, and eventually nicotine entering the body, which can reinforce both taking and asking.

Asking a friend, "May I have a cigarette?" is verbal behavior because the direct action of the friend, not the speaker, brings about the reinforcing change in the environment. Of primary importance in understanding verbal behavior is recognizing that verbal behavior is operant behavior, that is, it is controlled by its consequences and related environmental events. These events include reinforcement history, current discriminative stimuli, and establishing operations. Verbal response products, whether they are spoken, written, or signed, are stimuli that enter into the same kinds of environment-behavior relations as do non-verbal stimuli. Detailed analyses of these relations are provided elsewhere (e.g., Hayes, Hayes, Sato, & Ono, 1994; Michael, 1993; Skinner, 1957).

Skinner (1957) proposed a functional categorization of verbal operants that is of some value on understanding human language use. Two especially important relations that he described are the mand and the tact. In lay terms, a mand is a unit of verbal behavior that is controlled by what would be currently reinforcing for the speaker. A more precise definition is provided by Michael (1993): " The mand can be defined as a verbal operant in which the response is reinforced by a characteristic consequence and is therefore under the functional control of the establishing operation relevant to that type of consequence" (p. 100). The previously discussed request, "May I have a cigarette?" is a good example of a mand. So is "Give me a cigarette!" Both verbal operants specify the same consequence, and both are influenced by the same establishing operation (e.g., nicotine deprivation). Thus, both mands are members of the same operant response class.

In lay terms, tacts are "naming" responses. Unlike mands, tacts are controlled by the presence of nonverbal stimuli. Tacts characteristically are established and maintained through conditioned reinforcement. For example, the sight of an uncultivated marijuana plant may evoke the response "ditch weed" from a novice user. A more experienced user may then say "damned straight," thereby increasing the future frequency of the novice user tacting "ditch weed" in the presence of similar plants, which come to serve as discriminative stimulus for emitting the response "ditch weed."

Although the preceding examples are simple and contrived, they do serve to illustrate that what people say about drugs (or about anything else) is determined, in large part, by their experiences with an audience of listeners. Verbal behavior is learned behavior, and is therefore almost endlessly flexible. This is important to recognize, because verbal behavior of a special sort—specifically, rule-governed behavior—can play an important role in determining drug effects.

Rules specify relations among antecedent stimuli, responses, and consequences and alter behavior by changing the function of other stimuli. Because behavior analysts characteristically refer to relations among events as contingencies, rules can be accurately described as function-altering, contingency-specifying stimuli (Schlinger & Blakely, 1987). For example, giving a tired student who must study for an exam the rule, "If you take this pill, you'll feel wide awake," may alter the function of the pill from a neutral stimulus to that of a reinforcing stimulus.

Rules may enable previously neutral stimulus to serve functions similar to those of establishing operations and discriminative stimuli. They may also enable events too delayed to affect behavior directly to function as reinforcers (or punishers). To exemplify these effects, consider a hypothetical experiment described by Poling and LeSage (1992). Subjects are paid college students, each of whom smokes over a pack of cigarettes each day. They agree to reside on a residential ward for five consecutive days. Their access to various parts of that ward, to social interactions, and to cigarettes is controlled by the experimenter. Unless otherwise specified, each subject is given one cigarette every hour from 8 a.m. to 10 p.m., therefore, they are mildly cigarette deprived relative to their usual smoking levels.

Each day, beginning at nine in the morning, subjects sit at a console that contains a telegraph key, red and blue stimulus lights above the key, and a cigarette dispenser. A progressive-ratio 50 (PR 50) schedule of cigarette delivery is arranged for presses of the key and, once responding is initiated, the session continues until two consecutive minutes elapse without a response. The measure of interest is the breaking point, defined as the number of responses in the last ratio completed each session. Written instructions are provided on a note card taped above the key. Across five consecutive sessions, the following instructions appear on the card:

Day 1. You can earn cigarettes by pressing the key.

Day 2. You can earn cigarettes by pressing the key. Cigarettes are available only when the red light is on.

Day 3. You can earn cigarettes by pressing the key. The cigarettes that you earn by pressing the key will be the only ones available to you today.

Day 4. You can earn cigarettes by pressing the key. For each cigarette that you earn, you will be required to miss 15 minutes of the social period scheduled from 9 to 11 tonight.

Day 5. You can earn cigarettes by pressing the key. No cigarettes will be delivered now; they will be delivered at 8 tonight.

The day 1 instructions (rules) should establish responding similar to that produced by direct exposure to the contingencies described. On day 2, the red light should control responding in a manner similar to an S^D. That is, far more responding occurs when the light is on than when it is off. On day 3, one would expect a higher breaking point than that obtained on the other days; the statement concerning cigarette available serves as an establishing operation, increasing the reinforcing value of cigarettes. Assuming that social interaction is important to the subjects, relatively little responding would occur on day 4. Here, delayed aversive consequences reduce drug-seeking behavior. Considerable responding probably would occur on day 5, even though there is a substantial delay between responding and cigarette delivery. As with day 4, the provision of rules enables delayed consequences to affect behavior.

Contrast these performances with those likely to occur in the absence of rules. Sans rules, substantial key-press responding may or may not occur on day 1. If it did, the red light may have developed discriminative control over responding on day 2, although this would require a substantial period of time to occur. Behavior would not be affected by the restricted access arranged on day 3, or the delayed consequences in effect on days 4 and 5. Clearly, rules affect drug-related behavior in this hypothetical example. As illustrated in the chapters that follow, rules also can modulate drug actions in the everyday world.

Concluding Comments

Generating and following rules is operant behavior, acquired and maintained as a result of a long and complex history of interaction with other people. Whether a given person follows a particular rule depends, in large part, on her or his experience with similar rules and rule-givers. Thus, the capacity of rules to modify drug action is not fixed, but differs substantially across time and people. Rule-governed behavior is fundamentally orderly, but it is complex, and almost endlessly variable. Much the same is true of contingency-shaped behavior—that is, of responses controlled by direct exposure to their consequences.

Drug effects are always orderly, but that does not mean that they are simple or easy to understand. Principles of operant and respondent conditioning provide a useful conceptual framework for examining the behavioral effects of drugs, and the mechanisms through which those effects are produced. In general, expertise in behavior analysis is prerequisite for success in behavioral pharmacology: Only if one knows how behavior is controlled in the absence of drugs can one make sense of how drugs influence behavior. Of course, some understanding of basic pharmacological principles is also required. Chapter 3 introduces those principles.

References

de Villiers, P. (1977). Choice in concurrent schedules and a quantitative formulation of the law of effect. In W. K. Honig & J. E. R. Staddon (Eds.), *Handbook of operant behavior* (pp. 233-287). New York: Prentice-Hall.

Hayes, S. C., Hayes, L. J., Sato, M., & Ono, K. (1994). *Behavior analysis of language and cognition.* Reno, NV: Context Press.

Lattal, K. A., & Poling, A. (1981). Descriptions of response-event relations: Babel revisited. *The Behavior Analyst, 4,* 143-152.

Mackintosh, N. (1974). *The psychology of animal learning.* New York: Academic Press.

Malott, R. W., Whaley, D. L., & Malott, M. E. (1997). *Elementary principles of behavior.* Upper Saddle River, NJ: Prentice Hall.

Michael, J. L. (1975). Positive and negative reinforcement, a distinction that is no longer necessary; or a better way to talk about bad things. *Behaviorism, 3,* 33-44.

Michael, J. L. (1982). Distinguishing between discriminative and motivational functions of stimuli. *Journal of the Experimental Analysis of Behavior, 37,* 149-155.

Michael, J. L. (1993). *Concepts and principles of behavior analysis.* Kalamazoo, MI: Society for the Advancement of Behavior Analysis.

Poling, A., & LeSage, M. (1992). Rule-governed behavior and human behavioral pharmacology: A brief commentary on an important topic. *The Analysis of Verbal Behavior, 10,* 37-44.

Poling, A., & Ryan, C. (1982). Therapeutic applications of differential-reinforcement-of-other-behavior (DRO) schedules: A review. *Behavior Modification, 6,* 3-20.

Schlinger, H., & Blakely, E. (1987). Function-altering effects of contingency-specifying stimuli. *The Behavior Analyst, 10,* 41-45.

Skinner, B. F. (1953). *Science and human behavior.* New York: Macmillan.

Skinner, B. F. (1957). *Verbal behavior.* New York: Appleton-Century-Crofts.

Zeiler, M. (1977). Schedules of reinforcement: The controlling variables. In W. K. Honig & J. E. R. Staddon (Eds.), *Handbook of operant behavior* (pp. 201-232). New York: Prentice-Hall.

Chapter 3

Principles of Pharmacology

Alan Poling
and Thomas Byrne
Western Michigan University and
Massachusetts College of Liberal Arts

As discussed in Chapter 1, behavioral pharmacology makes use of principles of both behavior analysis and pharmacology in explaining the effects of drugs. Chapter 2 introduced fundamental principles of behavior analysis. The present chapter, which summarizes material discussed in more detail by Benet, Kroetz, and Sheiner (1996), Hollinger (1997), Julien (1998), Poling, Gadow, and Cleary (1991), and Ross (1996), overviews pharmacology.

Labeling and Classifying Drugs

A **drug** is any chemical that affects living processes, although the term often is restricted to substances introduced into, not produced by, the body (e.g., most people do not refer to neurotransmitters as drugs). Drugs that affect mood, thought processes, or overt behavior are called **psychoactive**, and drugs that are prescribed with the intent of improving mood, thought processes, or overt behavior are called **psychotropic**. The terms psychoactive drug and behaviorally-active drug are rough synonyms, as are behavior-change medication and psychotropic medication.

Although some drugs come from plants and animals, most are synthetic substances. The nomenclature used to describe drugs is rather confusing. All drugs have a chemical name, which provides a description of the molecule according to rules outlined in *Chemical Abstracts*. In addition to its chemical name, a new drug is usually given a code name by its manufacturer. If the drug is developed for clinical use, the drug will be given a United States Adopted Name (USAN) by a panel of experts. The USAN is a nonproprietary name and is often referred to as the **generic name** of the drug. When a drug is admitted to the *United States Pharmacopeia*, which lists therapeutic agents approved for use in the United States, the USAN becomes the official name. Nonproprietary (or generic) names are commonly used in pharmacology and will be used in this text.

After a drug is given an official name, it is assigned a **proprietary name** (also termed the trade, or brand, name) by the manufacturer. These names are protected by trademark laws, are usually easy to pronounce, and may suggest a drug's therapeutic action. Trade names are capitalized when they appear in print. A drug manufacturer patents a newly formulated agent and controls the right to manufacture it for 17 years. When the period of patent protection expires, any drug company can manufacture the drug and sell it either by its nonproprietary (generic) name or by a different trade name. Medications marketed by several manufacturers may have several trade names.

Most drugs that are used recreationally have slang names. Such names characteristically vary with time and place. Moreover, the same slang name may be used to refer to several different drugs. For instance, "speed" may refer to amphetamine, methamphetamine, or designer amphetamine derivatives. Table 3-1 shows the chemical, proprietary, nonproprietary, and slang names of a commonly abused drug.

Table 3-1. Chemical, Generic, Trade, and Slang Names of a Commonly Abused Drug

Chemical name	Generic name	Trade name	Slang name
Phencyclidine 1 (1-phencyclohexy) piperidine	Phencyclidine	Sernylan	Angel dust

A number of systems have been developed to classify drugs; none is entirely satisfactory. Drugs may be classified according to their chemical structure, their physiological actions, their behavioral effects, or their therapeutic usage. The usual mode of classification is on the basis of the most important clinical use of medicinal drugs, and on the most obvious behavioral effect of drugs not used medicinally. Thus, diazepam (Valium), chlordiazepoxide (Librium), and triazolam (Halcion) are grouped together as antianxiety agents (anxiolytics), whereas LSD, MDA, mescaline, and psilocybin are grouped together as hallucinogenic drugs (hallucinogens). Further categorization in terms of structure or mechanism of action sometimes occurs, as when mescaline and MDA are considered together as noradrenergic hallucinogens and LSD and psilocybin are grouped as serotonergic hallucinogens. Table 3-2 lists a number of drugs according to their usual therapeutic application or most pronounced behavioral effect in humans. Even though the behavioral effects of drugs from the same class might differ substantially, it is convention in pharmacology to emphasize a small number of prototypes in describing the effects of particular drug classes.

Pharmacokinetics

Pharmacokinetics refers to the absorption, distribution, biotransformation, and excretion of drug molecules. These four processes determine, in large part, the intensity and duration of drug effects. **Absorption** is the process whereby drug

Table 3-2. Generic and Trade Names of Several Common Drugs, Classified According to Primary Medical Use or Most Prominent Behavioral Effect

Anxiolytics

alprazolam (Xanax)
buspirone (Buspar)
chlordiazepoxide (Librium)
lorazepam (Ativan)
triazolam (Halcion)

Antidepressants

amitryptline (Elavil, Endep)
doxepin (Adapin)
imipramine (Janimine)
phenelzine (Nardil)
trazadone (Desyrel)

Psychomotor Stimulants

caffeine
cocaine
dextroamphetamine
methamphetamine
methylphenidate (Ritalin)

Opioid analgesics

codeine
heroin
meperidine (Demerol)
methadone (Dolophine)
morphine

Neuroleptics

chlorpromazine (Thorazine)
chlorprothixene (Taractan)
clozapine (Clozaril)
haloperidol (Haldol)
thioridazine (Mellaril)

Anticonvulsants

mephobarbitol (Mebaral)
carbamazepine (Tegretol)
diazepam (Valium)
phenytoin (Dilantin)
valproic acid (Depakene)

Hallucinogens

dimethyltryptamine
lysergic acid diethlamide
mescaline
psilocybin
scopolamine

molecules enter the bloodstream. **Distribution** involves the movement of drug molecules through the bloodstream to the site of action, the place where drug molecules affect protoplasm to produce an effect. **Biotransformation** refers to the changes in the structure of drug molecules characteristically produced by enzymatic action in the liver. Most drugs are converted into inactive metabolites, but some are changed to an active form. **Excretion** is the process responsible for the removal of drug molecules and metabolites from the body, usually in the urine.

Movement of Drug Molecules

From the time a drug enters the body until it exits, molecules of that drug characteristically are moving across membranes into various fluids, including the bloodstream, the urine, the extracellular fluid, and the intracellular fluid. For example, to be absorbed after oral ingestion, a drug in tablet or capsule form must dissolve in the fluids of the stomach. It then passes through the membranes that line the wall of the digestive tract, into the bloodstream. These membranes, and those that drug molecules must traverse to enter other bodily fluids, such as the urine or the extracellular fluid, are constructed of lipids (fats) and proteins. They are only about 0.0000032 inch in thickness (Julien, 1998) and are semi-permeable to drugs and endogenous substances. Membranes are semi-permeable in that they can be readily crossed by some molecules, but not by others.

Molecules move across membranes due to passive diffusion. That is, they move down a concentration gradient. An example of diffusion can be seen when one puts a drop of food dye in a glass of water. At first, the dye will be concentrated in a small portion of the water, which will be colored. Over time, the dye diffuses so that its concentration throughout the water is about equal, and the water is of a consistent color.

There are very small pores in the body's membranes, through which water and some water-soluble drugs, such as alcohol, can pass. Nonetheless, substances that are lipid soluble (soluble in fat) characteristically pass more readily across cell membranes than do substances that are water soluble. Ionized molecules (ions) carry an electrical charge and are water-soluble, therefore, they do not readily cross membranes. Unionized molecules do not carry an electrical charge, are lipid-soluble, and readily cross membranes. Molecules of most drugs exist as a mixture of ionized and unionized forms. The proportion of molecules in each form is not fixed, but depends on the pK_a of the drug and the relative acidity (pH) of the medium in which the drug is dissolved.

The pH is a number, ranging from 1 to 14, that represents the concentration of hydrogen ions (H+) in a solution. The lower the pH, the higher the concentration of H+. Solutions with a low pH (a high H+ concentration) are called acids; solutions with a high pH (a low H+ concentration) are called bases. The pK_a of a drug is the pH at which one-half of that drug's molecules occur in ionized form. The importance of pK_a and internal pH is readily apparent if one considers that weak acids (pK_a of 3 of 4) are well absorbed from the stomach, an acidic medium, whereas weak bases (pK_a of 8 or 9) are absorbed poorly from the stomach, but are absorbed more readily from the less acidic intestines.

When pH differs on two sides of a membrane, as between the bloodstream and the stomach, the ratio of water-soluble (ionized) to lipid-soluble (unionized) molecules will differ on the two sides. In this case, an equal concentration of lipid-soluble drug will be present on the two sides. But, because water-soluble molecules are unable to cross the membrane, the total amount of drug will be greater on the side with the higher ratio of water-soluble to lipid-soluble molecules.

In some cases, the size of drug molecules limits their ability to cross membranes; not surprisingly, small molecules characteristically cross membranes more readily than large ones. Molecules of a few drugs are actively transported across membranes. That is, energy-using systems move those molecules from one side of a membrane to the other.

Route of Administration

Obviously, a drug must enter the body before it can be absorbed. The method by which a drug enters an organism is called the **route of administration**. Most drugs are administered orally, parenterally (by injection), or by inhalation. A few are administered by being placed in contact with the skin, or with membranes in the mouth, nasal cavity, or rectum. The route of administration plays an important role in the rate and pattern of drug absorption, and consequently in the duration and intensity of the drug's effect. Figure 3-1 illustrates differences in the effects of a hypothetical drug when administered orally and by intravenous, intramuscular, and subcutaneous injection.

The oral route, in which the drug is swallowed, is convenient and commonly used with humans. Nonetheless, the route has some limitations. A few drugs, such as insulin, are inactivated by stomach enzymes, and others do not pass readily into

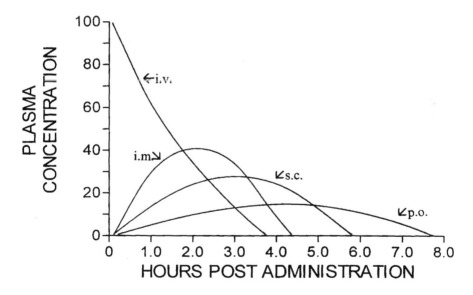

Figure 3-1. *Plasma concentration of a hypothetical drug as a function of route of administration and time following drug administraiton. Routes of administration are abbreviated as follows: IV = intravenous, IM = intramuscular, SC = subcutaneous, PO (oral). The general relations shown are typical of many drugs, although specific time courses of changes in drug blood level vary widely.*

the blood stream. Even for a drug that is absorbed relatively well, the amount that will enter the bloodstream may be difficult to estimate accurately. Individuals differ with respect to their natural speed of absorption, which (as discussed above) is also influenced by stomach and intestinal pH and by the presence of food or other drugs in the gut. Because food alters absorption, many medications are taken between meals. The usual exceptions are those agents that cause gastric upset if taken on an empty stomach.

The rate of absorption is determined, in part, by the form in which the drug is administered. Liquids are usually absorbed more readily than solids, although the two dosage forms sometimes are used interchangeably. Particulars of manufacture, such as the thickness of the pill coating, type of filler substances, and hardness of the tablet also alter the rate of absorption. Therefore, different brands of the same medication may be absorbed at different rates. This can be of clinical significance because the amount of drug in the blood is related directly to therapeutic (and other) responses.

In some cases, manufacturers intentionally prepare drugs in a form that slows absorption. For example, CIBA Pharmaceuticals markets methylphenidate (Ritalin) in the form of regular and sustained-release (Ritalin SR) tablets. Active drug is more slowly absorbed from the sustained-release tablets, which prolongs the duration of drug effects (Birhamer, Greenhill, Cooper, Fried, & Maminski, 1989). Because chewing sustained-release Ritalin tablets speeds absorption, patients are advised to swallow them whole.

Intravenous (IV) injection involves introducing the drug directly into the blood stream with the use of a hypodermic needle. Absorption is bypassed, the peak blood level occurs immediately and can be specified precisely, and the maximal drug effect occurs with very little delay. The rapid onset of drug action following IV injection can be of benefit, as when an injection of naloxone is used to reverse the effects of a heroin overdose. But this same characteristic can cause problems, because there is little time to counter untoward effects. For instance, a person who overdoses on heroin taken via IV injection is likely to be incapacitated so rapidly as to be unable to even call for help.

All parenteral routes can cause tissue damage and scarring. In addition, unless sterile techniques are used, a syringe can introduce microbes that produce infection. This can be seen in the high rates of HIV infection among heroin addicts. A few substances cannot be injected intravenously because they are not soluble in the bloodstream and may produce blood clots. Also, allergic reactions often are more pronounced when a drug is given IV than when it is administered via other routes.

Intramuscular (IM) administration involves injecting a drug into skeletal muscle tissue. Muscle tissue contains a high density of blood vessels, which allows for relatively rapid absorption. Of course, blood flow to a given muscle is not fixed. For example, muscle contraction increases blood flow, which causes faster absorption. The volume of the injection and the solubility of the drug also influence absorption.

Intraperitoneal (IP) administration involves injecting the drug into the peritoneal cavity. The peritoneal cavity is the area between the abdominal organs and the dermis. It is richly vascularized, hence, absorption following an IP injection is relatively rapid. IP injections are rarely used with humans, but are a common route for administering drugs to rats. Because of rats' small size, using IV or IM injections with them can be difficult. But IP injections also pose problems, in that the close proximity of the injection site to internal organs leads to the possibility of serious internal damage and infection. Care must be taken to insure sterility, and the injection itself must be quick and smooth to prevent lacerations.

Subcutaneous (SC) administration involves placing a drug under the skin; if a syringe is used, the injection is not deep enough to penetrate muscle tissue. This route allows for a slow and constant rate of absorption, which is useful when a sustained drug effect is desired. Subcutaneous administration may involve the insertion of a pellet or a dispenser that provides slow, steady absorption over a period of weeks or months. An example is Norplant, a contraceptive device that is surgically implanted under the skin of a woman's arm. The implant disperses progestin, a hormone that prevents pregnancy, for a period of up to five years.

Inhalation involves breathing in gases, aerosols, or small particles carried in a gas or smoke. Because the membranes that line the lungs are richly endowed with blood vessels, absorption of inhaled drug molecules that readily cross membranes (e.g., nitrous oxide, halothane) is very rapid.

Several other routes of administration are available, but will not be covered here. It is, however, important to realize that the duration and magnitude of a drug's effects depend critically on how that drug is administered. Although the general pattern of drug absorption (and drug effects) across time can be described for different routes, several variables influence absolute rates of absorption. Therefore, even when the route is fixed, the duration and magnitude of a drug's effects can differ markedly across individuals, or across situations in a given individual.

Distribution

Once a drug is absorbed, within about one minute it is distributed throughout the bloodstream. Drug molecules move through passive diffusion from the blood stream into other body fluids. Parts of the body that are richly perfused with blood vessels, such as the heart, liver, brain, and kidneys, receive most of the drug shortly after absorption; the drug may reach muscle, skin, and fat considerably later. As discussed in Chapter 4, drugs characteristically affect behavior by interacting with neurons located in the brain. To reach this site of action, drug molecules pass from the aorta to smaller arteries, then to the capillaries. Molecules then move through the capillary walls to the extracellular fluid, where they diffuse and eventually contact the cells that they affect.

At a given time, only a small fraction of the drug molecules present in the body are in the brain, producing an effect. The remainder are located in other parts of the body, and many of them never reach the brain. But they are important nonetheless, because the number of drug molecules that reaches the brain depends upon the total amount of drug in the body. In addition, even in the case of psychoactive drugs, actions on organs other than the brain are important. For instance, many of the side effects of psychotropic drugs, including the dry mouth and blurred vision associated with certain neuroleptic drugs (e.g., chlorpromazine, or Thorazine), are produced outside the brain. With some medications, such as vitamins and antibiotics, the primary therapeutic effects characteristically are produced outside the brain.

Molecules of many drugs combine with large protein molecules in the blood in a process called **protein binding**. Protein-bound molecules are unable to pass out of the blood stream and do not reach the site of action, but this process is not irreversible. As unbound molecules pass out of the bloodstream, bound molecules are released so that the ratio of bound to unbound molecules in the blood remains roughly constant. Although the maximal effect of a drug is reduced by protein binding, the process prolongs the effect of the drug by creating a reservoir of bound drug molecules that are released over time (Briant, 1978).

Depot binding, which occurs when drug molecules bind to parts of the body that they do not affect (so-called **silent receptors**), has the same effect. Silent receptors are located throughout the body in muscle, bone, and fat. The importance of depot binding as a determinant of drug effects is exemplified by the barbiturates, which have a high affinity for lipids and bind to silent receptors in fatty tissue. Because of this, these drugs produce weaker, but longer lasting, effects in obese people than in slim individuals.

In order for a drug to affect receptors in the brain, it must pass through the **blood-brain barrier**, which is a mechanism that protects the brain from harmful substances. In most capillaries outside the brain, there are clefts between cells of the capillary wall, as shown in Figure 3-2. Drug molecules can potentially pass through these spaces as well as through fenstrae (literally, "windows"), which are gaps in the capillary cell membranes. As also shown in Figure 3-2, capillaries in the brain do not have clefts between the cells, but are fused together in what are called tight junctions. Fenstrae are also absent in brain capillaries. Passage of drug molecules that are large, ionized, or water soluble is greatly impeded by the characteristics of capillaries in the brain. Thus, the same characteristics that enable drug molecules to enter the bloodstream with ease—that is, being small, unionized, and lipid

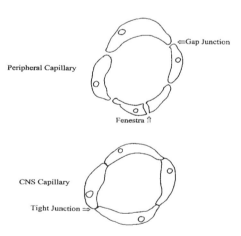

Figure 3-2. *Structural differences in peripheral and central nervous system (CNS) capillaries make it more difficult for drugs to exit the bloodstream in the CNS.*

soluble–also allow drug molecules to exit the blood stream and enter the brain with ease.

Comparing the effects of morphine and heroin illustrates the importance of these characteristics in determining drug effects. Both drugs affect the same receptors on neurons in the brain, and they have comparable behavioral effects. But heroin (diacetylmorphine), which is produced from morphine and closely resembles it (Figure 3-3), is more lipid-soluble than morphine, and as a consequence penetrates the blood-brain barrier more readily. Because of this, heroin is about three times as potent as morphine.

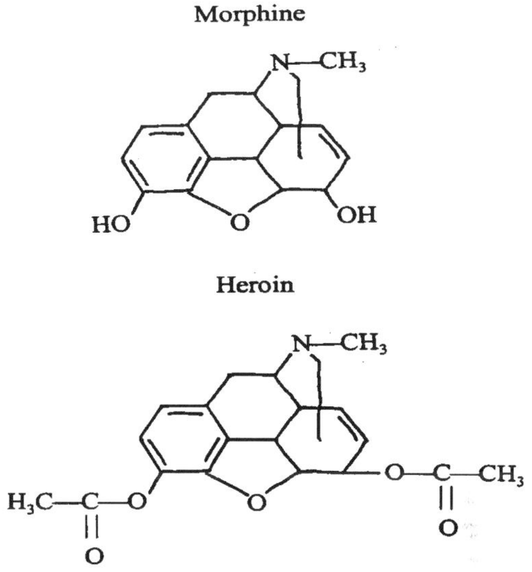

The placenta, which is a

Figure 3-3. *The chemical structures of heroin and morphine molecules.*

membrane that separates the blood stream of a fetus from that of its mother, is similar to other membranes in the body in its permeability. Therefore, small, lipid-soluble, unionized molecules - including molecules of many abused drugs and medications - cross it readily. Put simply, the placenta is not a effective barrier that protects the fetus from substances taken by its mother. Instead, similar concentrations are likely to be observed in both. This is of obvious concern in that some drugs are known to produce **teratogenic effects**, that is, they induce structural damage in the developing fetus. Other drugs damage the fetus by inducing respiratory depression.

Biotransformation

As they pass through the body, most drugs are changed into new compounds termed **metabolites**. Characteristically, drugs are eventually biotransformed into inactive metabolites (substances that do not affect biological processes), but it is not unusual for intermediate metabolites to produce biological effects. In a few cases, parent compounds themselves are not active, but their metabolites do produce behavioral effects. For example, chloral hydrate is rapidly metabolized to trichlorethanol, which is very similar to ethanol (beverage alcohol). It is trichlorethanol, not the parent drug, that is responsible for the sedative-hypnotic effects of chloral hydrate.

Substances within the cells of the liver, called **enzymes**, initiate and facilitate the chemical reactions that transform drugs into metabolites. In most cases an active drug is metabolized into a substance (or substances) that is water soluble and can be excreted through the kidneys. Some drugs, however, are not metabolized and pass from the body unchanged. Muscimole, which is a hallucinogenic drug found in the mushroom *Amanita muscaria*, does so. Specifically, it is excreted in urine, often at rather high concentrations. People native to parts of Siberia learned of this, and sometimes ingested their own urine after consuming *Aminita* mushrooms in order to attain greater psychoactive effects.

The chemical processes involved in biotransformation may involve the nonsynthetic reactions of oxidation, reduction, or hydrolysis, in which drug molecules are "broken down." Synthetic (conjugation) reactions, in which a drug or its metabolite combines with an endogenous (naturally occurring) substance, such as an amino acid, also contribute to biotransformation. All of these reactions are rather complex, and it is beyond our scope to cover them.

It is, however, important to understand that the systems through which drugs are metabolized typically are not selective. Instead, they act on several different drugs and endogenous substances. Because of this, there is competition for these systems, such that the presence of one drug may slow the biotransformation of a second one. When this occurs with drugs that are inactivated through biotransformation, the magnitude and duration of one drug's effects is increased by the presence of the second drug.

In many cases, repeated exposure to a drug causes the body to produce more of the enzymes that inactivate that drug. This process, called **enzyme induction**, is one mechanism through which tolerance develops. As discussed later, tolerance occurs when some effect of a drug is diminished in magnitude as a result of exposure to that drug. When the same enzyme system inactivates more than one drug, as is usually the case, enzyme induction produced by exposure to one drug typically leads to a degree of tolerance to the other drugs. This phenomenon is called **cross** (or crossed) **tolerance** and occurs, for instance, with heroin, morphine, and opium.

Because the liver is the primary site of biotransformation, which inactivates most drugs, conditions that impair hepatic (liver) function typically increase the magnitude and duration of drug effects. Because of this, people with liver disease (e.g., cirrhosis) often develop increased sensitivity to medications and recreational drugs. Because their livers are only beginning to function, newborn infants also are very sensitive to drugs. Elderly individuals may be as well, because hepatic function characteristically declines with advanced age.

Excretion

As mentioned previously, the kidneys are the most important organs for the elimination of drugs. The kidneys first nonselectively filter many different substances out of the blood, then they release lipid-soluble substances back into the blood. Special transport systems also return to the blood stream certain essential water-soluble molecules, such as glucose. Other molecules, including water-soluble molecules of drugs and their metabolites, are distributed to the bladder and eventually are discharged in urine.

Although most drugs or their metabolites are excreted in the urine, excretion can occur by other routes. Some substances may be eliminated in feces; this often occurs for orally-administered drugs that are not fully absorbed. Drugs may also be excreted in exhaled air, saliva, tears, or breast milk, or be sequestered in the hair or skin. For the most part, these routes are of minor importance. They may, however, be of special significance in some cases, as when human hair is used to screen for illicit drug use, or when hormones and antibiotics given to dairy cows are passed to humans in milk.

The rate of elimination of a drug depends on its physical properties, the amount administered (dose), the route of administration, and organismic variables that alter the body's response to the drug (e.g., age, disease). As mentioned earlier, the magnitude of a drug's observed effects is directly related to drug blood level. Therefore, it is common practice to describe the time course of action of a substance by referring to changes in drug blood level across time. Just as the rate of disappearance of a radioactive isotope is readily expressed as the time needed for one-half of it to decay (the half-life), the rate of disappearance of a drug may be described in terms of its biological half-life. The half-life, abbreviated as $T_{1/2}$, is calculated by measuring the time required for a given blood level to decline by 50%. With many drugs, this value does not change significantly as a function of initial drug blood lever or dosage, and such drugs are described as having **linear kinetics**. For such drugs, a constant fraction of drug is eliminated per unit time. Table 3-3 shows how a hypothetical drug with a half-life of 2 hours would be eliminated across time. In this table, it is assumed that the drug was administered intravenously, which would result in peak blood levels being reached immediately.

Table 3-3. Total Amount (Mg) of a Hypothetical Drug in Blood at Various Times after Intravenous Injection[a]

	Time after injection (hours)						
	0	4	8	12	16	20	24
Total drug (mg)	400	200	100	50	25	13	7
	800	400	200	100	50	25	13

[a]*This drug has a half-life of 4 hours and follows linear kinetics. Although the drug would remain in the blood at a low concentration for an extended period, observable effects would disappear well before all of the drug was eliminated (e.g., when total mg drug fell below 25)*

Close examination of Table 3-3 will reveal two important points. The first is that the decline in drug level describes an exponential decay curve. No matter how much drug is in the body, a given percentage of that amount is eliminated in a given amount of time. This percentage remains constant. The total amount of drug eliminated, however, is not fixed, but depends on the amount of drug present in the

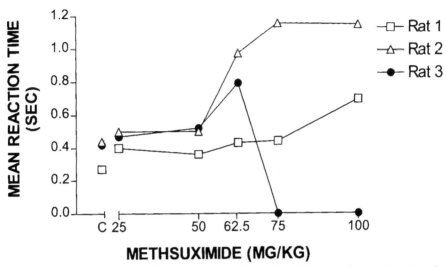

Figure 3-4. *The effects of methsuximide, an anticonvulsant drug, on the reaction time of two rats. Data are from Nickel, Alling, and Poling (1990).*

body. In fact, rate of elimination and the amount of drug in the body are directly related, such that doubling the dose increases the duration of action by one half-life. This is the second important point evident in the table. There is, of course, some limit to the maximal rate of drug elimination, and for all drugs linear kinetics hold only within a range of concentrations.

Some drugs have **nonlinear kinetics** at all concentrations, which means that the mechanisms that eliminate them are easily saturated, causing the relative rate of elimination to decrease (and the apparent half-life to increase) with dosage and concentration. The maximum rate of elimination for such drugs does not vary with the amount of drug in the body. For example, regardless of the amount of ethanol (beverage alcohol) ingested, the rate of metabolism in humans is constant at about 10 milliliters of absolute ethanol per hour. Ingesting more than 10 ml per hour, a relatively common behavior, will result in increasing ethanol concentration in the blood stream and in the brain, and corresponding behavioral effects. For ethanol and other drugs with nonlinear kinetics, there is a range of apparent half-lives for any individual, each affected by the dose and the initial concentration at which the $T_{1/2}$ is measured.

Even for drugs with linear kinetics, the rate of elimination varies across individuals as a function of genetics, physiological characteristics, and exposure to that and other drugs (i.e., drug history). For instance, changing the pH of urine can dramatically alter the rate of excretion of some drugs by changing the proportion of molecules that are ionized, and hence water soluble. As a case in point, changing the urinary pH from 6.4 to 8.0 changes the fraction of unionized salicylate, a strong acid and the active ingredient in aspirin, from 1% to 0.04% and increases the rate of excretion by 400-600% (Mayer, Melmon, & Gilmon, 1980). Because of this, administration of sodium bicarbonate (baking soda) to produce an alkaline urine and more rapid excretion is part of the treatment for children suffering from the real and common medical emergency of salicylate poisoning.

Because many different factors can influence drug elimination, half-life values are expressed only within rather broad ranges. Those values are, however, of importance in medicine. For example, a medication should be administered about once per half-life to maintain stable blood levels. Because it takes about five half-lives after the first administration to reach a stable blood level, evaluation of drug efficacy prior to that time will be inconclusive (Poling et al., 1991).

Given that the rate of disappearance of many drugs is exponential, detectable levels of drug (or metabolites) may be present well after detectable behavioral or physiological effects have disappeared. That is, some minimal concentration must be present at the site of action and, correspondingly, in the blood stream and elsewhere in the body, to produce an observable effect. Subthreshold levels, even if detectable, may be of no consequence with respect to the effects of interest.

If a drug is taken more rapidly than it can be inactivated, blood levels and overt effects increase over time. This phenomenon, known as **accumulation**, is a problem with many toxins, such as heavy metals, which enter the body in small amounts over the course of the lifetime, but are eliminated slowly, if at all. Accumulation also can be a problem when people receive chronic administrations of long-acting medications with variable half-lives. **Chronic** administrations are repeated administrations, characteristically given close enough together so that biologically active drug levels are constantly present in the body. Chronic administrations are contrasted with **acute administrations**, which are spaced far enough apart so that drug effects disappear between administrations.

Dose-Dependent Drug Effects

Drug **dose** refers to the amount of drug administered. The effects of all drugs are dose-dependent: the amount of drug that is administered determines both qualitative and quantitative aspects of its effects. At very low doses, all drugs fail to produce observable effects; at high enough doses, all doses produce toxic (harmful) reactions. For example, one is unlikely to detect any behavioral effects in an adult who has drunk a thimbleful of vodka over an hour. But one is likely to observe severe and general debilitation if the same person consumed a quart of vodka over the same period. Clearly, answering the question "What are the behavioral effects of vodka?" requires specification of the amount drunk.

Drug doses conventionally are expressed in metric units, usually in terms of milligrams (mg). One mg is approximately 1/28,000 of an ounce. In everyday clinical practice, physicians frequently ignore body weight in specifying dosage, and simply refer to mg/day. But, because humans (and other animals) vary substantially in size, and body size directly influences how much of a given amount of drug reaches the site of action, it is convention among researchers to express drug dosage in terms of units of drug (mg) per unit of body weight (kg). A kg equals 2.2 pounds. Thus, if two pigeons being used in an experiment, one weighing 1 kg and a second weighing 0.47 kg (i.e., 470 mg), were each to receive 3.2 mg/kg morphine, the former bird would receive 3.2 mg of drug (3.2 x 1), whereas the latter bird would receive 1.5 mg (3.2 x 0.47). Although not always formally stated in the specification of dosage, the time between administrations obviously is a powerful determinant of drug effects. If the pigeons just described received morphine once per day, their dosage could accurately be expressed as 3.2 mg/kg/day.

With some drugs, the amount administered correlates poorly with the level of drug in the blood. For those agents, a more useful measure than mg/kg is one that indicates how much drug is in the blood, which is often expressed as micrograms (mcg or ug) of drug per milliliter (mL) of blood.

Dose-response relations typically are depicted graphically. A **dose-response curve** plots a response measure across doses. The response measure characteristically is plotted on the vertical (y) axis and dosage is plotted on the horizontal (x) axis. Figure 3-4 is a dose-response curve showing the relationship between the dose of methsuximide, a drug used to treat epilepsy, and the reaction time of rats. This figure shows that methsuximide produced dose-dependent increases in reaction time. That is, reaction time increased as a direct function of drug dose.

The relation between drug dosage and the magnitude of effect is typically expressed in one of two ways. When the response measure of interest is continuous (i.e., capable of varying across a range of values), like reaction time, it is common to scale the magnitude of response on the y axis, as in Figure 3-4. When the response measure of interest is discrete (i.e., the response either occurs or fails to occur), it is common to present the dose-response relation in terms of the percentage of total exposed subjects that evidenced the response at each dose. Figure 3-5, which depicts the percentage of subjects who fell asleep within 15 minutes of receiving two hypothetical hypnotic drugs (A and B), shows such a relation.

From this figure, the **median effective dose** (ED_{50}) of each drug can be extrapolated. This is the dose at which 50% of the subjects evidenced the response of interest (sleep), and is indicated in Figure 3-5 by a dashed line. The maximal effectiveness, or **peak efficacy**, of each drug is also apparent. This is the largest effect produced by any dose of the drug. At its most effective dose, Drug B induced sleep in over 90% of the subjects, whereas no dose of Drug A induced sleep in more than 75% of the subjects. Therefore, Drug B has the greater peak efficacy. Peak efficacy is not, however, synonymous with potency. **Potency** technically refers to the amount of drug required to produce an effect of specified magnitude, frequently the ED_{50} dose. The ED_{50} dose of Drug A is lower than that of Drug B, therefore, Drug A is more potent.

Within reason, the amount of drug required to produce a given response is unimportant. For example, the usual oral antipsychotic dose range for haloperidol (Haldol) is 2 to 20 mg/day, whereas the usual dose of chlorpromazine (Thorazine) is 200 to 800 mg/day (Baldessarini, 1996). Usual doses of both drugs are small enough to take easily by mouth. Assuming equal therapeutic response to the two drugs, haloperidol would not be superior to chlorpromazine, despite the large

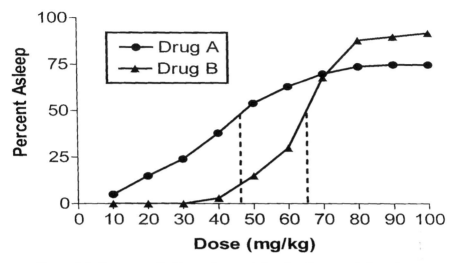

Figure 3-5. *Percentage of subjects who were induced to sleep at each dose of two hypothetical drugs. The ED$_{50}$ dose of each drug is illustrated by the dashed line and is the dose at which 50% of the subjects fell asleep within a specified period (e.g., 1 hour). The figure also shows that drug A is more potent, but drug B has greater peak efficacy.*

difference in potency. Potent drugs may appear to be especially powerful, but potency alone is a poor index of drug action.

Our discussion of the interpretation of dose response curves has thus far dealt primarily with a discrete response measure (percentage of subjects evidencing the effect). Interpretation is very similar when the response measure is continuous, except that the ED$_{50}$ dose would be defined as the dose that produced an effect equal to 50% of the maximal possible effect in the subject or group of subjects whose data were under consideration. As when a discrete response measure is used, peak efficacy would be defined in terms of the largest observed effect. It is, of course, often possible to convert continuous response measures into discrete ones, although the reverse usually is impossible.

Regardless of the kind of response measure used, adequate understanding of a drug's effects requires careful analysis of a range of doses and outcome measures. Summary measures, like the ED$_{50}$, are apt to be misleading. As a case in point, consider Figure 3-6, which depicts the desired effect and the lethality of two hypothetical drugs, C and D, that are being developed by a drug company for use in treating heartworms, which are dangerous parasites in dogs. The company's research has shown that the ED$_{50}$ for eliminating heartworms is 10 mg/kg, for Drug C and that at doses above 25 mg/kg it eliminates heartworms in all treated dogs. The ED$_{50}$ for Drug D is 25 mg/kg and it is effective in all subjects at doses above 75 mg/kg. As a measure of the relative safety of the two drugs, the **median lethal dose**

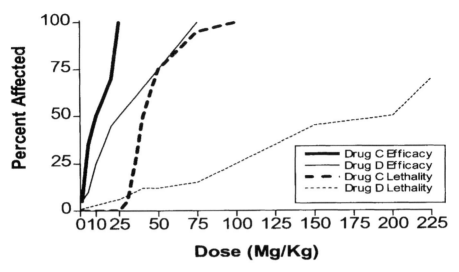

Figure 3-6. *Hypothetical data showing the desired and lethal effects of two drugs used to treat heartworms in dogs. ED_{50} and LD_{50} doses of each drug are indicated by dashed lines.*

(LD_{50}), which is the dose that kills 50% of subjects, also has been determined. The LD_{50} dose is 40 mg/kg for Drug C and 200 mg/kg for Drug D. Of course, comparing these doses is of no value in determining relative safety, because the two drugs differ in potency with respect to the desired, or therapeutic, effect (eliminating heartworms).

Following the logic that the relative safety of a drug increases as the distance between the dose required to produce the desired effect and the dose that produces adverse effects (death in our example) grows, one could calculate and compare Therapeutic Indices for the two drugs. The **Therapeutic Index** (TI) is a measure of relative drug safety that often is calculated by dividing the LD_{50} dose by the ED_{50} dose, although more conservative measures sometimes are used (e.g., $TI = LD_1 / ED_{90}$, where LD_1 is the dose that produced death in 1% of subjects and ED_{90} is the dose that produced the desired effect in 90% of subjects). If calculated accorded to the formula LD_{50} / ED_{50}, the TI would be 4 for Drug C and 8 for Drug D.

If the TI for the two drugs was the only information available, it would be tempting to conclude that Drug D is the safer of the two medication. Figure 3-6 suggests, however, that a small percentage of dogs receiving any therapeutic dose of Drug D will die. Although this is not evident in the figure, perhaps even at low doses the drug induces fatal allergic reactions in some animals, a reaction not unlike that observed in a small proportion of people who receive penicillin, or are stung by bees. Drug C, in contrast, seems to be unlikely to cause any deaths, even at doses that produce the desired effect in every dog. Drug C is actually the safer compound, and if dosage is regulated carefully it should never kill a dog and benefit each one that receives it.

Clearly, adequate understanding of the effects of any drug requires consideration of a full dose-response curve. Any of a wide variety of relations, linear or curvilinear, may be obtained between the amount of drug given and the magnitude and type of the resultant effect. In truth, it is difficult to predict the nature of a dose-response relation *a prior*, or following the administration of fewer than three appropriately-selected doses.

The foregoing examples, real and contrived, and the discussions accompanying them, have emphasized that: 1) all drugs have dose-dependent effects; 2) all drugs have multiple effects, and 3) all drugs have toxic (harmful) effects at sufficiently high doses. These statements hold so broadly, and are so important, that it is appropriate to view them as fundamental tenets of pharmacology. A fourth fundamental tenet, alluded to but not specifically stated in our discussion of pharmacokinetics, is that all drugs have time-dependent effects. That is, both qualitative and quantitative aspects of drug action depend on when effects are assessed relative to the time of drug administration. Table 3-4 lists these four fundamental tenets of pharmacology. Understanding them is prerequisite for making sense of the behavioral effects of any drug.

Table 3-4. Four Fundamental Tenets of Pharmacology

- All drugs produce dose-dependent effects.
- All drugs produce multiple effects.
- All drugs produce toxic effects at sufficiently high doses.
- All drugs produce time-dependent effects.

Tolerance and Physical Dependence

The effects of a drug often are influenced by the schedule of delivery. For instance, tolerance develops with chronic exposure to many drugs. **Tolerance** occurs when repeated administration of a given dose produces a smaller effect or when a higher dose is required to produce the same effect. Figure 3-7 illustrates the development of tolerance to the rate-reducing effects of morphine in pigeons responding under a progressive-ratio schedule of food delivery. After chronic exposure to the drug, a higher dose of morphine was required to produce a given degree of rate reduction than was required prior to chronic drug administration. Put differently, the dose-response curve shifted to the right as a function of chronic exposure. Measuring the degree of the rightward shift, for instance, by comparing pre- and post-chronic ED_{50} doses, allows the degree of tolerance to be quantified.

The rapidity with which tolerance develops and the extent to which it occurs depend upon the drug in question, the response being measured, and the conditions of exposure. For example, substantial tolerance develops to the euphoric and analgesic effects of morphine, but little or no tolerance develops to the constipation and pupillary constriction that the drug causes.

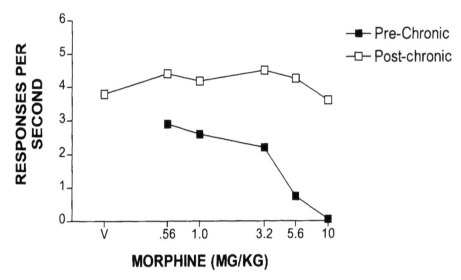

Figure 3-7. *Pre- and post-chronic dose-response curves showing the effects of morphine on the response rate of a single pigeon exposed to a progressive-ratio 25 schedule of food delivery. Because the dose-response curve was shifted to the right following chronic exposure, tolerance developed to morphine's rate-reducing effects.*

Pharmacologists conventionally differentiate **metabolic** (or kinetic) **tolerance** and **pharmacodynamic** (or cellular) **tolerance**. The former occurs when exposure to a drug increases the subsequent rate of its metabolism and excretion, a process that often involves enzyme induction, as previously discussed in the section on biotransformation. The latter is evident when adaptation to a drug occurs at a cellular level so that a given level of drug at the site of action produces weaker responses on subsequent exposures. One mechanism that contributes to pharmacodynamic tolerance, receptor up-regulation, is discussed in Chapter 4. Metabolic and pharmacodynamic tolerance are not mutually exclusive; they appear together with certain drugs, such as nicotine.

A third kind of tolerance, **behavioral tolerance**, occurs when responsiveness to a drug decreases only when a learned response has been emitted in the drug state; drug exposure *per se* is not sufficient for the development of tolerance (see Chapter 8). The existence of behavioral tolerance, which is a fairly easy to demonstrate, underscores the fact that drug-behavior interactions, not exposure to drug alone, determines drug effects.

Sensitization

In some cases, repeated exposure to a drug may increase its effects. This phenomenon is known as **sensitization**. With drugs that are activated in biotransformation, enzyme induction can lead to sensitization. Also, for drugs self-administered by humans, learning how to use the drug (e.g., to hold in marijuana smoke) and to detect its effects may contribute to greater effects with repeated use.

Physical Dependence

Tolerance is commonly discussed together with physical dependence, because the two often (but not inevitably) appear together. **Physical** (or physiological) **dependence** is present when a withdrawal (or abstinence) syndrome appears when exposure to the drug is terminated. A **withdrawal syndrome** involves changes in physiological status (e.g., seizures), overt behavior (e.g., increased drug seeking), or subjective state (e.g., reported dysphoria). The specific signs and symptoms that constitute the withdrawal syndrome vary in kind and intensity with drug type and dosage regimen. In some cases, the withdrawal syndrome is mild and only unpleasant, as when a person stops using caffeine and experiences headache. In other cases, the withdrawal syndrome is severe and life-threatening, as when a person stops drinking alcohol and experiences delirium and seizures.

One explanation of the withdrawal syndrome is that the continuous presence of a drug causes a physiological adaptation, which results from the activation of systems that compensate for the presence of the drug in the body. These compensatory systems continue to operate for a time after the drug is withdrawn, and it is their action that leads to the withdrawal syndrome. Consistent with this explanation, which also accounts for pharmacodynamic tolerance, is the observation that physiological and behavioral responses during withdrawal are characteristically in the opposite direction from responses produced by the drug. For that reason, they are sometimes called **rebound effects**. An example of a rebound effect is the explosive diarrhea that follows termination of chronic exposure to morphine, which produces constipation.

Although tolerance and physical dependence often occur together, and both can be explained, in part, in terms of the activation of systems that compensate for the physiological disruption produced by drugs, tolerance may occur in the absence of physical dependence. For instance, tolerance develops rapidly to the hallucinogenic effects of LSD, but the drug is not known to produce physical dependence. Even when physical dependence and tolerance occur together, they do not necessarily develop at the same rate and to the same degree (National Institute on Drug Abuse, 1978). Therefore, it appears that somewhat different processes control the two phenomena.

In any consideration of how the body reacts to drugs, it is crucial to realize that *drugs do not induce new physiological or behavioral processes*. That is, drugs produce their effects by interacting with systems that control bodily activities in the absence of drugs. Drugs can produce *quantitative* changes in the function of cells, and thereby produce levels of physiological or behavioral activity outside the usual, homeostatic, range. But they cannot produce *qualitative* changes in cellular function. Inevitably, the response to a drug is within the framework of normal physiological function and is limited by the capacity of the cell to respond. Given this, our understanding of drug effects at the physiological level is always limited by our understanding of normal physiological function.

Drug Interactions

Humans frequently take two or more drugs together, therefore, it is important to be aware of the possibility of **drug interactions**, which occur if the presence of one drug significantly alters the effects of another drug. For example, the analgesic acetaminophen (Tylenol) substantially increases the risk of liver damage in people who drink relatively large amounts of alcohol. For that reason, Tylenol bottles carry an alcohol warning.

Drugs can interact through a sizable number of mechanisms. In some cases, known collectively as pharmacokinetic interactions, one agent alters the absorption, distribution, biotransformation, or excretion of another. Consider, for instance, a situation in which Drug A inhibits the biotransformation of Drug B, which is inactivated by liver enzymes. This would result in higher blood levels of Drug B, and increased effects. If, in contrast, Drug A induced (increased the level of) the enzymes that inactivate Drug B, the result would be a decrease in the blood levels and the effects of Drug B.

In addition to pharmacokinetic interactions, drugs can interact by directly affecting the same physiological system, either by acting in parallel or opposite directions, or by altering different physiological systems that have a common end point. Drug interactions may be infra-additive, in which case the presence of one drug reduces the effects of another, or supra-additive (synergistic), which occurs when the presence of one drug increases the effects of another. Although the possibility of drug interactions is an important consideration with respect to both medications and drugs of abuse, many drugs do not interact in a significant way. Even when they do, the use of multiple medications is often unavoidable for patients who have two or more disorders, each of which requires a different medication.

Concluding Comments

Although the effects of drugs are lawful and can in principle be predicted accurately, drugs are not "magic bullets" that selectively and inevitably alter particular behaviors. All drugs are to some extent nonselective in their actions, and the actions of all drugs are modulated by many variables. Thus far, we have introduced several variables that influence drug action, including drug dose, route and frequency of administration, and past or current presence of other drugs in the body. The age of the person taking the drug and the presence of disease are other determinants of drug actions that were introduced. Although not specifically mentioned, genotype can influence the action of certain drugs, as can gender. All of these variables are important in trying to make sense of the variability of drug effects across people and situations.

Although knowing the general classes of variables that influence drug action is an essential part of mastering pharmacology, fully understanding the effects of any drug requires knowledge of its mechanisms of action, that is, the general processes through which it produces its effects. As mentioned in Chapter 1, pharmacologists often seek to explain the effects of drugs in terms of the neurochemical changes that those substances explore. The following chapter explores neurochemical mechanisms of drug action, and considers the importance of such mechanisms for behavioral pharmacology.

References

Baldessarini, R. D. (1996). Drugs and the treatment of psychiatric disorders: Psychosis and anxiety. In J. G. Hardman, L. E. Limbard, P. B. Molinoff, R. W. Ruddon, & A. G. Gilman (Eds.), *The pharmacological basis of therapeutics* (pp.399-430). New York: McGraw-Hill.

Benet, L. Z., Kroetz, D. L., & Sheiner, L.. B. (1996). Pharmacokinetics. In J. G. Hardman, L. E. Limbard, P. B. Molinoff, R. W. Ruddon, & A. G. Gilman (Eds.), *The pharmacological basis of therapeutics* (pp. 3-27). New York: McGraw-Hill.

Birhamer, B., Greenhill, L. L., Cooper, T. B., Fried, J., & Maminski, B. (1989). Sustained release methylphenidate: Pharmacokinetic studies in ADHD males. *Journal of the American Academy of Child and Adolescent Psychiatry, 28,* 768-772.

Briant, R. H. (1978). An introduction to clinical pharmacology. In J. S. Werry (Ed.), *Pediatric psychopharmacology: The use of behavior modifying drugs in children* (pp. 3-28). New York: Brunner/Mazel.

Hollinger, M. A. (1997). *Introduction to pharmacology.* Washington, DC: Taylor & Francis.

Julien, R. M. (1998). *A primer of drug action.* New York: Freeman.

Mayer, S.E. Melmon, K.L., & Gillman, A.G. (1980). Introduction: The dynamics of drug absorption, distribution, and elimination. In A.G. Gilman, L.S. Goodman, & A. Gilman (Eds.), *The pharmacological basis of therapeutics* (pp. 1-27). New York: Macmillan.

National Institute on Drug Abuse. (1978*). Behavioral tolerance: Research and treatment implications.* Washington, DC: U.S. Government Printing Office.

Nickel, M., Alling, K., & Poling, A. (1990). Effects of methsuximide on the reaction time of rats. *Life Sciences Advances, 9,* 745-748.

Poling, A., Gadow, K. D., & Cleary, J. (1991). *Drug therapy for behavior disorders: An introduction.* New York: Pergamon.

Ross, E. M. (1996). Pharmacodynamics. In J. G. Hardman, L. E. Limbard, P. B. Molinoff, R. W. Ruddon, & A. G. Gilman (Eds.), *The pharmacological basis of therapeutics* (pp. 29-41). New York: McGraw-Hill.

Chapter 4

Neuropharmacology

Lisa Baker, Thomas Morgan, and Alan Poling
Western Michigan University

Neuroscience is one of the most popular and fastest growing fields of study in recent years. The Society for Neuroscience, an organization dedicated to advancing knowledge of the nervous system, has grown from a membership of 500 when first founded in 1970 to over 25,000 in 1998. Its popularity is in no small part due to the fact that research on the nervous system has greatly advanced our understanding and treatment of several neurological and neuropsychiatric disorders. Neuroscience research, specifically research in neuropharmacology, has also begun to clarify the physiological mechanisms through which drugs produce their behavioral effects. **Neuropharmacology** is the specialization of neuroscience concerned with drug-induced modifications of nervous system functions. As noted in Chapter 3, behaviorally-active drugs characteristically alter neuronal activity, and their effects at this level constitute physiological mechanisms of action. To understand how the body reacts to a drug, one must understand these mechanisms, as well as the processes of absorption, distribution, biotransformation, and excretion.

Knowledge about the nervous system is essential for making sense of the neuropharmacological actions of psychoactive drugs. You will recall from Chapter 3 that drugs do not induce novel physiological activities. Instead, they alter normal physiological processes. Given this, understanding how the nervous system functions in the absence of drugs is a prerequisite for understanding drug effects. This chapter provides a general overview of the nervous system, describes the processes of electrical and neurochemical transmission in nerve cells (neurons), and provides examples of how psychoactive drugs modify neurochemical transmission.

The Nervous System

One of the major functions of the nervous system is the production of behavior. A second important function is the detection of environmental stimuli. By convention, systems that are responsible for movement (i.e., behavior) are called **motor systems**; they contain **efferent** neurons. Those that are responsible for detecting (i.e., sensing) environmental stimuli are termed sensory systems; their neurons are **afferent**. The two main structural divisions of the nervous system are the central nervous system (CNS), which comprises the brain and spinal cord, and the peripheral nervous (PNS), which comprises all nerves outside the spinal cord. Figure 4-1 diagrams the divisions of the nervous system. As noted in Chapter 3, most drugs

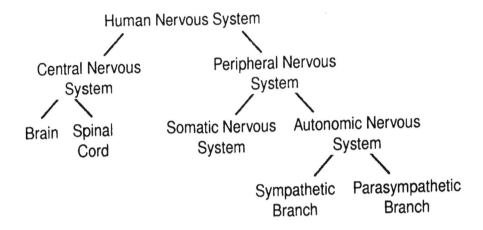

Figure 4-1. *Divisions of the human nervous system.*

produce their effects by altering CNS activity. Although a drug's actions in the central nervous system are of primary importance for understanding its behavioral effects, peripheral actions also are important. For example, some medications alter heart rate and respiration through their actions on the autonomic nervous system (see below). These peripherally-mediated drug actions may be annoying side effects for some users.

The Peripheral Nervous System

The branch of the PNS that is directly affected by the sensory organs and that controls the skeletal muscles is called the **somatic nervous system**. The branch that regulates the cardiac muscle and the smooth muscles and glands is called the **autonomic** (meaning self-governing) **nervous system** (ANS). There are two divisions of the ANS, sympathetic and parasympathetic, which operate in an opposing fashion to maintain homeostatic balance in several bodily systems. Both divisions are necessary for survival. Activation of the **sympathetic** division naturally occurs in the context of "fight or flight" situations, which are situations in which the body must expend energy. Increased heart rate and respiration, increased blood flow to skeletal muscles, elevated blood sugar, pupil dilation, and sweating are all signs of sympathetic arousal. The **parasympathetic** division is involved in activities that conserve the body's energy. Relatively slow heart rate, secretion of digestive fluids, and increased blood flow to the digestive system are associated with parasympathetic activation. Drugs that activate the sympathetic division of the ANS are termed **sympathomimetic**. Most stimulant drugs (e.g., amphetamine, cocaine) and some hallucinogens (e.g., LSD, mescaline) produce sympathomimetic effects.

The PNS is relatively simple in structure and is more easily accessed than the CNS. Neurons in the somatic nervous system synapse directly on the muscles that they affect; the neurotransmitter in this system is acetylcholine and the receptors are nicotinic (**neurotransmitters** are naturally-occurring substances that allow cells to interact with one another; neurotransmitters and their receptors subtypes are discussed subsequently). A **synapse** is the junction between two neurons, or between a neuron and an effector cell (e.g., a muscle). When activity passes from one neuron to another at a synapse, the former neuron is termed **presynaptic**, the later **postsynaptic**. Synaptic transmission is further discussed in a later section of this chapter.

In both the sympathetic and parasympathetic branches of the autonomic nervous system, preganglionic neurons exit the spinal cord and synapse with postganglionic neurons, which in turn synapse on effectors. Acetylcholine is the neurotransmitter released by both preganglioinic and postganglionic neurons in the parasympathetic branch (i.e., at both pre- and postganglionic synapses). Acetylcholine also is released by postganglionic neurons in the parasympathetic branch, but norepinephrine is released by preganglionic neurons in this system. As Hoffman, Lefkowitz, and Taylor (1996) relate, "The concept of chemical neurotransmission was developed primarily to explain observations relating to the transmission of impulses from postganglionic autonomic fibers to effector cells" (p. 109). Over time, this concept has been extended to explain CNS activity and, as emphasized in this chapter, drug effects thereon.

The Central Nervous System

The brain comprises a very complex set of subsystems or networks organized in a hierarchical manner. The details of brain organization are not of critical importance for the purpose of this chapter, although the main components of the brain are summarized in Table 4-1. Some of the brain structures listed in this table will be mentioned later in the context of specific drug actions. Before those actions can be considered, however, we must review the essentials of neuronal communication.

Neurons: Structural Units of the Nervous System

The human brain contains over 100 billion nerve cells, or **neurons**. Neurons have two general functions (Julien, 1992). One is conducting electrical impulses over long distances. The other, as Julien (1992) notes,

> [I]s their ability to carry out specific input and output relations with both other nerve cells and other tissues of the body, the functions of which the neurons may control. The input-output connections determine the function of a particular neuron and, in turn, the patterns of behavioral response that neuronal activity may elicit. (p. 376)

The structure of neurons allows these functions to occur, and will be considered initially.

Neurons come in many shapes and sizes, some specific to a particular brain region, but the basic structure of all nerve cells is the same. Several important components of neurons are illustrated in Figure 4-2.

Table 4-1. Major Divisions of the Brain and Their Primary Functions

Division	Subdivision	Structures	Primary Functions
Forebrain	Telencephalon	Cerebral Cortex	sensation and perception, motor control, complex mental processes
		Basal Ganglia	motor control, sensorimotor integration
		Hippocampus	learning and memory
		Amygdala	emotions
	Diencephalon	Thalamus	sensory processing
		Hypothalamus	homeostatic regulation: feeding and metabolism temperature regulation, reproductive behaviors
Midbrain	Mesencephalon	Tectum	
	Inferior colliculus	Superior colliculus	oculomotor and orientation reflexes
		auditory relay	
		Tegmentum	
		Periaqueductal gray	sensory processing, pain relay
		Red nucleus	postural reflexes, motor control
		Substantia nigra	postural reflexes, motor control
Hindbrain	Metencephalon	Cerebellum	motor coordination, learning
		Pons	autonomic regulation, sleep
	Myelencephalon	Medulla oblongata	autonomic control, some reflexes: respiration, heart rate, blood pressure, vomiting, coughing

The **soma,** or cell body, contains the nucleus and other structures that maintain the life of the cell. The **cell membrane** defines the cell's boundaries. It consists of a double layer of phospholipid molecules, with numerous proteins scattered throughout. Some of these proteins are especially important in the neuron's capability for receiving and transmitting messages. Although a neuron may receive messages from other neurons at any place along the cell membrane, the **dendrites** are extensions of the neuron that are specialized for receiving chemical messages. Dendrites branch out from the soma in various directions. The number and extent of the dendritic branches varies among neurons. Dendrites contain numerous protrusions called **spines**. Embedded in the membrane of the dendritic spines are complex protein molecules which contain receptor sites for chemical messengers called **neurotransmitters**. Neurotransmitters are discussed in a later section of this chapter.

The **axon** is another extension from the soma. Most axons divide and branch out in several directions. However, only one axon extends from the soma, whereas numerous dendrites may originate from the soma. The beginning of the axon is called the **axon hillock**. It is at this location that the nerve impulse, or action potential, is initiated. The endings of each axonal branch are called **axon terminals**. At the end of each terminal is a knob called a **terminal button** (bouton). It is from the terminal buttons that neurotransmitters are released into the synaptic cleft. The synaptic cleft is the gap between two neurons that form a synapse.

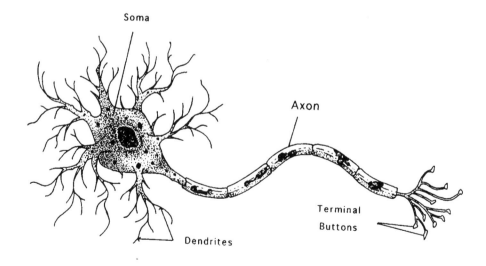

Figure 4-2. *A typical neuron with the soma, dendrites, axon, and terminal buttons labeled.*

Electrical Transmission within Neurons

The electrical signals conducted by neurons are termed nerve impulses, or **action potentials**. The action potential occurs as a result of a series of alterations in the cell membrane that permit the exchange of charged particles between the fluid inside the cell (intracellular fluid) and the fluid surrounding the cell (extracellular fluid). The easiest way to understand the nerve impulse is to compare it to electricity flowing along a wire. Electricity moves along a wire due to the flow of negatively charged particles (electrons) toward positively charged particles (protons). Similarly, the nerve impulse results from the movement of charged particles, such as sodium (Na+) and chloride (Cl-), called ions. The flow of ions in and out of the cell is regulated by the cell membrane.

Across the cell membrane is a small difference in electrical charge; the inside of the cell is electrically negative with respect to the outside. This difference is called the membrane potential. All cells have a membrane potential, but neurons and muscle cells have the unique ability to change the membrane potential rapidly under certain circumstances. When a neuron is electrically inactive, the membrane potential is referred to as the **resting potential.** The generation and maintenance of the resting potential is dependent on the selective permeability of the membrane and the unequal distribution of ions across the membrane. The semi-permeability of the cell membrane arises from the selectivity of ion channels, which allow some ions but not others to pass through the membrane. Membrane permeability in neurons is not fixed, however, but changes due to the actions of protein molecules, which function as channels or gates through which ions pass between the intracellular and extracellular fluid. Some times these channels are open, other times they are closed.

The unequal distribution of ions across the cell membrane arises from two passive forces that act on ions: electrostatic pressure and diffusion. **Electrostatic pressure** refers to the fact that opposite charges attract and like charges repel. As noted in Chapter 3, **diffusion** refers to the tendency of molecules to distribute equally, or move from areas of higher concentration to areas of lower concentration. When the membrane is in its resting state, there is a higher concentration of sodium (Na^+) and chloride (Cl^-) ions outside the cell, whereas potassium (K^+) and large protein molecules (A^-) are more heavily concentrated inside the cell. The cell membrane is easily crossed by K^+ but not by Na^+, because most K^+ channels are open and most Na^+ channels are closed. The force of diffusion pushes K^+ toward the extracellular fluid. But as K^+ leaves the cell, electrostatic pressure tends to push K^+ back into the cell. Thus, the total movement of K^+ toward the outside of the cell (efflux) is equal to the total movement of this ion toward the inside of the cell (influx). This is also true for Na^+ and Cl^- ions. The membrane is not completely impermeable to Na^+; small amounts are allowed in. However, through the actions of an active transport mechanism, which requires energy, Na^+ is pumped out of the cell, while K^+ is pumped into the cell at a ratio of 3 to 2. It is important to note that while the Na^+-K^+ pump contributes to the long term maintenance of the resting membrane potential, it contributes relatively little to this steady state from moment to moment.

Rather, it is a balance of the influx and efflux of ions across the membrane that determines the resting membrane potential.

A resting membrane potential is present in all cells. But only in neurons are resting potentials converted to action potentials. This occurs because voltage-dependent Na^+ channels are present in neurons. When the cell is electrically inactive during the resting potential, most Na^+ channels are closed. A local graded change in voltage across the membrane causes these channels to open briefly, and Na+ moves toward the intracellular fluid due to the passive forces of diffusion and electrostatic pressure. This event is followed by the opening of K^+ channels, and K^+ moves outside the cell. The Na^+ channels are then inactivated for a brief period while K^+ channels remain open. This alteration in the membrane conductance for Na^+ and K^+ ions is what causes the action potential, which is a wave of electrical activity that moves down the axon until it reaches the axon terminals. Metaphorically, the action potential resembles a flame traveling along a fuse. Arrival of the action potential at the axon terminals initiates the release of neurotransmitter molecules into the synaptic cleft. Those molecules adhere to, and affect the characteristics of, the postsynaptic neuron's membrane, as described in the next section.

Opening of voltage-dependent ion channels is triggered by depolarization (a reduction in the magnitude of the resting potential). One way that the membrane is depolarized is through the action of **neurotransmitter-dependent sodium channels**. These channels open when neurotransmitter molecules combine with receptors located in the membrane, as discussed in the following section. A few drugs alter neuronal communication by interfering with the exchange of ions responsible for the action potential. For example, local anesthetics block sodium channels and prevent the propagation of nerve impulses (Julien, 1992). Most psychoactive drugs, however, produce their actions through the modification of chemical transmission between neurons. The next section describes the details of neurochemical transmission.

Neurochemical Transmission

Synaptic transmission occurs when events in one neuron alter activity in a second neuron (or effector). Synaptic transmission occurs both electrically and chemically. Although electrical synapses are more common in both vertebrate and invertebrate organisms, neurochemical synapses have received considerably more attention, particularly in neuropharmacology. It is generally thought that chemical synapses provide for diversity and plasticity not afforded by electrical synapses. Chemical synapses involve the release of **neurotransmitters** from **presynaptic** neurons. Neurotransmitters bind to receptors on **postsynpatic** neurons, and may influence their electrical activity. Neurotransmitters also bind to **autoreceptors** on the presynaptic neuron, and are capable of modulating various biochemical processes therein. Several important neurotransmitters, and the abbreviations used to refer to them, are listed in Table 4-2. This list keeps growing, as previously unrecognized neurotransmitters are isolated. In general, the following criteria must be met for a chemical found in the CNS or PNS to be considered as a neurotransmitter (Julien, 1992):

1) The proposed neurotransmitter must be synthesized within the neuron and be present in the presynaptic neuron.
2) The proposed neurotransmitter must be released when the presynaptic neuron is stimulated electrically.
3) The proposed neurotransmitter must mimic the action that normally occurs at the synapse.
4) There must be a mechanism for inactivation of the proposed neurotransmitter.
5) Drugs that block the actions of the proposed neurotransmitter must also block the effects produced by stimulating the presynaptic neuron.

Although relatively simple in concept, these criteria are difficult to apply in empirical tests. Therefore, although many neurotransmitters have been identified with near certainty, researchers are less confident regarding the status of other endogenous substances, which may or may not be neurotransmitters.

Table 4-2. Selected Neurotransmitters

Amino Acids	**Peptides**
Gamma-aminobutyric acid (GABA)	Morphine-like sub-stances
Glycine	Endorphins
Glutamate	Enkephalins
Monoamines	Somatostatin
Catecholamines	Substance P
Dopamine (DA)	**Others**
Epinephrine (E)	Acetylcholine (Ach)
Norepinephrine (NE)	Adenosine
Indolamines	Histamine
Serotonin (5-hydroxytryptamine, 5-HT)	

While it was once believed that a given neuron contained only one kind of neurotransmitter, more recent findings indicate that this is untrue. The axon of a single neuron may contain more than one neurotransmitter, as well as other substances that affect neurotransmission but are not themselves neurotransmitters (Feldman, Meyer, & Quenzer, 1997). For example, **neuromodulators** influence the action of neurotransmitters by altering their synthesis, release, interactions with receptors, or inactivation. Given the practical difficulties of studying living brains and the multitude of endogenous chemicals found in them, our present understanding of neurochemistry is rudimentary. Nonetheless, it is adequate to allow for a meaningful description of the neuropharmacological mechanisms of action of many psychoactive compounds. To understand those actions, one needs to understand the essential steps in neurotransmittion, which are well understood.

Obviously, production of the neurotransmitter is the necessary first step in the process of neurochemical transmission. The precursor molecules for most neurotransmitters are derived from the organism's diet. For example, the precursor molecule for the neurotransmitter dopamine is the amino acid tyrosine and the precursor for serotonin is another amino acid, tryptophan. Acetylcholine is derived from acetate, the anion found in vinegar, and choline, a substance derived from the breakdown of fats. Precursor molecules are transported into neurons, then neurotransmitters are synthesized from them by enzymes inside the neuron. Neurotransmitters are synthesized both in the cell body and in the terminal buttons. These substances are packaged in small synaptic vesicles, which are produced from recycled membrane material by the Golgi apparatus and the cisternae in the cell body, then transported to the terminal buttons.

The synaptic vesicles cluster around the release zone of the presynaptic membrane. The arrival of an action potential at the axon terminal initiates a cascade of events that leads to neurotransmitter release. Based on several studies in a variety of species, Almers (1990) has suggested the following model to describe how this process occurs. Initially, protein molecules in the membrane of the synaptic vesicles attach to protein molecules in the presynaptic membrane. When the presynaptic membrane is depolarized by the arrival of an action potential, voltage-dependent calcium channels in the presynaptic membrane open. Calcium ions (Ca^{2+}) enter the terminal button and bind with protein molecules that join the presynaptic membrane and the synaptic vesicles. The cluster of protein molecules then moves apart, creating a fusion pore, through which the neurotransmitter is dumped into the synaptic cleft. We know that the entry of calcium ions is an essential step in this process. If neurons are placed in a solution containing no calcium ions, an action potential will not cause the release of the neurotransmitter (Carlson, 1998).

Once released into the synaptic cleft, neurotransmitter molecules diffuse across the cleft and attach to binding sites on protein molecules that are embedded in the postsynaptic membrane. These binding sites are called **receptors**. The attachment of neurotransmitters to receptors involves chemical bonding that characteristically is reversible and noncovalent, such as ionic or electrostatic interactions, hydrogen bonding, and hydrophobic interactions mediated by van der Walls forces (Feldman et al., 1997). These are complex, but common, chemical interactions. For our purposes, it is sufficient to recognize that the structure of a neurotransmitter (or drug) molecule and the structure of a given receptor determine if and how they interact. The notion of structure-activity relations is central to neuropharmacology, and often is explained by a **lock-and-key analogy**.

For instance, as discussed later, neuroleptic (or antipsychotic) drugs such as thioridazine (Mellaril) and chlorpromazine (Thorazine) appear to produce their therapeutic effects by blocking receptors that respond to the neurotransmitter dopamine. When the lock-and-key analogy is used to explain the action of such drugs, the dopamine receptor is envisioned as a lock, and molecules of dopamine and the neuroleptics as similar but not identical keys. The dopamine key matches the receptor lock perfectly and will unlock it, thereby affecting the neuron on which the receptor is located. The neuroleptic key, in contrast, matches the receptor lock imperfectly. The neuroleptic key will enter the lock, but will not unlock it. Therefore, when neuroleptic molecules combine with dopamine receptors, cellular activity is not directly affected. But, just as ill-fitting keys prevent matching keys from entering and opening locks, neuroleptic molecules prevent dopamine molecules from combining with receptors and affecting the activity of the neuron.

As noted previously, the binding of a neurotransmitter molecule to a receptor in the postsynaptic membrane causes the opening of an ion channel, which allows particular ions to either enter or leave the postsynaptic cell. There are two ways that the binding of a neurotransmitter to a receptor can cause the opening of an ion channel. Some neurotransmitters open ion channels directly by binding with **ionotropic** receptors. This type of receptor is an ion channel that consists of a neurotransmitter binding site. When the neurotransmitter binds to the receptor, the ion channel opens.

The second type of receptor is called **metabotropic** because several metabolic steps are involved in the opening of ion channels. The cascade of biochemical events initiated by the binding of neurotransmitters to metabotropic receptors is rather complicated. These receptors are located near other proteins in the cell membrane called G proteins. When the neurotransmitter binds to the receptor site, the receptor activates a G protein. A portion of the G protein then breaks away and activates an enzyme which is also located in the cell membrane. The activated enzyme then stimulates the production of a chemical in the cytoplasm of the cell. This chemical is often referred to as a **second messenger**. The second messenger then initiates a series of chemical events, culminating with the opening of an ion channel. A common second messenger is cyclic adenosine monophosphate (AMP). Besides opening ion channels, second messengers are involved in a number of other biochemical processes within the cell. Thus, in addition to producing postsynaptic potentials, neurotransmitters are capable of regulating a variety of biochemical functions.

The electrical activity that results from a neurotransmitter binding to a postsynaptic receptor depends on what type of ion channel is opened. As discussed previously, the influx or efflux of particular ions changes the local membrane potential of the postsynaptic cell. The postsynaptic membrane potential may be depolarized by the opening of Na^+ channels or hyperpolarized by the opening of K^+ or Cl^- channels. Depolarization (which occurs when the membrane potential is reduced) increases the likelihood that the neuron will generate an action potential and is therefore considered an excitatory process. Hyperpolarization decreases the likelihood that a neuron will generate an action potential and is an inhibitory process. It is important to recognize that it is the type of ion channel associated with the receptor site and not the neurotransmitter itself that determines the type of postsynaptic potential that occurs at a particular synapse. Thus, the same neurotransmitter substance can have both excitatory and inhibitory actions, depending on the ion channels linked to the receptor sites with which it binds. For most neurotransmitters, there are multiple receptor subtypes. Examples will be discussed in a later section describing drug effects at receptor sites.

Postsynaptic potentials are terminated when the neurotransmitter is deactivated. Neurotransmitters are deactivated by two different processes. Most neurotransmitters are deactivated through a process called **reuptake**, in which transport molecules located on the presynaptic membrane rapidly remove the neurotransmitter from the synaptic cleft. The other process through which postsynaptic potentials are terminated is through **enzymatic deactivation**. The postsynaptic potentials caused by acetylcholine are terminated in this way. The postsynaptic membrane at cholinergic synapses contains an enzyme called acetylcholinesterase. This enzyme destroys acetylcholine, thereby terminating the postsynaptic potential.

Neuropharmacological Mechanisms of Drug Action

Most psychoactive drugs produce their effects by modifying synaptic transmission. Now that you have a basic understanding of the multiple steps involved in neurochemical transmission, you can appreciate the mechanisms through which drugs can modify this process and ultimately influence behavior. At the most general level, drugs can either mimic or block the effects of a particular neurotransmitter. Drugs that facilitate or mimic the actions of a neurotransmitter are called **agonists**. Drugs that block or inhibit the actions of a neurotransmitter are called **antagonists**. There are several ways that drugs can produce either of these effects. The following section describes examples of the mechanisms through which psychoactive drugs may act.

Drug Effects on Synthesis of Neurotransmitters

Drugs can either facilitate or inhibit the synthesis of neurotransmitters. Drugs that increase the rate of synthesis are considered indirect agonists, while drugs that interfere with synthesis are indirect antagonists. The rate of neurotransmitter synthesis may be increased by administering the precursor of a transmitter substance. One common example is the dopamine (DA) precursor L-DOPA, which is used in the treatment of Parkinson's disease (L-DOPA is the active isomer of the DA precursor DOPA). The symptoms of this motor disorder are caused by the selective degeneration of DA neurons in a region of the midbrain called the substantia nigra. Drugs that increase DA activity alleviate these symptoms. DOPA is the first product in the biosynthesis of dopamine. The amino acid tyrosine is converted to DOPA by the enzyme tyrosine hydroxylase. DOPA is then converted to dopamine by the enzyme DOPA decarboxylase. The administration of L-DOPA elevates DA synthesis and increases the amount of DA released by dopaminergic neurons. This action ensures that the dopaminergic neurons that remain intact in a person with Parkinson's disease function optimally.

Another way that drugs may affect this step in neurochemical transmission is by acting on the enzymes involved in the biosynthesis of transmitters. For example, p-chlorophenylalanine (PCPA) interferes with the synthesis of serotonin (5-HT) by inhibiting the activity of the enzyme tryptophan hydroxylase. PCPA has been shown in rats to reduce motor activity and food intake, and to produce a period of sedation followed by a prolonged period of insomnia (Borbely, Neuhaus, & Tobler, 1981). Another drug, *a*-methyl-*p*-tyrosine (AMPT), interferes with dopamine synthesis by inactivating the enzyme tyrosine hydroxylase. Because dopamine is converted to norepinephrine, this drug also interferes with norepinephrine (NE) synthesis. Although AMPT has no clinical use, it is used as a research tool to investigate how DA and NE systems control behavior.

Drug Effects on Storage of Neurotransmitters

Drugs may modify synaptic transmission by interfering with the storage of neurotransmitter substances in synaptic vesicles. A popular example of a drug that produces its actions through this mechanism is reserpine. Reserpine prevents the storage of all monoamines (DA, NE, 5-HT) by blocking transporters in vesicle membranes. When an action potential reaches the terminal button, these neurotransmitter substances are not released because the vesicles are empty. Thus, reserpine is an indirect monoamine antagonist. Reserpine is derived from a root of a shrub that grows in India. Thousands of years ago it was discovered to be useful in the treatment of snakebite. Due to its actions on noradrenergic synapses in the peripheral nervous system, reserpine decreases blood pressure. In fact, this drug was a common treatment for high blood pressure until it was replaced by newer drugs that produce fewer side effects. Because its actions are relatively nonselective, reserpine produces many significant side effects, including depression.

Drug Effects on Release of Neurotransmitters

There are a number of drugs that modify neurotransmitter release. The venom of the black widow spider is an indirect cholinergic agonist because it stimulates the release of acetylcholine (ACh). The botulinum toxin produces the opposite effect by preventing the release of ACh. This toxin is produced by bacteria that grow in improperly canned food and is a dangerously potent poison. As noted previously in discussing the somatic nervous system, ACh is the neurotransmitter released at the neuromuscular junction (synapses between nerve and muscle). Too little ACh at these synapses causes paralysis, while too much ACh at these synapses can produce seizures. Either effect can be fatal.

A number of psychotropic drugs also produce their actions by modifying transmitter release. *d*-Amphetamine (Dexedrine) and methylphenidate (Ritalin) are stimulants used in the treatment of Attention Deficit Hyperactivity Disorder. These drugs facilitate the release of both DA and NE. Fenfluramine, an appetite suppressant, enhances 5-HT release. Amphetamine also acts on 5-HT release and has been used clinically as an appetite suppressant in attempts to treat obesity. Because of its high abuse potential and the rapid development of tolerance to its appetite suppressant effects, however, amphetamine is not a good drug for this use. Another amphetamine-like compound, phenteramine, was combined with fenfluramine in the diet medication called Phen-Fen. This drug combination was recently removed from the market due to potentially fatal cardiac reactions.

Drug Effects on Receptors for Neurotransmitters

Thus far, we have described examples of agonists and antagonists that indirectly alter the effects of neurotransmitters. Drugs also can mimic the actions of a neurotransmitter by binding to the same receptors and exerting similar actions. That is, they can be direct-acting agonists or antagonists. For example, nicotine mimics the actions of ACh by binding to a subtype of ACh receptors. These receptors are actually called nicotinic receptors, named after nicotine. Muscarine, a chemical found in a poisonous mushroom, binds to another subtype of ACh receptors, called muscarinic.

Atropine is another substance found in nature that binds to muscarinic receptors. Unlike muscarine, atropine is a cholinergic antagonist. It exerts its actions by preventing the binding of ACh with muscarinic receptors. Atropine and another anticholinergic substance, scopolamine, are both found in the Belladonna plant, sometimes called the "deadly nightshade," and in another plant called Jamestown Weed, or "Jimson Weed." Atropine and scopolamine can produce hallucinatory and dissociative experiences. While under the influence of these substances, a person may experience confusion for several hours, and upon recovery will have little memory for events that occurred during the period of intoxication. Due to its sedative properties, scopolamine once was an ingredient in some over-the-counter sleep-aid medicines. In small doses, atropine may be used as an antidote to some nerve gases, which are known to increase synaptic levels of ACh by blocking its enzymatic deactivation. Atropine also is used by opthamologists and optometrists to dilate the pupils.

Curare is a cholinergic antagonist that exerts its actions on nicotinic receptors. Like the botulinum toxin, curare causes paralysis of skeletal muscles. Curare is extracted from several species of plants found in South America. For centuries, native tribes of South America have coated the tips of hunting arrows with extracts from these plants. Today, curare has some medical use. It sometimes is given prior to surgery to relax muscles so they will not contract when cut. Curare does not render one unconscious or insensitive to pain, so an anesthetic is also required. Additionally, the patient must be respirated because curare makes breathing difficult or impossible.

A number of psychotherapeutic drugs are known to bind with DA receptors. As previously mentioned, antipsychotic drugs used in the treatment of schizophrenia are dopamine antagonists. They occupy DA receptor sites and prevent dopamine from exerting its actions. The receptor pharmacology of this drug class is actually more complicated than revealed in our earlier discussion. Most of these drugs bind to a particular subtype of DA receptors and may also bind to receptor subtypes for other monoamines. The receptor classification for the dopamine system is fairly complicated. Recent advances in molecular biology have identified at least five different dopamine receptor subtypes. They are classified into two subfamilies: the D1 subfamily includes both D_1 and D_5 subtypes while the D2 subfamily consists of the D_{2short}, D_{2long}, D_3, and D_4 subtypes (Civelli et al., 1991; Sibley & Monsma, 1992).

The first antipsychotic drugs developed were primarily D2 receptor antagonists. For example, chlorpromazine (Thorazine) and haloperidol (Haldol) were two of the earliest drugs used to treat schizophrenia, and they block D2 receptors. Due to this action in a region of the basal ganglia called the neostriatum, these neuroleptics produce side effects that resemble Parkinson's disease. (As an aside, consider whether L-DOPA could be used to treat neuroleptic-induced Parkinsonian symptoms. The answer is "no," because the mechanism through which these drugs produce their therapeutic effects (reducing dopaminergic activity by blocking receptors) is the same mechanism that produces the motor disturbance. To the extent that L-DOPA is effective in increasing dopaminergic activity, thereby reducing Parkinsonian symptoms, it should also be effective in countering the antipsychotic effects induced by neuroleptics.

In addition to producing motor disturbances that resemble those associated with Parkinson's disease, the long-term use of neuroleptics causes **tardive dyskinesia** in some people. This disorder is characterized by spontaneous and uncontrollable movements, particularly of the facial muscles, which interfere with eating and speaking. Other side effects result from the anticholinergic and antiserotonergic activity of common neuroleptic drugs (Poling, Gadow, & Cleary, 1991).

Over the last four decades, pharmaceutical chemists and neuropharmacologists have worked to develop antipsychotic drugs that do not produce significant side effects. One of the more recently developed antipsychotic drugs is clozapine (clozaril), which exerts its actions primarily on D_4 receptors in the nucleus accumbens and not on D_2 receptors in the neostriatum. Clozapine does not produce Parkinsonian side effects or tardive dyskinesia. Other compounds currently under development for the treatment of schizophrenia act on D_3 receptors.

Determining whether a drug acts as an agonist or antagonist is not always easy, and some drugs appear to have both effects. For example, at high doses apomorphine stimulates postsynaptic D_2 receptors and is considered a DA agonist. But at low doses, apomorphine is considered an indirect antagonist because it activates presynaptic autoreceptors, which inhibits the synthesis and release of DA. Like the dopamine system, the noradrenergic and serotonergic systems are complicated by the fact that there are multiple receptor subtypes for these neurotransmitters. Four subtypes of adrenergic receptors and at least nine subtypes of serotonergic receptors have been identified in the CNS. Lysergic acid diethylamide (LSD) and several other hallucinogens appear to exert their behavioral effects by interacting with serotonin receptors. LSD is another drug that is both an agonist and an indirect antagonist. For years researchers believed that LSD exerted its behavioral effects by stimulating somatic and dendritic autoreceptors in the raphe nuclei. However, recent investigations indicate that LSD is also a direct agonist at postsynaptic 5-HT_{2A} receptors in the forebrain and it is likely that these actions are responsible for its behavioral effects (Carlson, 1998).

GABA (gamma-aminobutyric acid) is an inhibitory neurotransmitter with two receptor subtypes: $GABA_A$ and $GABA_B$. $GABA_A$ receptors are ionotropic and control chloride ion channels. $GABA_B$ receptors are metabotropic and control K^+

channels. The GABA$_A$ receptors contain at least five different binding sites and various drugs bind to the different sites. For example, benzodiazepines such as chlordiazepoxide (Librium), diazepam (Valium), and triazolam (Halcion) bind to one of these sites and facilitate the inhibitory actions of GABA. The benzodiazepines are widely used in medicine and have all but replaced the similarly effective but somewhat more dangerous barbiturates. Both benzodiazepines and barbiturates are classified as CNS depressants, and each chemical group includes substances useful in the treatment of anxiety disorders, insomnia, and epilepsy.

Opioid analgesics also exert their actions through direct receptor activation. These drugs consist of agents derived from the opium poppy, such as morphine and codeine (termed opiates, whereas all drugs that produce morphine-like effects are termed opioids), as well as synthetic derivatives of these compounds, such as heroin, methadone, meperidine (Demorol), and hydromorphone (Dilaudid). These drugs exert their actions through specific receptors in the brain and spinal cord. Opiate receptors were first discovered in 1973 by Pert and Snyder. Shortly after this discovery, other researchers identified endogenous ligands (endogenous substances that combine with receptors) for these receptors. These endogenous ligands are the peptide substances known as the **endorphins** (named for endogenous morphine) and **enkephalins** (Greek translation: in the head). These endogenous peptides are part of the body's defense system against pain. They are released in response to painful and stressful stimuli. Interestingly, the ancient Chinese treatment for pain, acupuncture, appears to involve the release of endorphins; its effects are blocked by the opiate antagonist naloxone (Mayer, Prince, & Rafii, 1977).

There are at least four opiate receptor subtypes: mu, kappa, delta, sigma. Both mu and kappa receptors appear to be involved in the analgesic effects of opiates. Mu receptors are also involved in the mood-enhancing effects that contribute to the abuse liability of these drugs. Little is known about delta and sigma receptors, although it has been suggested that sigma receptors may mediate some of the dissociative effects (e.g., "out of body" hallucinations) produced by these drugs.

In some cases, protracted exposure to an agonist reduces the number of receptor sites available to the neurotransmitter (and exogeneous drugs). That is, receptors other than those activated by the agonist are actually inactivated by the presynaptic neuron (Feldman et al., 1997). This process, called **down-regulation**, partially compensates for the effects of the agonist. **Up-regulation**, in which the number of available receptors increases due to an absence of agonist activity, also occurs. For example, when 6-hydroxydopamine (which destroys presynaptic noradrenergic neurons) was used to reduce the amount of NE that reached beta-adrenergic receptors, the number of such receptors (as indexed by binding assays) increased in some parts of rats' brains, but not in others (Johnson, Wolfe, & Molinoff, 1989). Up- and down-regulation are homeostatic mechanisms, and their existence indicates that the neurochemical effects of a drug may be far more complicated than they initially appear to be. For instance, an agonist drug might initially increase electrical activity in a particular neuronal pathway. If, however, significant down-regulation occurred, activity could eventually return to at or below pre-drug levels, leading to tolerance. Regardless of the level of analysis, drugs have multiple effects.

Drug Effects on Deactivation of Neurotransmitters

The last step in neurochemical transmission is deactivation of the neurotransmitter. Several drugs exert their actions by inhibiting this process. Acetylcholine is deactivated by the enzyme acetylcholinesterase (AChE). Neostigmine and physostigmine are AChE inhibitors used in the medical treatment of a hereditary, and ultimately fatal, autoimmune disorder called myasthenia gravis. For reasons not well understood, in people with this disorder the skeletal muscle ACh receptors are attacked by the immune system. With the progressive loss of these receptors, there is a gradual weakening of the muscles, eventually paralysis, and finally death. As a temporary treatment, AChE inhibitors prolong the effects of the ACh on the remaining receptors, thereby strengthening muscle contractions.

Several drugs are known to interfere with the deactivation of monoamines. Many of these drugs are used to treat depression and other affective (or mood) disorders. The synaptic actions of the monoamine transmitters (DA, NE, 5-HT) are deactivated by reuptake. Synaptic levels of these neurotransmitters are also regulated by the enzyme monoamine oxidase. This enzyme is found in presynaptic terminal buttons of monoaminergic neurons, where it destroys excessive amounts of these transmitter substances. The major classes of antidepressant drugs include the tricyclic antidepressants (e.g., imipramine, desipramine), which block monoamine reuptake, and the MAO inhibitors (e.g., iproniazid, deprenyl), which block monoamine oxidase. More recently developed antidepressants are the selective serotonin reuptake inhibitors (SSRIs) such as fluoxetine (Prozac) and paroxetine (Paxil). These drugs are widely prescribed for a number of disorders including depression, obsessive compulsive disorder, and some anxiety-related disorders such as bulimia and premenstrual syndrome

Cocaine, too, modifies monoaminergic transmission by blocking reuptake. Amphetamine, which was mentioned above as a monoamine releaser, also blocks reuptake of these neurotransmitters. The effects of these stimulants on DA reuptake is of particular interest to researchers. Dopamine pathways originating in the ventral tegmentum project diffusely to several regions in the forebrain, including the prefrontal cortex and nucleus accumbens. As discussed later, several studies indicate that these mesocortical and mesolimbic pathways are critically involved in the reinforcing properties of stimulants, such as cocaine and *d*-amphetamine.

Drugs and Biological Models of Mental Illness

As discussed above, blocking dopaminergic activity with neuroleptic medication provides relief of symptoms in most patients diagnosed as schizophrenic. Moreover, prolonged exposure to drugs that increase dopaminergic activity (e.g., amphetamine) produces changes in behavior that closely resemble those characteristic of schizophrenia. These findings led to the speculation that schizophrenia resulted from metabolic errors leading to either (a) overproduction of dopamine in the limbic system or cortex of the brain, or (b) production of an endogenous amphetamine-like compound. Similarly, the finding that drugs useful in treating depression increased monaminergic activity suggested that depression results from a deficit in serotonergic and/or noradrenergic activity (Baldessarini, 1996b).

These and related biological models of mental illness continue to be popular, despite the fact that attempts to document metabolic differences in humans diagnosed as schizophrenic or depressed have yielded inconclusive results (Baldessarini, 1996b). Moreover, genetic studies have suggested that inheritance can account for only a portion of the causation of these disorders. Finally, the role of environmental variables in generating schizophrenia and depression is widely recognized (Baldessarini, 1996a). Given these considerations, it is not presently possible to explain either condition in terms of neurochemical events. It is nonetheless interesting that the biological models of mental illness that have been proposed are "pharmacocentric," (Baldessarini, 1996b, p. 402), that is, based on drug effects in people with the disorders. That this is so illustrates an important point, namely, that drugs are useful tools for studying the processes that control behavior.

Neuropharmacology and Behavioral Pharmacology

Behavioral events have physiological correlates, and it is reasonable to determine the extent to which a given variable, pharmacological or otherwise, influences events at these two fundamentally different levels of analysis. Of course, for a behavior analyst, it is not *necessary* to do so. Whether it is profitable to do so is open to debate. In general, a strong argument can be made to the effect that humanity's knowledge of physiological processes is not currently adequate to explain the kinds of behavioral phenomena that are of interest to behavior analysts. Therefore, it is more profitable to search for explanations in terms of relations among environmental and behavioral variables.

It can also be argued, however, that much is known about the neurochemical effects of drugs, and such knowledge is relevant to predicting and controlling their behavioral effects. For example, drugs with similar neuropharmacological actions often produce similar subjective effects as revealed in drug discrimination and self-report studies. In addition, drugs that increase dopaminergic activity in certain parts of the brain are apt to serve as positive reinforcers. Given such findings, it is clear that some behavioral effects of drugs can be accurately predicted given their neurochemical actions.

Nonetheless, drugs with different neuropharmacological actions can produce equivalent behavioral effects. Such an outcome is evident in an elegant study by Mansbauch, Harrod, Hoffmann, Nader, Lei, Witkin, and Barrett (1988). Those researchers examined the effects of four anxiolytic drugs on punished and unpunished keypeck responding in pigeons. A push-pull perfusion technique was used to collect samples of cerebrospinal fluid (CSF) from the birds while they responded. Levels of the metabolites of norepinephrine (3-methoxy-4-hydroxyphenlethyleneglycol, dopamine (homovanillic acid and dihydroxyphenylacetic acid), and serotonin (5-hydroxyindoleacetic acid) in the CSF were determined. By measuring levels of metabolites, which result from the enzymatic inactivation of neurotransmitters, levels of neurotransmitter activity could be estimated. Their primary finding was that certain doses of each drug selectively increased the rate of punished responding (such antipunishment effects are characteristic of anxiolytic drugs), but the changes in neurotransmitter metabolites produced by the four drugs differed greatly. Thus, drugs with different neurochemical actions produced comparable behavioral effects.

The study by Mansbauch et al. (1988) demonstrates that neuroscientists have developed techniques that allow for the direct measurement of neurochemical events that are occurring while animals perform relatively complex behaviors in the presence and absence of drugs. Although it is beyond our scope to cover them here, these and other sophisticated techniques are partially responsible for the remarkable advances that have occurred in neuropharmacology in recent years. These techniques are summarized by Barrett (1991) and by Feldman et al. (1997).

Despite ever-increasing technological sophistication, however, current knowledge of brain function is not sufficiently detailed to account for drug effects on even simple learned behaviors. Consider, for instance, that the same rat could be trained through differential reinforcement to go to the right in an electrified T-maze following injections of atropine, d-amphetamine, morphine, or chlordiazepoxide. In this case, each drug would serve as a discriminative stimulus (S^D) for turning right, even though their neurochemical actions are very different. On the other hand, one drug, perhaps morphine, could be established as a discriminative stimulus for two different behaviors, for instance, turning right in one rat and turning left in a second one. As best we know, morphine exerts its effects as a discriminative stimulus primarily by acting as an agonist at mu receptor sites, and would have such an effect in both rats. Nonetheless, it controls different behaviors in these animals, and it would reliably control neither turning left or right in a rat with no history of differential reinforcement in the presence of morphine. Although it is plausible to assume that morphine somehow produces different effects in the brains of the three rats, the nature of that difference is unknown. The point, of course, is that current understanding of the relation of brain function to behavior is incomplete.

Given this, simple neurochemical models of complex drug effects—which are especially likely to appear in articles written for nonspecialists—should be viewed with caution. For example, as related in a recent *Science* article (Wickelgren, 1997), experiments have shown that a) withdrawal from marijuana produces emotional stress that is mediated by corticotropin-releasing factor (CRF), which also mediates the stress produced by withdrawal of heroin (and other drugs), and; b) tetrahyrocannabinol (THC), one of the primary active drugs found in marijuana, causes release of dopamine in the brain's "reward pathway," as does heroin (and other drugs). After discussing possible interpretations and implications of these findings, the article ends as follows (Wickelgren, 1997):

> [B]oth papers should help revise the popular perception of pot as a
> relatively - although not completely - safe substance to something substantially more sinister. "I would be satisfied if, following all this evidence,

people would no longer consider THC a 'soft' drug," says Di Chiara [one of the researchers who conducted the study described in b above]. "I'm not saying it's as dangerous as heroin, but I'm hoping people will approach marijuana far more cautiously than they have before. (p. 61)

In truth, Di Chiara's findings tell us absolutely nothing about the dangerousness of THC. As discussed below, many different positive reinforcers—including those necessary for human survival, such as food, water, and sexual activity—increase dopaminergic activity in the "reward pathway." But these reinforcers are not generally construed as sinister. The finding that emotional stress occurs and CRF is released during withdrawal from a variety of drugs is interesting, and it may be that stress generally serves as an establishing operation during withdrawal, increasing the reinforcing effectiveness of all drugs that produce physical dependence. But this shared mechanism by no means indicates that different drugs, such as heroin and marijuana, have comparable abuse potential. Drug abuse is a *behavioral* problem, not a neurochemical one. Therefore, the only way to determine the dangerousness of marijuana (or THC) relative to other drugs is to examine how people use those substances and the problems that they experience.

As noted in discussing the *Science* article, it is well established that many drugs that serve as positive reinforcers, including nicotine, alcohol, heroin, and marijuana, ultimately increase dopaminergic activity in the nucleus accumbens system that runs through the medial forebrain bundle (Gandner, 1992). So, too, do other positive reinforcers. This is an interesting finding, and it may well be that inherited or acquired differences in dopaminergic activity in the absence of drugs influence the likelihood that a person will become pathologically involved in drug self-administration. Neuroscientists are evaluating this possibility from a variety of perspectives, and their findings may contribute to the treatment as well as the explanation of drug abuse. Nonetheless, it is meaningless to say that "people abuse drugs because they increase dopaminergic activity," a message commonly advanced in the media. For instance, a recent (Nash, 1997) article in *Time* magazine begins with the heading "Addicted: Why do people get hooked? Mounting evidence points to a powerful brain chemical called dopamine." Insofar as increased dopaminergic activity is prerequisite for a drug to serve as a positive reinforcer, then such an increase may well be necessary for addiction to occur. But it certainly is not sufficient, insofar as not everyone who experiences such an effect becomes addicted.

Moreover, insofar as dopamine may in some sense be responsible for all positive reinforcement, an equally valid article could be written under the heading "Little angels: Why do some kids work hard and do well? Mounting evidence points to a powerful brain chemical called dopamine." Such an article is unlikely to appear. Dopamine, it seems, is more interesting when offered as a simple explanation of why people get into trouble with drugs than for why they repeat any behaviors at all.

Concluding Comments

The 1990s have been called the "Decade of the Brain." In this decade, neuroscientists have perfected the use of several noninvasive techniques that allow them to study the living human brain, as well as more invasive procedures suited for use with animals. Through the use of these techniques, they have begun to discover *how* drugs produce their effects in terms of elementary physiological processes. Questions about *why* drugs produce particular effects, however, are better answered in terms of genetic and environmental variables.

In general, physiological explanations of behavior are reductionistic. The term **reduction** (or reductionism) is used to refer to attempts to explain phenomena in terms of simpler phenomena. Physiological explanations of behavior are inevitably reductionistic. As Carlsen (1988) points out, a physiological psychologist "may explain the movement of a muscle [which produces behavior] in terms of changes in the membrane of muscle cells, the entry of particular chemicals, and the interactions among protein molecules within the cells" (p. 11). He goes on to explain that the process of reduction can be taken further, as when a molecular biologist "explains these events in terms of the forces that bind various molecules together and cause various parts of the molecules to be attracted to one another" (p. 11). Different levels of analysis define, in part, different disciplines. There is no one level of analysis (degree of reduction) that best explains a phenomenon, but reductionism becomes counterproductive when it ceases to allow for the prediction and control of the events to be explained. For example, no matter how much one knows about the forces that bind molecules, that knowledge will not allow for the accurate prediction or control of any kind of behavior.

As emphasized throughout this chapter, knowledge of the neurochemical effects of a drug allows one to predict some, but by no means all, of its behavioral effects. Many variables discussed in the balance of this book influence a drug's behavioral effects, and the actions of these variables cannot presently be explained at the neurochemical level. For the present, and for the foreseeable future, behavioral mechanisms of drug action offer a viable alternative to neurochemical mechanisms for explaining the behavioral effects of drugs. The coming decade has been designated as the "Decade of Behavior," and behavioral mechanisms of action are emphasized in this book.

References

Almers, W. (1990). Excocytosis. *Annual Review of Physiology, 52*, 607-624.

Baldessarini, R. J. (1996a). *Chemotherapy in psychiatry: Principles and practice.* Cambridge, MA: Harvard University Press.

Baldessarini, R. J. (1996b). Drugs and the treatment of psychiatric disorders: Psychosis and anxiety. In J. G. Hardman, L. E. Limbird, P. B. Molinoff, R. W. Ruddon, & A. G. Gilman (Eds.), *The pharmacological basis of therapeutics* (pp. 399-430). New York: McGraw-Hill.

Barrett, J. E. (1991). Behavioral neurochemistry: Application of neurochemical and neuropharmacological techniques to the study of operant behavior. In I. J. Iversen & K. A. Lattal (Eds.), *Experimental analysis of behavior* (Part 2, pp. 79-116). New York: Elsevier.

Borbely, A. A., Neuhaus, H. U., & Tobler, I. (1981). Effect of p-chlorophenylalanine and tryptophan on sleep, EEG and motor activity in the rat. *Behavior and Brain Research, 2*, 1-22.

Carlson, N. R. (1988). *Foundations of physiological psychology*. Needham Heights, MA: Allyn and Bacon.

Carlson, N. R. (1998). *Physiology of behavior*. Needham Heights, MA: Allyn and Bacon.

Civelli, O., Bunzow, J. R., Grandy D. K., Zhou. Q-Y, & Van Tol, H. H. M. (1991). Molecular biology of the dopamine receptor. *European Journal of Pharmacology, 207*, 277-286.

Delcomyn, F. (1998) *Foundations of neurobiology*. New York: W. H. Freeman and Company.

Feldman, R. S., Meyer, J. S., & Quenzer, L. F. (1997). *Principles of neuropsychopharmacology*. Sunderland, MA: Sinauer.

Gardner, E. L. (1992). Cannabinoid interactions with brain reward systems–The neurobiological basis of cannabinoid abuse. In L. Murphy & A. Bartke (Eds.), *Marijuana/cannabinoids neurology and neurophysiology* (pp. 275-336). Boca Raton, FL: CRC Press.

Hoffman, B. B., Lefkowitz, R. J., & Taylor, P. (1996). Neurotransmission: The autonomic and somatic motor nervous systems. In J. G. Hardman, L. E. Limbird, P. B. Molinoff, R. W. Ruddon, & A. G. Gilman (Eds.), *The pharmacological basis of therapeutics* (pp. 105-140). New York: McGraw-Hill.

Johnson, E. W., Wolfe, B. B., & Molinoff, P. B. (1989). Regulation of subtypes of adrenergic receptors in rat brain following treatment with 6-hydroxydopamine. *Journal of Neuroscience, 9*, 2297-2305.

Julien, R. M. (1992). *A primer of drug action*. New York: Freeman.

Mansbach, R. S., Harrod, C., Hoffmann, S. M., Nader, M. A., Lei, Z., Witkin, J. M., & Barrett, J. E. (1988). Behavioral studies with anxiolytic drugs v. Behavioral and neurochemical analyses in pigeons of drugs that increase punished responding. *Journal of Pharmacology and Experimental Therapeutics, 246*, 114-120.

Mayer, D. J., Price, D. D., & Rafii, A. (1977). Antagonism of acupuncture analgesia in man by the narcotic antagonist naloxone. *Brain Research, 121*, 368-372.

Nash, J. M. (1997). Addicted: Why do people get hooked? *Time*, May 5, 68-76.

Pert, C. B., & Snyder, S. H. (1973). Opiate receptor: Demonstrated in nervous tissue. *Science, 179*, 1101.

Poling, A., Gadow, K. D., & Cleary, J. (1991). *Drug therapy for behavior disorders: An introduction*. New York: Pergamon.

Sibley, D. R., & Monsma, J. R. (1992). Molecular biology dopamine receptors. *Trends in Pharmacological Sciences, 13*, 61-69.

Wickelgren, I. (1997). Marijuana: Harder than thought? *Science*, June 27, 1967-1968.

Chapter 5

Assessing Drug Effects in Nonhumans

Alan Poling and Thomas Byrne
Western Michigan University and
Massachusetts College of Liberal Arts

Most behavioral pharmacologists ultimately are interested in drug effects in humans and, as discussed in Chapters 6 and 7, they have developed sound procedures for conducting research with humans. There are, however, ethical and practical restrictions that limit the kind and number of drug studies that can be conducted with our own species. Even when research with humans is possible, it may prove difficult to control conditions well enough to allow for an uncontaminated assessment of drug action. In view of these considerations, many studies in behavioral pharmacology have used nonhuman subjects, including rats, pigeons, mice, and nonhuman primates. Research with such animals is conducted in the belief that results will generalize to humans.

Many disciplines, including medicine, genetics, pharmacology, and physiology, make heavy use of nonhuman research subjects. The experimental analysis of behavior has long done so, and its subjects and procedures have been readily adopted by behavioral pharmacologists. As discussed in Chapter 1, Skinner (1953) provided a clear rational for the use of nonhuman subjects in the experimental analysis of behavior and, by extension, in behavioral pharmacology. As also discussed there, he acknowledged that the processes that account for nonhuman behavior might be inadequate to account fully for human behavior. He contended, however, that whether or not processes demonstrated in nonhumans are applicable to humans should be determined by empirical means. Over time, many studies have shown that the basic processes of operant and respondent conditioning are similar across many species, including humans. This is reassuring for those who wish to generalize drug effects from nonhumans to humans, insofar as behavioral pharmacology emphasizes that drugs often produce their effects by influencing processes of operant and respondent conditioning. The primary purpose of this chapter is to introduce some of the strategies that behavioral pharmacologists use to study drug effects in nonhumans.

General Research Strategies

As described in Chapter 1, behavioral pharmacologists are interested in behavioral loci and mechanisms of drug action, and in the variables that influence drug effects. They pursue these interests in many different ways, using a wide range of experimental tactics and strategies. There are, however, some common features of many studies, and those are outlined below.

Subjects

Behavioral pharmacologists study several nonhuman species, although rats, pigeons, mice, and various nonhuman primates are favored. Precedent, cost, size, ease of maintenance, characteristic lifespan, and the nature of the experimental question are among the variables that influence the species selected for study. Although certain general standards of animal husbandry apply to all laboratory animals, different species obviously require different treatment. Ator (1991) provides a good summary of the proper treatment of common laboratory animals, and lists many resources that will be of value to researchers who study animals. Proper treatment is ethical treatment, and researchers who study drug effects in nonhumans are subject to national, state, and local laws and regulations designed to ensure animal welfare. Prior to conducting research with nonhumans, investigators must have the proposed procedures approved by an appropriate Institutional Animal Care and Use Committee (IACUC).

Equipment

In most studies, nonhuman subjects are confined in an **operant chamber** (sometimes known as a Skinner Box), which is a small box-like structure where conditions can be arranged to control and measure behavior. Figure 5-1 illustrates an operant chamber for use with pigeons. A typical chamber contains at least one object (called the operandum or manipulandum) that is manipulated by the subject to perform the operant response of interest. In typical chambers designed for pigeons, round plastic buttons, termed **keys**, are pecked inward; rat and mouse chambers contain levers that are pressed downward. Monkey chambers often contain levers or response chains that are pulled. Appropriate movement of an operandum operates an electrical switch, and a response is recorded.

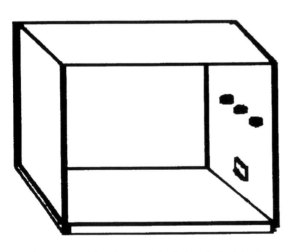

Figure 5-1. *Line drawing depicting the inside of a typical operant chamber for pigeons. Three response keys and an aperture through which birds can gain access to food are shown on the front wall.*

Chambers also contain devices for delivering reinforcers. Liquids are delivered via dippers or drinking tubes, foods by pellet dispensers or magazines that are raised to allow access. In drug self-administration studies, subjects may be fitted with chronically indwelling catheters that allow injection by means of an infusion pump. In addition to reinforcers, other stimuli may be presented in the operant chamber. For example, visual stimuli (e.g., different colors) could appear on keys or on translucent windows, and auditory stimuli could be delivered via speakers. In some studies, provision is made for delivering electric shock to subjects, either through electrodes or through a metal grid floor.

Operant chambers appropriate for use with nonhuman subjects are commercially available, although researchers often build their own equipment, or modify commercial units to meet special needs. In most studies, the same computer that records data arranges experimental events. Specialized computer programs are available for behavioral research, as discussed by Perone (1991).

Of course, operant chambers are not the only apparatus used by behavioral pharmacologists. A researcher interested in drug effects on learning might use a radial-arm or a water maze, for instance, or someone interested in analgesia might use a hot plate or tail-flick apparatus. Ideally, a researcher tailors equipment to the experimental question, although there is certainly a tendency for most people to use what is currently available and familiar.

Dimensions of Behavior

Although human observers are occasionally used to record nonhumans' responses, as in studies of aggressive behavior (Kemble, Blanchard, & Blanchard, 1993), response measures in nonhuman behavioral pharmacology characteristically are quantified mechanically. Whether quantified by humans or machines, behavior can be measured along several dimensions. Among those commonly reported in behavioral pharmacology studies are:

Rate, which is expressed as responses per unit time (e.g., responses per minute) and is calculated by dividing frequency by time. If, for example, a smoker inhaled through a cigar 17 times in a 4-minute observational period, the rate of inhaling would be 4.25 inhalations per minute (17/4). Response rate is determined by **interresponse time** (IRT), which is the time elapsed between two consecutive responses.

Duration specifies the time that elapses from the beginning to the end of a behavior. Another time-based measure, **latency,** designates the time that passes from the onset of a stimulus to the onset of a response. Reaction time is a latency measure.

Accuracy specifies the extent to which a given behavior is appropriate to the current stimulus conditions. For example, "X = 4" is an accurate (correct) response to solving the equation "X = 6 - 2." An answer of "8" would be inaccurate (incorrect).

Choice is often indexed as the percentage (or proportion) of responses (or time) allocated to one alternative relative to total responses (or time). For example, consider a person who often buys drinks from a vending machine that dispenses either cola or root beer. If the person purchases cola 7 times out of 10 trips to the machine, then cola is preferred on 70% of the purchasing opportunities.

Permanent products are tangible items or environmental effects that result from the occurrence of a particular behavior. Products sometimes may be measured when the behavior of interest can not be readily measured. For example, Pavlov did not actually measure the behavior of salivary glands secreting. Instead, he measured saliva, the product of salivation.

Experimental Arrangements

There is no mystery to evaluating the behavioral effects of any drug: One determines whether any independent variable (including a drug) affects a behavior of interest by comparing levels of behavior (the dependent variable) when the independent variable is and is not operative, or is operative at different levels (e.g., doses). Factors other than the independent variable that are likely to affect the dependent variable (i.e., extraneous variables) are eliminated or held constant across conditions. Therefore, if levels of the dependent variable differ when drug is and is not present (or is present at different doses), it is logical to assume that there is a drug effect.

There is no one best way to evaluate the behavioral effects of a drug. As noted in Chapter 1, behavioral pharmacologists generally prefer within-subject experimental designs and visual data analysis. But most of them do not hesitate to use between-subjects designs and inferential statistics when the nature of the experimental question or the data collected make it appropriate to do so. In general, the manner in which a researcher conducts a study and analyzes its results depend upon 1) her or his training and experience, 2) the experimental question, 3) available resources, 4) ethical considerations, and 5) the proposed audience. Many researchers rely on a relatively small number of experimental procedures and conduct the majority of their studies in similar fashion, although they may be conversant with, and accepting of, other approaches.

Most studies in behavioral pharmacology examine the effects of drugs on steady state behavior, which is behavior that in the absence of perturbation does not change its characteristics over time (Sidman, 1960). Such behavior is **stable,** that is, it exhibits little variability (bounce) or trend (progressive change in level) across time. For example, if a woman runs three miles every evening and over the past three months has always finished in between 18.6 and 20.2 minutes, with no trend across time, most people would consider her running speed to be stable.

When behavior occurs in a steady state, the effects of drugs or other environmental variables on behavior should be readily apparent, because the steady state will be disrupted. For example, one Saturday evening our hypothetical runner drinks four beers in an hour, then takes 23 minutes to traverse her usual route. Two weeks later, she drinks the same amount and runs three miles in 23.4 minutes. Compared to her running times when not drinking, these data suggest that drinking alcohol substantially slowed running.

The value of studying steady state behavior is readily apparent if one considers the difficulty in measuring the effects of drinking four beers on running if the person's times for traversing three miles ranged from 15 to 30 minutes in the absence

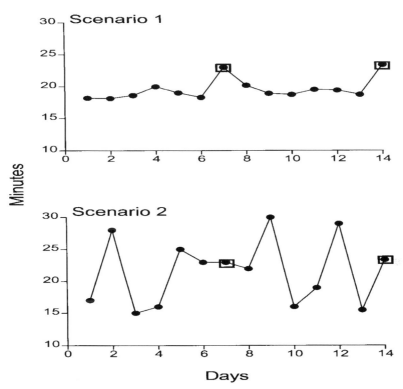

Figure 5-2. *Hypothetical data showing the time required for a woman to run three miles in the presence (boxes) and absence (no boxes) of alcohol. Stable baseline data are depicted in the upper frame, where the effects of drinking four beers are readily apparent. Unstable baseline data are shown in the lower frame, where no obvious drug effect is apparent.*

of alcohol. In this case, running times of 23 and 23.4 minutes after drinking four beers would be hard to interpret, because they fall within the range observed in the absence of drug. Figure 5-2 depicts these two scenarios.

Although not a formal experiment, the scenario of the runner illustrates the logic of probe experimental designs, which are often used by behavioral pharmacologists. In a **probe design**, brief exposures to an independent variable are superimposed on otherwise constant conditions (Poling, Methot, & LeSage, 1995). Actual data collected using a probe design are shown in Figure 5-3, which depicts the effects of 1.8 and 3.2 mg/kg doses of morphine on pigeons' rates of key-pecking under a fixed-ratio (FR) 25 schedule of food delivery. Here, during one-hour sessions conducted each day, every 25th key peck produced 3-second access to grain.

To generate the data in Figure 5-3, the pigeons were injected with morphine 30 minutes prior to every sixth session. Doses of 1.8 and 3.2 mg/kg were administered once each. Prior to every fifth session, the birds received an injection of isotonic saline solution (the substance with which morphine was combined for injection, i.e.,

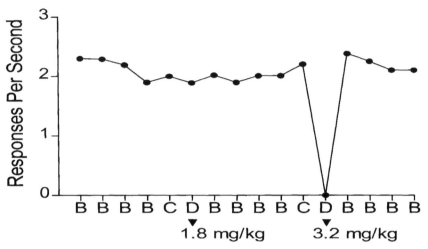

Figure 5-3. *Mean response rates of two pigeons under an FR 25 schedule of food delivery during 1-hour sessions in which no injections, vehicle injections, or morphine (1.8 or 3.2 mg/kg) injections were given. Data are unpublished findings from our laboratory.*

its **vehicle**) 30 minutes prior to testing. Saline injections allowed the experimenters to determine if any change in behavior was due to the injection itself (an extraneous variable), rather than the drug. In the shorthand commonly used to describe experiments, this arrangement would be labeled a BBBBCD design, where B represents baseline, C represents vehicle control, and D represents morphine injections.

As can be seen in the graph, response rates in the absence of drug were stable, and vehicle injections had no effect. Morphine completely suppressed responding at a dose of 3.2 mg/kg, but 1.8 mg/kg had no apparent effect. The graph also shows that responding returned to baseline levels during the sessions following exposure to 3.2 mg/kg. Thus, it appears that acute administration of morphine produced response-rate reductions that were both dose dependent and reversible.

Although Figure 5-3 adequately portrays the outcome of a very simple experiment, its level of detail is excessive for depicting the results of a more complicated study. Most research in behavioral pharmacology evaluates several drug doses, and the conventional way to show the behavioral effects of more than one dose of a drug is with a dose-response curve. Dose-response curves are covered in detail in Chapter 3. Figure 5-4 shows a dose-response curve from an experiment in which the acute and chronic effects of morphine were examined in a pigeon performing under an FR 75 schedule of food delivery.

After the overall rate of responding stabilized in the absence of drug, several doses of morphine were administered according to a BBBBCD design, as described above. In this study, doses were administered in an ascending sequence, where the initial dose was quite low, and the dose was increased in quarter-log units until the response rate fell to below 10% of the pre-drug level. After initial dose-response testing, the subject received 5.6 mg/kg morphine each day for 30 days. Finally, a second (post-chronic) dose-response curve was determined by substituting other doses of morphine for the chronic (3.2 mg/kg) dose. Thus, the design was more complicated than a simple probe design, although similar logic was employed.

Figure 5-4 shows the effects of morphine by depicting response rates during drug sessions as a percentage of mean response rates during vehicle sessions. For example, a value of 100 indicates that the response rate in the presence of that dose of drug was equivalent to the mean response rate when vehicle was injected. That is, the drug did not affect response rates. A value of 50 indicates that the drug response rate was 50 percent of the mean vehicle response rate.

It is evident from Figure 5-4 that morphine produced generally dose-dependent decreases in response rates when administered before or after chronic exposure. Comparing pre- and post-chronic dose-response curves shows that substantial tolerance developed to this effect. Clearly, summary graphs depicting dose-response curves are relatively easy to interpret, especially when data are represented as a percentage of control (non-drug) levels. It is, however, true that potentially useful information is always lost when data are summarized. In some cases, conclusions supported by summary data are not equivalent to those supported by more detailed presentations.

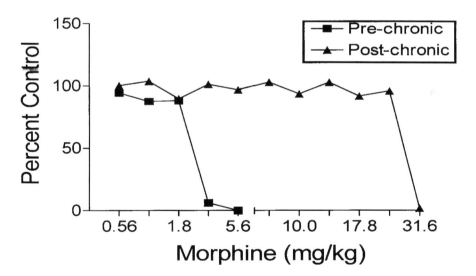

Figure 5-4. *Mean response rates of a pigeon under an FR 75 schedule of food delivery during 1-hour sessions in which the indicated dose of morphine was administered prior to and after the birds were given 30 days of chronic exposure to 5.6 mg/kg morphine. Each indicated dose was administered once. Drug rates are expressed as a percentage of vehicle control rates. Data are unpublished findings from our laboratory.*

Interpreting Drug Effects

Different dimensions of the same behavior often are not affected in the same way by a given drug. Therefore, care should be taken to ensure that primary attention is paid to dimensions that are of theoretical or practical importance. The simple fact that a drug changes some dimension of a nonhuman's behavior does not mean that the effect is important, or can be related in any meaningful way to humans. Consider, for example, a case in which a researcher is evaluating an environmental contaminant found in the Great Lakes. The substance appears in low concentrations in humans and other animals living nearby and is feared to be toxic, but its actual effects have not been investigated. Given these considerations, the researcher decides to examine the effects of the drug in food-deprived rats responding under a fixed-interval (FI) 2-minute schedule of food delivery. Under this schedule, the first response in each session is followed by food delivery. Thereafter, the first response emitted after two minutes have elapsed from the preceding food delivery produces food; responses prior to that time have no programmed consequence.

In the absence of drug, this schedule usually engenders relatively low overall response rates, with most responding occurring towards the end of each 2-minute interval. Assume that this pattern is evident in each of four rats, whose behavior is stable. At that point, the researcher begins to administer drug. The starting dose is a very low one, and does not alter the rate of responding. Every Friday, the dose is doubled. Every Thursday, a vehicle control injection is administered. As doses increase, response rates fall, and a dose is finally reached at which responding ceases altogether. What can be made of these findings?

Obviously, the drug is behaviorally active. Also obviously, it is toxic at sufficiently high doses, insofar as the animals ceased responding, and thereby lost the opportunity to obtain food. This is a harmful outcome, because the animals are food deprived and operating at a caloric deficiency. But what about the rate decreases at lower doses? So long as the rate and pattern of responding is adequate to obtain the available reinforcers, they are not harmful. If anything, they are in a small way beneficial, in that they prevent calorically-deprived organisms from wasting energy in emitting unnecessary lever presses.

Following this logic, it appears that the drug is toxic in this assay only at the highest dose tested. That dose, let us assume, produced a blood level far in excess of levels reported in humans and other animals from the Great Lakes region. The same is true of all doses that were behaviorally active. It may, therefore, be the case that the doses being evaluated are so large as to be meaningless. Water is toxic at sufficiently high doses, and may even cause death, but to say that water is a dangerous toxin is ludicrous. Perhaps asserting that the contaminant is dangerous is also ludicrous.

But perhaps not. It is well established that different species differ dramatically with respect to their sensitivity to drugs and that smaller animals generally are less sensitive than larger ones. Moreover, the rats' exposure to the drug was very brief, but humans and other animals in the natural environment may be exposed to it repeatedly over many years. Therefore, the harmful effects observed in rats may well suggest that the drug poses the risk of disrupting behavior in individuals who encounter it in their everyday world. There is, in fact, no way to determine which of these interpretations is correct.

Examining values of an independent variable outside the range encountered in the natural environment makes it easier to detect the effects of that variable, but also makes it more difficult to generalize with confidence from the experimental setting to the natural environment. In the case of our hypothetical environmental contaminant, further research would be required before one could make any strong assertions about its safety. *No single experiment is adequate to index the behavioral effects of a drug.*

There are, of course, behavioral assays that far surpass the FI schedule in generating results that are readily extended to humans. For example, nonhuman self-administration procedures yield data that accurately predict abuse potential in humans. In short, any drug that nonhumans self-administer has abuse potential, although a few drugs that nonhumans do not self-administer (e.g., LSD) are at least occasionally abused by humans (Griffiths, Bigelow, & Henningfield, 1980; Meisch & Lemaire, 1993; Young & Herling, 1986). Given this, it is easier for most people to see the significance of studies of drug self-administration than to see the significance of studies of the effects of drugs on schedule-controlled behavior. That this is so does not, however, mean that studies of the latter sort are of no value.

In fact, as discussed later in this chapter, studies of drug effects under various schedules of reinforcement have yielded a wealth of information about the classes of variables that modulate drug effects. Different procedures have different uses, and over the years behavioral pharmacologists have developed assays suitable for examining behavioral loci and mechanisms of drug action, and variables that modulate drug effects. The balance of this chapter introduces some of the assays that are frequently used in studies with nonhumans. Before considering those assays, however, it is worthwhile to examine further how drug doses are selected in nonhuman studies, and strategies for relating those doses to human exposure levels.

In the initial examination of a drug's behavioral effects, doses are selected empirically. That is, the researcher usually begins with what she or he believes to be a subthreshold dose and increases dosage systematically until effects ranging from just-perceptible changes in behavior to general and nonsystematic disruption of performance are observed. After a behaviorally-active range of doses initially is established for a given species and route of administration, subsequent studies characteristically examine similar doses. There appears to be no alternative to this strategy, which has been used widely and productively. As noted, however, it does pose difficulties for generalizing effects to humans, who may receive very different doses.

This problem can be overcome in some instances by determining in nonhumans whether a drug disrupts behavior at doses that produce the therapeutic effect for which the drug is used with humans. For example, with opioid analgesics, doses that reduce sensitivity to "painful" stimulation (e.g., heat applied to the paws) can be compared to doses that produce other behavioral effects. Or, with anticonvulsant drugs, doses that reduce seizures can be compared to those that affect operant behavior. If behavioral disruption is observed at analgesic or anticonvulsant doses, similar disruption might be observed in human receiving therapeutic drug doses. Although the actual doses that produce analgesia or anticonvulsant effects may differ substantially across species, these doses do provide a meaningful benchmark for comparing drug effects in humans and other animals. Unfortunately, with many drugs there are no objective measures that correlate the dose range in laboratory animals with the therapeutically relevant human range. Because of this, extrapolations from nonhumans to humans must be made cautiously.

Common Assays in Behavioral Pharmacology

As previously indicated, many methods are used to study the behavioral effects of drugs. These methods are summarized in a book edited by van Haaren (1993), which is nearly 700 pages in length. Obviously, it is beyond our purposes to even list, let alone describe, all of the assays covered there. Instead, we simply introduce a number of important assays, and point out the kinds of experimental questions that they are used to answer.

Repeated Acquisition of Behavior Chains and Other Measures of Learning

Several procedures are available for assaying drug effects on learning. One, the repeated acquisition of behavior chains (or, simply, repeated acquisition) procedure is often used by behavioral pharmacologists (e.g., Thompson & Moerschbaecher, 1979). The **repeated acquisition procedure** requires the subject to learn a sequence of responses (usually spatially defined) that varies from one test session to the next. For example, in one of our studies (Picker & Poling, 1984), pigeons received food dependent upon the completion of a four-response chain (sequence). Three response options were available during each component (i.e., left-key peck, right-key peck, center-key peck), and the correct response for each component was defined by spatial locus. Each component in the chain was correlated with a different key color. That is, all keys were (for example) red until the first correct response occurred, blue until the second correct response occurred, white until the third correct response occurred, and green until the fourth correct response occurred, at which time food was delivered. After this, the sequence began again. Incorrect responses darkened the test chamber for a brief period. The sequence of responses designated as correct changed on a daily basis. On Monday, for instance, the correct sequence might be peck right, peck left, peck right, peck center, whereas the sequence center, left, center, right might be correct on Tuesday. Sessions ended after 70 food deliveries or one hour, whichever occurred first.

After extensive training under the repeated acquisition procedure in the absence of drug, the percentage of total responses that are incorrect varies relatively little across test sessions. At that point, drug effects can be evaluated. In the Picker and Poling (1984) study described above, after responding stabilized acute administrations of various doses of five anticonvulsant drugs (clonazepam, valproic acid,

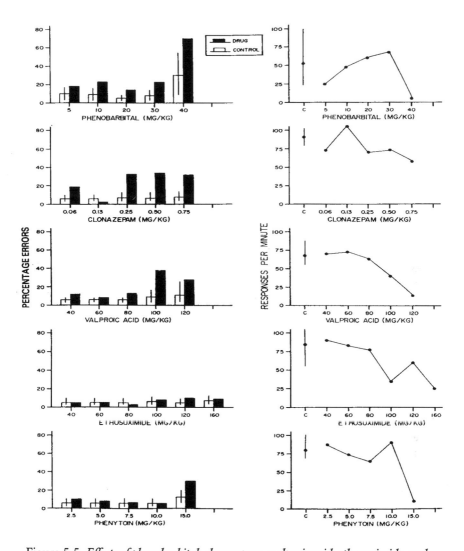

Figure 5-5. *Effects of phenobarbital, clonazepam, valproic acid, ethosuximide, and phenytoin on response rate and percentage of errors for one pigeon exposed to a repeated acquisition procedure. White bars in the left frame represent mean error percentages during control sessions; the vertical lines represents ranges across these sessions. Error percentages for control sessions reflect performance during pre-drug sessions until a number of reinforcers equal to that obtained during the following drug session was earned. Dark bars in the left frame represent mean percentages of errors during initial exposure to the listed drug and dose. Data presented at C (right frames) indicate the mean rate of responding during control sessions; vertical lines represent the range across these sessions. Data are from Picker and Poling (1984).*

ethosuximide, phenobarbital, and phenytoin) were examined. Results for one bird are summarized in Figure 5-5. This figure depicts the percentage of total responses that were correct during vehicle control sessions and during sessions when the indicated dosage of each of the five drugs was administered. It also depicts rate of responding.

Acute administrations of clonazepam, valproic acid, ethosuximide, and phenytoin produced generally dose-dependent decreases in rate of responding, while phenobarbital had little consistent effect on response rate. Phenobarbital and clonazepam produced dose-dependent increases in error rates. Although valproic acid and phenytoin generally increased errors relative to control values, this effect was not directly dose dependent or consistent across subjects. In contrast to the other anticonvulsants studied, ethosuximide had little effect on error rates, suggesting that there are qualitative as well as quantitative differences in the effects of antiepilepsy drugs under the repeated acquisition procedure. These data are consistent with preclinical and clinical evidence indicating that the majority of anticonvulsant medications can adversely affect learning, although this effect reportedly is not a major problem with ethosuximide at therapeutic doses (Picker & Poling, 1987).

Of course, as noted previously, the repeated acquisition procedure is not the only assay that is useful for studying learning in nonhumans. For instance, researchers interested in learning under respondent conditioning procedures might compare the number of trials (CS-US pairings) required for a CS to elicit a CR reliably in groups of animals exposed to drug and vehicle control conditions. The results of one such study (Schindler, Gormezano, & Harvey, 1985) are shown in Figure 5-6. In this study, a puff of air directed into the eye of restrained rabbits, which reliably elicits movement of the nictitating membrane (UR), served as the US. Tone and light presentations (CS) preceded the US in groups of rabbits that received control injections and in other groups that received 5 mg/kg morphine or 0.013 mg/kg LSD. At these doses, LSD facilitated learning, insofar as animals that received this drug acquired CRs faster and reached higher asymptotic levels than vehicle control animals. Morphine, in contrast, interfered with learning.

These results are not intrinsically more or less interesting or important than are results obtained under repeated acquisition procedures. But they are certainly not equivalent. Morphine typically has little effect on, or slightly decreases, accuracy under repeated acquisition procedures, that is, it does not strongly interfere with learning. There is no evidence that LSD facilitates learning under repeated acquisition procedures. Thus, the effects of morphine and LSD on "learning" are determined, in part, on how "learning" is measured. That this is so is neither surprising nor problematic, but it does call attention to two important points:

1)   Terms from the vernacular, like "learning" and "memory," are so general as to be of limited use in a science of behavior. They are, nonetheless, commonly and appropriately used by scientists when they attempt to explain the significance of their findings to laypeople.

2)   In their experiments, scientists (including behavioral pharmacologists) inevitably define terms like "learning" and "memory" **operationally,**

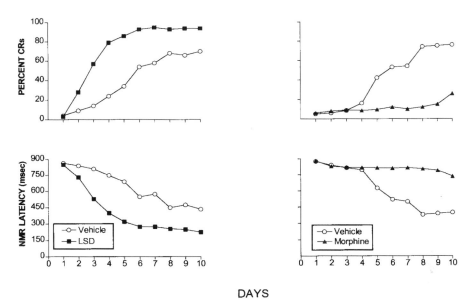

DAYS

Figure 5-6. *Effects of 5 mg/kg morphine and 0.013 mg/kg LSD on the acquisition of nictitating membrane conditional responses in rabbits. Data indicate the percentage of trials on which a conditional response was observed. Trials with tone and light conditional stimuli are combined in this figure, as are morphine and LSD controls. Data are from Schindler et al. (1985) and reproduced by permission.*

that is, with respect to how they measure the phenomena. Results obtained with one assay may or may not be similar to those obtained with another assay of what is labeled as the same general phenomenon.

Delayed Matching to Sample and Other Measures of Memory

Like repeated acquisition, delayed matching to sample is a discrete-trials procedure. Under the **delayed-matching-to-sample (DMTS) procedure**, on each trial a subject is presented with one of a number (e.g., two) of sample stimuli that differ in some physical aspect (e.g., in color). Some time after presentation of the sample stimulus ends, two or more comparison stimuli are presented. A response to the comparison stimulus that matches (i.e., is physically equivalent to) the sample stimulus is reinforced; errors end the trial without reinforcement (and, in many procedures, initiate a timeout during which the opportunity for reinforcement is lost). DMTS allows for an evaluation of drug effects on the performance of a complex conditional discrimination and provides a tenable assay of drug effects on "short-term memory."

A study by Picker, White, and Poling (1985) provides an example of the use of a DMTS procedure to study drug effects. In this study, pigeons were required to match stimuli (key colors) separated by 0.5, 1, 2, 4, or 8 seconds, with each delay interval presented equally often during daily sessions. To provide an index of response rate, five responses were required to extinguish the sample stimulus and (eventually) present the comparison stimuli. As shown in Figure 5-7, when administered acutely clonazepam, valproic acid, ethosuximide, phenobarbital, and phenytoin reduced rate of responding to the sample stimulus, whereas phenobarbital increased response rate. In this study, as in the previously-described study of the effects of the same drugs on repeated acquisition (Picker & Poling, 1984), the primary purpose of recording response rates was to determine that a behaviorally-active range of doses was evaluated. This was the case for all drugs, in both studies.

Phenobarbital, clonazepam, and valproic acid produced generally dose-dependent reductions in overall accuracy (i.e., accuracy summed across delay values). With these drugs, the relative magnitude of the accuracy decrement did not vary systematically with delay interval. Ethosuximide and phenytoin did not generally reduce overall accuracy, although the later drug did so in some instances. These findings suggest that there are substantial differences in the effects of anticonvulsant drugs on short-term memory.

Other assays of memory include passive avoidance tests and water mazes. In passive avoidance, an animal (usually a rat or mouse) is placed in a chamber containing two compartments. Characteristically, one is dark and the other lighted. The subject is placed in the lighted area and the time elapsed until the darkened area is entered (rats and mice naturally prefer darkened areas) is recorded. Upon entering the darkened area, the animal receives a foot shock. This is sufficient to increase the latency of movement to the darkened area on a subsequent trial, and the difference in latency from the first to the second trial is considered to reflect passive avoidance. By exposing groups of rats to different drug conditions before the second trial, drug effects on memory can be assessed. For example, under this procedure, diazepam produces generally dose-dependent impairment of passive avoidance (Lenègre, Chermat, Avril, Steru, & Porsolt, 1988). That is, drug-treated animals enter the darkened compartment significantly more quickly than do control rats that are not given drug.

The **Morris water maze** is a third assay of memory. In this assay, rats or mice are placed into a circular tank containing opaque water. The tank contains a platform just beneath the water's surface, and subjects can escape from the water (and the necessity of swimming) by finding and mounting the platform. Performance in the water maze is potentially controlled by a variety of stimuli, including the subjects' orientation in the environment. Over trials, latency to escape from the water (i.e., the time required for the subject to mount the platform) decreases, assumedly because the subject "remembers" stimuli from prior trials and responds to them appropriately. By examining how latency to escape changes over trials in animals that are and are not given drugs, and by separating trials by brief or long periods, researchers can assess drug effects on what cognitive psychologists call short-term and long-term memory (Porsolt, McArthur, & Lenègre, 1993). This assay is simple to use and is sensitive to many drugs. For example, atropine disrupts memory in the

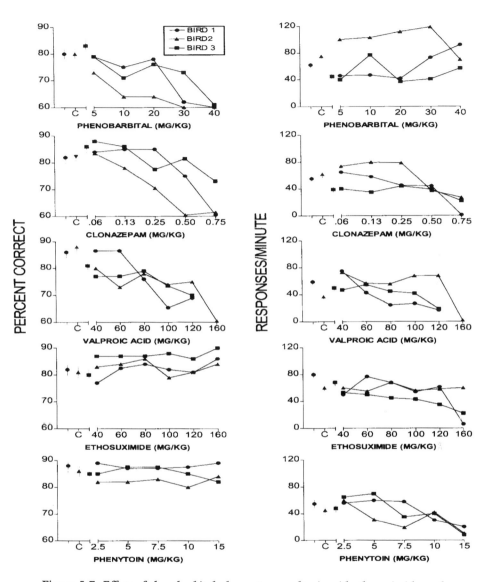

Figure 5-7. *Effects of phenobarbital, clonazepam, valproic acid, ethosuximide, and phenytoin on percentage of correct responses and rate of responding to the sample stimulus for individual pigeons. For the panels on the left, control data (indicated by C) are expressed as the mean percentage of correct responses averaged across five delays for the 10 sessions that preceded drug administration; vertical lines represent the standard error of the mean. Drug data are expressed as the percentage of correct responses for the two determination at each dose and are averaged across all five delays. The panels on the right shown the mean rate of responding to the sample stimulus during the 10 sessions that preceded drug administration (vertical lines represent the standard error of the mean) and during the two administrations of each dose. Data are from Picker et al. (1985).*

Morris water maze, and its effects are in some ways similar to those of aging (Lindner & Schallert, 1988).

Of course, all of the procedures described in this section could be considered measures of learning, as well as of memory. This is always the case. What we commonly term "learning" and "memory" are related phenomena and, as discussed earlier, neither has a precise meaning apart from the assay used to measure it.

Schedules of Reinforcement

Schedules of reinforcement specify relations among stimuli, responses, and the passage of time (see Chapter 2). Schedules of reinforcement have, as Morse (1975) noted, "fundamental as opposed to a practical significance for drug action" (p. 1869). The schedule of reinforcement under which behavior is maintained exercises powerful control over the rate and temporal pattern of responding. With many drugs, observed effects are rate dependent, as discussed in Chapter 8. That is, the direction and magnitude of their effects are determined by the rate of responding in the absence of drugs, which may be controlled by the schedule under which responding is maintained. Such an effect is evident in an early study by Dews (1955).

In this study, Dews examined the effects of pentobarbital on pigeons' rate of key pecking under a multiple FR 50 FI 15-minute schedule of food delivery. Under this schedule, the FR 50 and FI 15-minute components alternated, and each was correlated with a unique exteroceptive stimulus (key color). Food was delivered following every fiftieth response under the FR 50 schedule. Under the FI 15-minute schedule, the first response emitted at least 15 min after the preceding food delivery produced food; other responses had no consequence. When performance stabilized in the absence of drug, the FR schedule generated a much higher rate of responding than did the FI schedule. At this point, Dews evaluated the acute effects of six doses of pentobarbital. Results are shown in Figure 5-8.

Although pentobarbital is a prototypic depressant drug, it did not simply depress (reduce) response rates under both schedules. Instead, when drug rates were compared to control rates, the drug produced "depressant" effects (reduced rates) under the FI schedule, but it produced "stimulant" effects (increased rates) under the FR schedules. The fact that the schedule of reinforcement modulated the *qualitative* effects of pentobarbital was surprising and provided clear evidence that the manner in which a given behavior is maintained is a primary determinant of drug action.

Schedules of reinforcement provide useful tools for examining the effects of variables other than response rate as determinants of drug action. For example, the extent to which external discriminative stimuli influence drug action can be determined by comparing drug effects under different versions of a **fixed-consecu-tive-number (FCN) schedule**. Under the FCN schedule, subjects are required to respond a fixed number of times on one (work) operandum and then respond once on a second (reinforcement) operandum. Responding on the reinforcement operandum before the response requirement on the work operandum is completed resets the response requirement. Under one variant of the schedule (FCN-S^D), an external discriminative stimulus is correlated with completion of the response

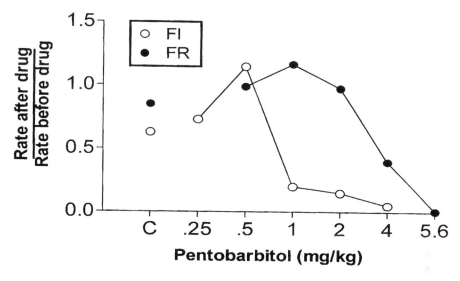

Figure 5-8. *Effects of pentobarbital on the mean response rates of pigeons responding under a multiple schedule of food delivery comprising FR 50 and FI 15-min components. Redrawn from Dews (1955).*

requirement on the work operandum, whereas no external stimulus change is programmed under the other variant (FCN). Accuracy levels, as measured by the proportion of response sequences that are long enough to meet the response requirement on the work operandum, are increased considerably by the addition of the external discriminative stimulus.

Comparing drug effects under FCN and FCN-S[D] schedules allows one to ascertain whether the addition of a discriminative stimulus influences drug effects. As a rule, drug effects are larger under an FCN schedule than under a comparable FCN-S[D] schedule. Such an effect is evident in Figure 5-9, which compares the effects of various doses of clonazepam and ethosuximide on the accuracy of two groups of pigeons, one exposed to an FCN 8 schedule, the other to an FCN 8-S[D] (Picker, Leibold, Endsley, & Poling, 1986). Under these schedules, the birds received food for responding between 8 and 12 times on one key, then responding once on a second key. Under the FCN 8-S[D], but not the FCN 8, the key changed color when the bird responded 8 times.

Clonazepam produced large decreases in reinforced response runs (accuracy) and rates of responding (not shown). The magnitude of these accuracy- and rate-decreasing effects were smaller in the group with the external discriminative stimulus. Ethosuximide also decreased rates of responding under both the FCN and the FCN-S[D] schedule. This drug, however, only reduced accuracy under the FCN schedule. These data suggest that the addition of an external discriminative stimulus attenuates the disruptive behavioral effects of anticonvulsant drugs. Similar modulation of drug action by discriminative stimuli occurs with many other drug classes.

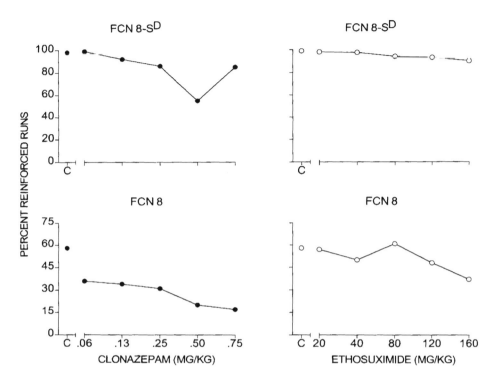

Figure 5-9. *Effects of clonazepam and ethosuximide on the mean percentage of reinforced runs by groups of pigeons responding under FCN 8 and FNC 8-S^D schedules of food delivery. Data are from Picker et al. (1986).*

The potential uses of schedules of reinforcement to examine drug action, and the variables that affect it, are nearly limitless. For example, punishment can be arranged for a scheduled operant response in some conditions and not in others, allowing punishment to be examined as a determinant of drug action (see Chapter 8). Doing so reveals that sedative-hypnotic drugs, but not drugs from other classes, characteristically increase punished behavior.

Behavioral history provides an example of another potential determinant of drug action than can be examined using schedules of reinforcement. In an early study in this area, Urbain, Poling, Millam, and Thompson (1978) examined the effects of *d*-amphetamine in two groups of rats bar pressing under an FI 15-second schedule of food delivery. One group had a history of responding under an FR 40 schedule, the other group had a history of responding under an interresponse-time-greater-than-11-second (IRT > 11-second) schedule.

The effects of acute injections of *d*-amphetamine under the FI schedule depended on the rats' behavioral history. Low to moderate doses increased response rates relative to control levels in rats with IRT > t histories, but the same doses consistently decreased response rates in animals with FR histories. Thus, the *qualitative* effects of the drug varied as a function of behavioral history. Urbain et al. (1978) explained these results in terms of rate dependency. In the absence of drug, rats with IRT > t histories responded much slower under the FI schedule than did rats with FR histories. Amphetamine characteristically reduces high-rate operants at doses that increase low-rate operants, and the results reported by Urbain et al. are consistent with such a rate-dependent effect. Note that the rate-dependent effects of *d*-amphetamine differ from those of pentobarbital, which increases high-rate operants relative to control values at doses that decrease or have no effect on low-rate operants.

Drug Self-administration Procedures

Behavioral pharmacologists have developed procedures that allow drugs to be delivered to laboratory animals via intraveneous, intragastric, intracranial, intracebroventricular, intramuscular, pulminary, and oral routes (Meisch & Lemaire, 1993). The intravenous route appears to be most commonly used in studies of drug self-administration, although the oral route is also common. The main advantages of the intravenous route are that precise quantities of drug can be administered and that drug effects occur with little delay, hence, delay of reinforcement is not a problem. On the down side, the intravenous route requires invasive surgical procedures and the duration of the procedure is limited. The oral route is free of these problems, and allows subjects to be studied for years. Onset of drug effects is delayed, however, and this factor coupled with the aversive taste of many drug solutions makes it harder to establish drugs as reinforcers via the oral route than via the intravenous route. That does not mean, however, that one route is better than the other. As Meisch and Lemaire (1993) point out, "The issue is not whether one route is better than another, for that depends upon the goals of an experiment: different routes have different profiles of advantages and disadvantages and may be selected to suit particular purposes" (p. 276).

Regardless of route of administration, schedules of reinforcement characteristically are useful for evaluating the reinforcing effects of drugs, and the variables that affect drug self-administration. For example, Nader and Woolverton (1992) gave rhesus monkeys a choice between cocaine (0.01-1.0 mg/kg/injection) and food under a discrete-trials procedure. When an FR 30 schedule was arranged for each reinforcer, the percentage of trials on which cocaine was chosen over food increased with cocaine dose. Increasing the response requirement for cocaine, but not food, decreased the percentage of trials on which cocaine was selected. When the schedule for cocaine delivery was FR 480, food was always preferred regardless of cocaine dose. Similarly, when the FR for cocaine was held constant and the FR for food was increased, cocaine self-administration increased. These results indicate that the availability of alternative reinforcers, and the schedule under which those reinforcers are available, strongly influence cocaine self-administration. Other variables that affect drug self-administration are discussed in Chapters 7, 8, and 10.

Drug Discrimination Procedures

Drug discrimination procedures demonstrate that drugs produce effects that subjects can detect. In essence, a drug is established as a discriminative stimulus by reinforcing one response (e.g., a right-key peck by a pigeon) in the presence of that drug and reinforcing another response (e.g., a left-key peck) when drug is not administered, and one demonstrates that the drug is serving as a discriminative stimulus by showing that the response previously reinforced in the drug state occurs reliably when the drug is administered but not when it is withheld. This basic procedure can be elaborated so that discriminations can be established among two or more drugs.

For example, Makhay, Young, and Poling (1998) established in pigeons a discrimination among injections of 5.6 mg/kg morphine, 5.6 mg/kg of the experimental drug U50,488H, and isotonic saline solution. The discrimination was established by alternating in a random sequence the three kinds of injections, and reinforcing (with food) pecks of, for example, the left key following morphine, the right key following U50,488H, and the center key following saline solution.

Morphine is an agonist at mu receptor sites in the brain, whereas U50,488H is a kappa agonist. In animals trained to discriminate a mu agonist from vehicle, or a kappa agonist from vehicle, there is some cross-generalization between mu and kappa agonists. That is, when a mu agonist (e.g., morphine) is substituted for the kappa agonist used in training (e.g., U50,488H), some responding occurs on the kappa-appropriate operandum. Similar cross-generalization occurs when a kappa agonist is substituted for a mu agonist used in training. These results suggest that the subjective effects of mu and kappa agonists are similar. That is, in mentalistic terms, morphine and U50,488H make animals "feel the same way." Another possibility, though, is simply that the two-response drug discrimination procedure is not very sensitive. To test this second possibility, Makhay, Young, and Poling (1998) administered various doses of both morphine and U50,488H to their subjects. In all cases, U50,488H engendered only U50,488H -appropriate responding, and morphine engendered only morphine-appropriate responding. Thus, there was no overlap in the subjective effects of mu and kappa agonists when those effects were assessed in a sensitive assay.

As this example illustrates, drug discrimination procedures can be used to examine correlations between neurochemical and behavioral effects of drugs. As discussed in Chapter 8, understanding that drugs may serve as discriminative stimuli also helps to account for the variability in drug effects observed across people and situations.

Other Assays

Although some procedures are used repeatedly, behavioral pharmacologists are innovative in developing assays that provide desired information. For example, during the 1980s our laboratory was involved in profiling the behavioral effects of anticonvulsant drugs in nonhumans. The purpose of that research was to provide

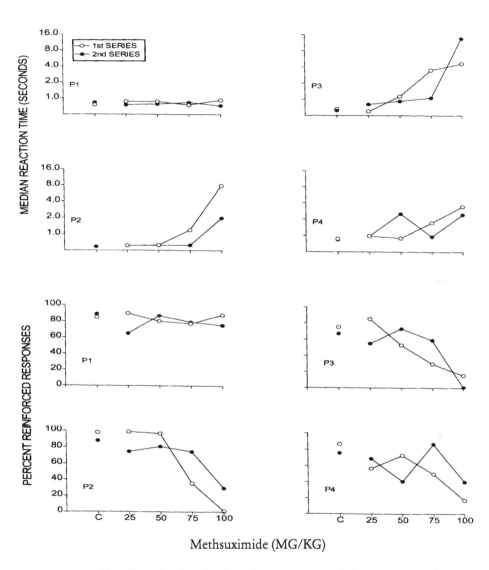

Figure 5-10. *Effects of methsuximide on the reaction time of pigeons. Data are from Blakely et al. (1989).*

information relevant to the probable behavioral side effects of these drugs when used to treat epilepsy in humans. Pursuant to that end, we examined drug effects on learning and memory, as previously described. We also examined drug effects in several other assays, including one that evaluated reaction time. Because much of our work had been done with pigeons, we decided to use the birds as subjects. No prior reports of drug effects on reaction time in pigeons had appeared, but a general procedure for assessing reaction time in rats had been described. We modified the procedure for use in drug studies with pigeons (e.g., Blakely, Starin, & Poling, 1989). In brief, each chamber was fitted with a plastic treadle that protruded from the front wall a short distance above the floor. A translucent panel that could be lighted in white or red was located just above the treadle. Through shaping, birds were trained to stand on the treadle when the panel was lighted in white. They also were trained to step off of the treadle when the panel turned red. Stepping off the panel terminated panel illumination. The time elapsed from the onset of red illumination until the bird stepped off the treadle was recorded, and constituted the reaction time. If the bird stepped down within two seconds of the change in illumination, it earned food. If it stepped down before the change in illumination, which occurred within 0.5 to 3 seconds after the panel was illuminated in white (with the specific interval selected at random), or after more than two seconds had elapsed after the change, the trial ended without food delivery. On average, trials were separated by one minute. Daily sessions ended after 40 food deliveries, 45 minutes, or 100 trials, whichever occurred first.

After protracted training, reaction times stabilized and birds earned food on almost all trials. At this time, the effects of acute injections of mephenytoin and methsuximide were examined. Results for methsuximide are summarized in Figure 5-10. In brief, both drugs produced generally dose-dependent increases in reaction times, and the increase was large enough to cause a loss of reinforcement at higher doses.

The extent to which these results can be safely generalized to epileptic humans who take mephenytoin or methsuximide is difficult to determine, but it is clear that the assay was adequate for providing an answer to the question, "What are the effects of mephenytoin and methsuximide on reaction time in pigeons?" That we developed a tenable assay of an effect of interest is unsurprising, for behavioral pharmacologists constantly develop new assays, and modify old ones, to provide desired information. Some prove valid and reliable and are generally adopted; others fade from popularity. Always, the question to ask in evaluating a procedure is "What, if anything, of importance can it tell us?"

Concluding Comments

The information that nature reveals to us depends on the questions that we ask, and the manner in which we attempt to secure answers to those questions. Controlled experiments with animals have proven valuable in quantifying the behavioral effects of a wide range of drugs and in isolating the variables that modulate drug action. Although other approaches to experimentation are sometimes necessary and useful, the tactics and strategies characteristic of the experimental analysis of behavior are especially valuable in analyzing drug effects.

As Branch (1991) points out, however, the relation between the experimental analysis of behavior and behavioral pharmacology is reciprocal. Demonstrating that drugs have (or can acquire) functional stimulus properties has been a real boon to behavior analysis, and a few studies have used drugs as tools in understanding behavioral processes. Both behavioral pharmacology and the experimental analysis of behavior are relatively young disciplines, and new findings and methods in one field are apt to have important implications for theory and practice in the other.

References

Ator, N. (1991). Subjects and instrumentation. In I. H. Iversen & K. A. Lattal (Eds.), *Experimental analysis of behavior* (Part 1, pp. 1-62). Amsterdam: Elsevier.

Blakely, E., Starin, S., & Poling, A. (1989). Effects of mephenytoin and methsuximide on the reaction time of pigeons. *Pharmacology Biochemistry and Behavior, 31*, 787-790.

Branch, M. (1991). Behavioral pharmacology. In I. H. Iversen & K. A. Lattal (Eds.), *Experimental analysis of behavior* (Part 2, pp. 21-77). Amsterdam: Elsevier.

Dews, P. B. (1955). Studies on behavior: I. Differential sensitivity to pentobarbital of pecking performance in pigeons depending on the schedule of reward. *Journal of Pharmacology and Experimental Therapeutics, 115*, 343-401.

Griffiths, R. R., Bigelow, G. E., & Henningfield, J. E. (1980). Similarities in animal and human drug-taking behavior. In N. Mello (Ed.), *Advances in substance abuse* (Vol. 1, pp. 1-90). Greenwich, CT: JAI Press.

Kemble, E. D., Blanchard, D. C., & Blanchard, R. J. (1993). Methods in behavioral pharmacology: Measurement of aggression. In F. van Haaren (Ed.), *Methods in behavioral pharmacology* (pp. 539-559). Amsterdam: Elsevier.

Lenègre, A., Chermat, R., Avril, I., Steru, L., & Porsolt, R. D. (1988). Specificity of piracetam's antiamnesic activity in three models of amnesia in the mouse. *Pharmacology Biochemistry and Behavior, 29*, 625-629.

Lindner, M. D., & Schallert, R. (1988). Aging and atropine effects on spatial navigation in the Morris water task. *Behavioral Neuroscience, 102*, 621-634.

Makhay, M., Young, A., & Poling, A. (1998). Establishing morphine and U50-488H as discriminative stimuli in a three-choice assay with pigeons. *Experimental and Clinical Psychopharmacology, 6*, 3-9.

Meisch, R. A., & Lemaire, G. A. (1993). Drug self-administration. In F. van Haaren (Ed.), *Methods in behavioral pharmacology* (pp. 257-300). Amsterdam: Elsevier.

Morse, W. H. (1975). Schedule-controlled behaviors as determinants of drug response. *Federation Proceedings, 34*, 1868-1869.

Nader, M., & Woolverton, W. (1992). Effects of increasing response requirement on choice between cocaine and food in rhesus monkeys. *Psychopharmacology, 108*, 295-300.

Perone, M. (1991). Experimental design in the analysis of free-operant behavior. In I. H. Iversen & K. A. Lattal (Eds.), *Experimental analysis of behavior* (Part 1, pp. 135-171). Amsterdam: Elsevier.

Picker, M., & Poling, A. (1984). Effects of anticonvulsants on learning: Performance of pigeons under a repeated acquisition procedure when exposed to phenobarbital, clonazepam, valproic acid, ethosuximide, and phenytoin. *Journal of Pharmacology and Experimental Therapeutics, 230*, 307-316.

Picker, M., Leibold, L., Endsley, B., & Poling, A. (1986). Effects of clonazepam and ethosuximide on the responding of pigeons under a fixed-consecutive-number schedule with and without an external discriminative stimulus. *Psychopharmacology, 88,* 325-330.

Picker, M., White, W., & Poling, A. (1985). Effects of phenobarbital, clonazepam, valproic acid, ethosuximide, and phenytoin on the delayed-matching-to-sample performance of pigeons. *Psychopharmacology, 84,* 494-498.

Poling, A., Methot, L., & LeSage, M. (1995). *Fundamentals of behavior analytic research.* New York: Plenum Press.

Poling, A., & Picker, M. (1987). Behavioral effects of anticonvulsant drugs. In T. Thompson, P. B. Dews, & J. Barrett (Eds.), *Neurobehavioral pharmacology* (pp. 157-192). Hillsdale, NJ: Lawrence Erlbaum.

Porsolt, R. D., McArthur, R. A., & Lenègre, A. (1993). Psychotropic screening procedures. In F. van Haaren (Ed.), *Methods in behavioral pharmacology* (pp. 23-51). Amsterdam: Elsevier.

Schindler, C. W., Gormezano, I., & Harvey, J. A. (1985). Effects of morphine and LSD on the classically conditioned nictitating membrane response. *Pharmacology Biochemistry and Behavior, 22,* 41-46.

Sidman, M. (1960). *Tactics of scientific research.* New York: Basic Books.

Skinner, B. F. (1953). *Science and human behavior.* New York: Macmillan.

Thompson, D. M., & Moerschbaecher, J. M. (1979). Drug effects on repeated acquisition. In T. Thompson & P. B. Dews (Eds.), *Advances in behavioral pharmacology* (Vol. 2, pp. 229-260). New York: Academic Press.

Urbain, C., Poling, A., Millam, J., & Thompson, T. (1978). *d*-Amphetamine and fixed-interval performance: Effects of operant history. *Journal of the Experimental Analysis of Behavior, 29,* 285-292.

Van Haaren, F. (1993). *Methods in behavioral pharmacology.* Amsterdam: Elsevier.

Young, A. M., & Herling, S. (1986). Drugs as reinforcers: Studies in laboratory animals. In S. R. Goldberg & I. P. Stolerman (Eds.), *Behavioral analysis of drug dependence* (pp. 69-122). Orlando, FL: Academic Press.

Chapter 6

Basic Research With Humans

Susan Snycerski, Sean Laraway, and Alan Poling
Western Michigan University

Since the earliest days of the discipline, behavioral pharmacologists have studied human as well as nonhuman subjects (e.g., Dews & Morse, 1958; Higgins, Bickel, & Hughes, 1993). The primary advantages of studying humans are that problems of generalizing results across species are avoided and that variables unique to humans that may modulate drug action can be examined. The primary disadvantage is that ethical and practical considerations limit the kind and number of investigations that can be performed with human participants.

It is convenient to distinguish three general areas of research in human behavioral pharmacology. One investigates the loci and mechanisms of action of psychoactive substances (most often, drugs of abuse) and determines the variables that modulate their effects. The second investigates the clinical utility of psychotropic drugs. The third investigates the success of drug abuse treatments. This chapter summarizes methods used in the area of research listed first. Put differently, it considers basic research methods. Chapter 9 examines clinical drug assessment and Chapter 10 deals with drug abuse and its treatment.

Basic Research Procedures

Whether studying drugs of clinical value or drugs of abuse, approval to use human subjects in research must be granted from a Human Subject Institutional Review Board (HSIRB). To secure such approval, a proposal describing in detail the experimental design, the drug(s) to be studied, the duration of the study, and any risks that subjects may encounter is submitted by the principal investigator to the HSIRB. If approval is obtained to conduct the study, each subject is required to sign an informed consent agreement indicating that they are aware of (1) any risks involved with participating in the experiment, and (2) their right to end participation at any time.

Subjects and Settings

When drugs without abuse potential are of interest, it is feasible for researchers to study people who have not had previous exposure to the substances, although they do not always do so. When studying drugs of abuse, however, ethical considerations characteristically limit subject selection to adults who have previously used the substance(s) to be studied. Regardless of whether subjects are initially drug-naive, they may either reside in the setting where the experiments are conducted, or live outside that setting and come for scheduled testing. The former arrangement is more costly, but allows for greater experimental control. The latter arrangement is cheaper and may allow experiments to be conducted over longer periods of time, but subjects may miss sessions, take unscheduled drugs, or engage in other activities that confound experimental findings.

Much basic research takes place in a laboratory setting and involves subjects performing arbitrary operants (e.g., pressing designated keys on a computer keyboard). Some research, however, takes place in more naturalistic settings, which may allow for social interactions. Social interactions and other complex behaviors may not be readily quantified by automated equipment. When this occurs, human observers are used to quantify dependent variables.

Experimental Arrangements

As in animal studies, within-subject experimental designs are favored in human behavioral pharmacology. Although the same tactics and strategies are appropriate for human and nonhuman research, practical and ethical considerations limit how human studies are conducted. For example, humans obviously cannot be exposed to dangerously high drug doses. Therefore, only a rather limited range of doses, characteristically in the low-to-moderate range, are studied in human behavioral pharmacology. Moreover, because the time available to study each person characteristically is limited, it may not be possible to utilize robust stability criteria, or to evaluate each dose on multiple occasions. These limitations, coupled with the subject heterogeneity that is inevitable in human research, might be expected to reduce the orderliness and meaningfulness of obtained results. This does not, however, appear to be the case; researchers in the area of human behavioral pharmacology have generated a substantial, and orderly, data base.

As with the procedures used to study drug effects in nonhumans, the procedures used with humans are too numerous, too complex, and used in too many ways to be covered in a single chapter. No attempt will be made to review them here. Instead, we will overview several common procedures, and provide examples of how they are used to examine behavioral loci and mechanisms of drug action. Procedures described in this chapter, as well as a number of other procedures commonly used in human behavioral pharmacology, are listed in Table 6-1. This table distinguishes procedures that directly evaluate the behavioral effects of drugs from those that provide indirect measures. It also distinguishes "cognitive" and "motoric" measures, although the distinction is rather arbitrary. In general, the former index what most people term learning and memory, the latter the performance of well-learned responses.

Physiological Measures

It is noteworthy that physiological measures are often reported as correlates of behavior in drug studies with humans, although this is rarely the case in nonhuman behavioral pharmacology. Common physiological measures taken with humans

Table 6-1. Procedures Commonly Used in Behavioral Pharmacology

Direct Behavioral Measures	Examples
Arousal	Electroencephalograph (EEG)
	Skin Temperature
	Skin Resistance
	Heart Rate
Perceptual Performance	Critical Frequency of Fusion (CFF)
Cognitive Performance	Repeated Acquisition (RA)
	Delayed Matching-to-Sample (DMTS)
	Digit-Symbol-Substitution-Test (DSST)
	Vigilance Tasks
Motor Performance	Reaction Time
	Tapping Rate
	Hand Steadiness
	Pursuit Rotor
	Driving
Self-Administration	Progressive-Ratio Schedules (PR)
	Concurrent Schedules
	Discrete-Trials
	Concurrent Choice
	Single-Access Procedures
Motivation	Progressive-Ratio Schedules (PR)
	Contingent Activity Procedures
Drug Discrimination	Two-Choice Procedures
	Three-Choice Procedures
	Stimulus Equivalence

Indirect Behavioral Measures	Examples
Arousal, Mood, and Activity	Profile of Mood States (POMS)
	Addiction Research Center Inventory (ARCI)
	Visual Analog Scale (VAS)
	Beck Depression Inventory (BDI)

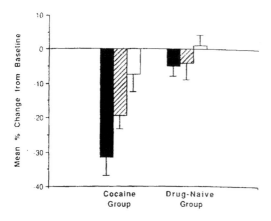

Figure 6-1. *Mean percent change from baseline skin resistance (±SEM) averaged over the video and task presentations in the cocaine (solid bar), opiate (striped bar), and non-drug sessions (open bar). Data are from Ehrman et al. (1992) and reproduced by permission.*

include heart rate, skin resistance, and skin temperature. For example, Ehrman, Robbins, Childress, and O'Brien (1992) recorded these measures, as well as self-reports of drug craving, in a study that assessed conditioned responses to cocaine-related stimuli in cocaine abusing patients. In this study, experimental subjects with a history of smoking free-base cocaine resided in a drug-dependency ward. Subjects with no prior use of cocaine served as a control group. All subjects were exposed to three conditions that comprised three components each. In the opiate condition, the first and second components required subjects to listen

to an audio tape, then watch a videotape portraying people talking about buying, selling, and injecting heroin. The third component required subjects to perform a task where they had to dissolve a white powder that resembled heroin, fill a syringe, then "tie off" as if they were going to inject the "heroin."

In the cocaine condition, the audio and videotapes portrayed people discussing experiences related to procuring, free-basing, and smoking cocaine. The task required subjects to heat a powder resembling cocaine and place it in a pipe as if they were going to smoke it. In the non-drug condition, subjects listened to an

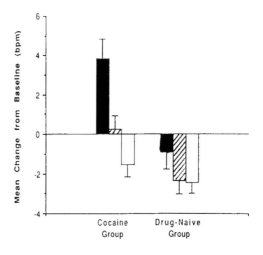

Figure 6-2. *Mean change from baseline heart rate (±SEM) averaged over the video and task presentations in the cocaine (solid bar), opiate (striped bar), and non-drug sessions (open bars). Data are from Ehrman et al. (1992) and reproduced by permission*

audio tape that provided instructions on how to operate a word processing program, watched a nature documentary, and played the video game "Pong." Physiological measures were recorded for each subject under all conditions.

When exposed to cocaine-related stimuli, cocaine-experienced subjects exhibited a decrease in skin temperature not evident in control subjects. As depicted in Figure 6-1, cocaine-experienced subjects also exhibited a greater decrease in skin resistance than did drug-naive subjects. Furthermore, as shown in Figure 6-2, the cocaine-related stimuli caused a greater increase in heart rate in the cocaine-experienced group than in the drug-naive group. Subjects in the experimental group reported craving for cocaine and symptoms of withdrawal when viewing cocaine-related stimuli, whereas those in the control group reported neither effect.

When subjects were exposed to the opiate-related stimuli, there were no significant physiological or self-reported changes in either the experimental (cocaine-experienced) or the control group. These findings demonstrate how both physiological and self-reported measures can detect changes in the body that occur in cocaine users when they are exposed to cocaine-related stimuli. They also are consistent with the results of several other studies, which demonstrate that stimuli historically paired with drug administration elicit conditioned and subjective responses (for reviews, see Baker, Morse, & Sherman, 1987; O'Brien, Ehrman, & Ternes, 1986; Robbins & Ehrman, 1992; Sherman, Jorenby, & Baker, 1988). The fact that such conditioning occurs has implications for treating drug abuse (Ehrman et al., 1992).

Subjective Evaluations

Subjects' craving for cocaine was an important dependent variable in the Ehrman et al. (1992) study. "Craving" is a **subjective** event, insofar as it can be directly detected only by the person in whom it occurs. **Objective** events, in contrast, are those that can be directly detected by multiple observers. Put differently, subjective events are **private events**, whereas objective events are **public events**. Many studies in human behavioral pharmacology, including several discussed later in this chapter, report both subjective and objective measures of drug effects. In principle, subjective measures provide information about "how drugs make people feel," whereas objective measures provide information about how drugs influence overt behavior.

Several more-or-less standardized instruments are frequently used to index the subjective effects of drugs. According to Higgins et al. (1993):

> Visual-analog scales, the short-form of the Addiction Research Center Inventory (ARCI) (Haertzen, 1966) and the Profile of Mood States (POMS) (McNair et al., 1971) [all of which are subjective measures] are three of the most frequently used procedures in human behavior pharmacology. The visual-analog scales in these studies are typically 100-point scales marked at opposite ends with terms such as "not at all" and "extremely." The questions posed might refer to drug effects, mood, or other items of interest to the experimenter. The ARCI short form is a 49-item true/false question-

naire that has been empirically separated into the following five subscales associated with different groups of abused drugs: amphetamine (A) and benzedrine (BG) scales designed to measure stimulant effects, the morphine-benzedrine group scale (MBG) putatively measuring euphoric effects, the pentobarbital-chlorpromazine-alcohol group scale (PCAG) designed to measure sedative effects and the lysergic-acid scale (LSD) designed to measure psychotomimetic effects. The POMS consists of 72 adjectives describing mood states and separated into the following empirically derived clusters: anxiety, depression, vigor, fatigue, confusion, friendliness. (p. 485)

As discussed in Chapter 1, radical behaviorists acknowledge the existence and potential importance of private events, which are stimuli and responses that occur "within the skin." They believe that people learn to describe these events in the same way that they learn to describe public events, that is, by virtue of the actions of their verbal community. Because private events are not directly accessible to other people, however, precise stimulus control by private events over verbal descriptions is very difficult to establish. Therefore, the simple fact that two or more people report a particular subjective state, for example, feeling anxious and confused, does not mean they are experiencing precisely the same private events. The fundamental nature of subjective effects makes it impossible to determine the extent to which they are being reported accurately, in a manner reflecting consistent stimulus control of verbal behavior by internal events. This is an important methodological limitation.

Of course, some private events may have associated **collateral responses** (Skinner, 1945). These are overt (public) changes in behavior or physiological status that occur in conjunction with a private event. When collateral responses are consistent with subject-reported data, the credibility of the latter are considerably enhanced. For example, in the study by Ehrman et al. (1992), changes in heart rate, skin temperature, and skin resistance reliably accompanied subject-reported craving for cocaine. These physiological measures parallel self-reports of craving in providing evidence of an altered internal environment in cocaine-experienced subjects.

Regardless of whether or not collateral responses are present, if a particular drug condition consistently evokes a particular subject-reported feeling state within and across individuals, it is clear that a) the condition does reliably engender detectable private events, and b) the individuals being tested have histories such that they react consistently to those events. Therefore, the subject-reported data are a reliable index of some aspects of drug action. For instance, in the Ehrman et al. (1992) study, viewing cocaine-related stimuli consistently engendered self-reported craving for cocaine only in people with a history of cocaine use. This is interesting information. But it also is imprecise information. In truth, only people who have viewed cocaine-related stimuli after having used the drug know "how it feels."

None of the foregoing considerations render subject-reported data meaningless or unscientific. They do, however, emphasize the value of not relying solely on subject-reported data as an index of drug action. Behavioral pharmacologists rarely do so. In fact, it is common for them to collect and report subjective data as an adjunct to other, more objective, indices of drug action (Higgins et al., 1993).

Drug Effects on Learning and Memory

As discussed in Chapter 5, terms like "learning" and "memory" are very general, and have no precise behavioral referent. Nonetheless, these terms are widely used, and procedures that assess what most people call "learning" and "memory" are common in behavioral pharmacology. One learning assay, **repeated acquisition** (of response chains), is favored with humans and nonhumans alike, and can be used to contrast drug effects on learning and the performance of well-learned responses. Under this procedure, acquisition of a new response chain each session is considered "learning" and repeating the same response chain every session is considered "performance." For instance, in the learning component, to earn a reinforcer a person might be required to press the number keys on a computer keyboard in the sequence 1, 2, 3, 2, 3, 1, 2, 3, 1, 2, on Monday, in the sequence 2, 3, 1, 2, 3, 2, 2, 1, 2, 2 on Tuesday, and in other sequences on subsequent days. In the performance component, the correct sequence might be 3, 2, 1, 2, 3, 3, 2, 2, 1, 3 every day. Over time, error rates would stabilize in both components, but they would be substantially lower in the performance component.

A study by Higgins, Rush, Hughes, Bickel, Lynn, and Capeless (1992) demonstrates the use of such procedures to determine drug effects in humans. This study examined the effects of alcohol and cocaine, both alone and in combination. Considering that surveys indicate that more than 90% of persons in the United States reporting current cocaine use also report current alcohol use (Grant & Harford, 1990), it surely is worthwhile to ascertain how the combination of these two drugs affects learning and performance.

In this study, healthy subjects who occasionally used cocaine and lived outside the experimental setting came to a laboratory for testing. They were asked to refrain from using drugs outside the experimental session, and were tested to ensure that they complied. In both the acquisition and performance components, operant responses were numeric key presses on a computer keyboard and the putative reinforcer was money. Subjects were given 20 trials to learn a new 10-response sequence in the acquisition component, then 20 trials to perform an unchanging 10-response sequence in the performance component. The words "learning" and "performance" appeared on the computer screen during those respective components. Together, the two components comprised 40 trials, which subjects finished in approximately 3 to 5 minutes.

Subjects were tested absent drug to obtain baseline measures and were given drug only when responding appeared stable. The doses for alcohol (95% ethyl alcohol) were 0.0 (placebo), 0.5 and 1.0 g/kg of body weight. Each dose was in 6 drinks consumed within a 30-minute period. Placebo drinks had 1 milliliter of alcohol floating on top to prevent subjects from knowing they were not getting alcohol. Cocaine was prepared by subjects in "lines" using a small mirror and a straight edge razor and was administered intranasally with a plastic straw. Doses of cocaine were 4, 48, and 96 mg/70 kg of body weight. The 4 mg/70 kg dose was used as a placebo because it was shown to produce a numbing sensation in the nasal membranes without producing noticeable levels of cocaine in the bloodstream. All doses of each drug were tested alone. All possible combination doses also were tested. Drug dosing was random, although alcohol and cocaine were always administered alone before any combination doses were tested, and the highest dose of cocaine was

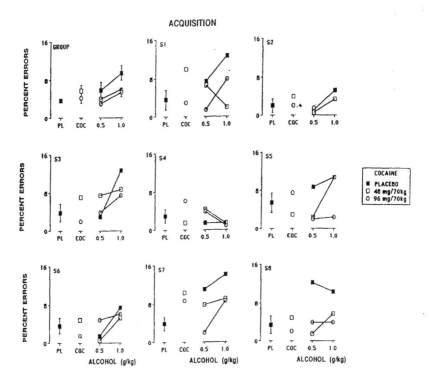

Figure 6-3. *Overall percentage of errors in the acquisition component are shown for subjects as a group (upper left panel) and for individual subjects as a function of alcohol dose. Data points above PL represent placebo-control values. Data points above COC represent the effects of cocaine administered alone. Connected data points represent the effects of the two alcohol doses alone (closed squares), and in combination with the 48mg/ 70kg (open squares) and 96mg/70kg (open circles) doses of cocaine. Data points across all dose conditions except PL represent peak effects (i.e., largest changes from predrug values). Data points above PL represent the midpoint of the range of values observed with individual subjects during placebo-control sessions. Brackets in the group function represent ± SEM, and those in the individual-subject functions represent the range of placebo-control values. Data are from Higgins et al. (1992) and reproduced by permission.*

administered only after subjects had been exposed to lower doses, and shown that they could safely tolerate them.

As shown in Figure 6-3, results from the acquisition component revealed that the overall percentage of errors increased over baseline levels when both doses of alcohol (0.5 and 1.0 g/kg) were administered. That is, learning impairment was evident when subjects ingested alcohol compared to when they had no drug. Cocaine alone did not affect accuracy relative to control levels. When cocaine (48 and 96 mg/70 kg) and alcohol (0.5 and 1.0 g/kg) were administered together, significantly fewer errors occurred than when the same doses of alcohol were administered alone. Thus, cocaine attenuated the learning impairment produced by alcohol. As depicted in Figure 6-4, regardless of whether they were administered alone or in combination, alcohol and cocaine had relatively little effect on accuracy under the performance component.

The finding that drug effects were smaller under the performance component than under the learning component is consistent with the general finding that degree

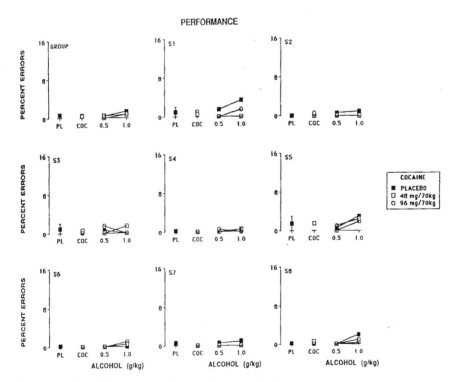

Figure 6-4. *Overall percentage of errors during peak effect in performance component are shown for subjects as a group (upper left panel) and for individual subjects as a function of alcohol dose; all else is the same as Figure 6-3. Data are from Higgins et al. (1992) and reproduced by permission.*

of stimulus control modulates drug action, as discussed in Chapters 5 and 8. The fact that cocaine attenuated ethanol-induced learning impairment is interesting, and suggests that the combination may be popular, in part, because cocaine reduces the disruptive behavioral effects of alcohol.

Although the repeated acquisition procedure is commonly construed as a measure of learning, it also indexes memory, insofar as it requires current performance to be influenced by past events. Another procedure that does likewise is **delayed matching to sample** (DMTS). As noted in Chapter 5, the DMTS procedure is commonly used to assess drug effects on short-term memory in laboratory animals. It can also be used for the same purpose with human subjects, as illustrated in a study by Wysocki, Fuqua, Davis, and Breuning (1981).

Wysocki et al. (1981) studied the effects of thioridazine (Mellaril) under a variation of the DMTS procedure termed **titrating delayed matching to sample**. In this variant, termination of the sample stimulus is followed by a predetermined delay, after which the comparison stimuli are presented. The length of delay varies according to the accuracy of the subject's performance on previous trials; correct responses increase the delay, whereas incorrect responses decrease it. In the study by Wysocki et al., four adults with mental retardation who had received daily doses of thioridazine for at least 150 days prior to the study served as subjects. A multiple-baseline across subjects design (see Chapter 9) was used to evaluate the effects of withdrawing thioridazine.

Initially, while still on medication, subjects were trained under a matching-to-sample procedure with no delay. Each trial began with presentation of a sample stimulus (illuminated red, blue, or green square) projected on the center of a response panel (plastic screen). When the subject depressed the center of the response panel (indicating that they were observing), the sample stimulus disappeared and the comparison stimuli (one square colored the same as the sample and a second sample randomly selected from the other two colors) were immediately presented. Correct responses, that is, touches of the comparison stimulus that matched the sample stimulus, were reinforced with food. Incorrect responses resulted in a 10-second timeout during which the response panel was dark and food was not available. Training continued until all subjects obtained 90 percent accuracy across two consecutive sessions.

After subjects had mastered the matching-to-sample discrimination, they were exposed to a titrating DMTS procedure. It was similar to the training arrangement, except that each session began with a 0-second delay, which was incremented following every fourth consecutive correct response at a given delay value. Delays were increased through the progression of 0, 1, 2, 3, 4, 5, 6, 8, 10, 12, 15, 18, 21, 24, 27, 30, 35, 40, 45, 50, 55, 60, 65, 70, 75, 90, and 105 seconds. When an incorrect response occurred, the delay for the next trial was decreased to the previous value (e.g., a 6-second delay would decrease to a 5-second delay). Sessions lasted until the first error made after 30 minutes. Subjects were tested twice each week under conditions where their daily dosage of thioridazine was gradually decreased under

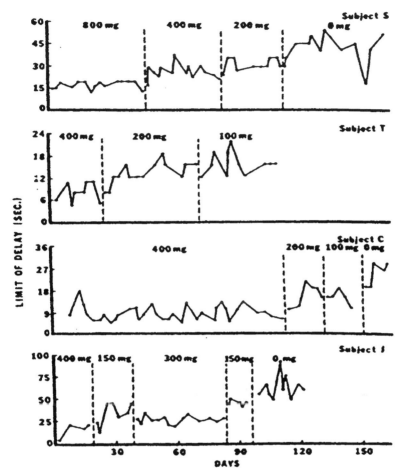

Figure 6-5. *Limit of delay reached each session by each subject as a function of daily thioridazine dose. Data are from Wysocki et al. (1981) and reproduced by permission.*

a multiple-baseline arrangement, as shown in Figure 6-5. For subject J, a dosage increase also was arranged.

The primary dependent variable was the maximum delay reached in each session. Figure 6-5 shows the maximum delay reached each session, by each subject, as a function of daily thioridazine dose. For all subjects, as the dose of drug decreased, maximum delay increased, with the highest delays reached at the lowest dose, which was 0 mg/day for 3 of the 4 people. Data from subject J provide an especially compelling demonstration of the functional relation between drug dose and maximum delay. For this subject, as the dose was decreased, the maximum delay increased; then, when the dose was increased, the maximum delay decreased. Insofar as the maximum delay reached under a titrating DMTS procedure is an index of memory, these data indicate that thioridazine impaired the memory of all subjects. Such an effect, if evident in the subjects' everyday environment, would constitute a significant adverse action of the drug. Thus, unless the drug produced clear, offsetting benefits, its use with these subjects could not be justified. In this regard, it is noteworthy that Wysocki et al. (1981) reported that:

> Standardized institutional data-collection procedures indicated no systematic changes in the frequency of inappropriate behavior for any of the subjects. Within 90 days of the completion of the experiment (the time of this writing), none of the subjects had been placed back on thioridazine or any other psychotropic drug, and there were no plans to do so. (p. 544)

The Wysocki et al. (1981) study is important for two reasons. First, it illustrates that procedures commonly used to index drug effects in nonhumans can be readily adapted for use with humans. Second, it shows that laboratory procedures may provide clues to clinically significant drug effects. Procedures for clinical drug assessment are covered in detail in Chapter 9.

Of course, many procedures in addition to DMTS and repeated acquisition can be used to examine drug effects on learning and memory in humans, and they do not necessarily yield equivalent results. The DMTS and repeated acquisition procedures are simple and sensitive, and they allow results obtained with humans to be compared with those obtained in other species. They do not, however, capture all of the complex interactions between behavior and the environment that are encompassed by the terms "learning" and "memory," and the results that they yield may not generalize to situations of clinical or practical concern. In general, when selecting a procedure for examining drug effects in any species, researchers should consider issues of precedent, practicality, and ecological validity. **Ecological validity** refers to the extent to which results obtained in a test situation generalize to a situation of practical or clinical concern.

Drug Self-Administration

The study of drug self-administration is directly related to drug abuse and has been studied extensively in nonhumans (e.g., Meisch & Lemaire, 1993). Within the last 30 years behavioral pharmacologists have also begun to study self-administration with human subjects (Higgins et al., 1993). Two general procedures are used to do so: (a) **single-access procedures**, in which one infers that a drug is a reinforcer if it is self-administered at a higher rate than placebo on different occasions; and (b) **concurrent (or choice) procedures**, in which one infers that a drug is a reinforcer if it is self-administered at a higher rate than placebo when both are available on the same occasion (Higgins et al., 1993).

Concurrent procedures may involve either **discrete-trials** or **free-operant** arrangements. In the former arrangement, operant responses can only occur at particular times, which are correlated with the presentation of particular stimuli. In the latter arrangement, such responses can occur at any time. One limitation of discrete-trials procedures is that they characteristically do not yield graded measures of preference. That is, one outcome is likely to be chosen on nearly every trial, as long as there is some meaningful difference between the outcomes. Graded measures of preference are readily obtained under concurrent free-operant procedures, which is a point in their favor. In addition, results obtained under such schedules can be readily quantified in terms of the generalized matching equation, which is the cornerstone of quantitative analysis in behavior analysis (see Davidson & McCarthy, 1988; deVilliers, 1977).

A useful single-access procedure for determining a drug's relative reinforcing value is the **progressive-ratio (PR) schedule** of reinforcement, which was introduced in Chapter 5 (for a review of the use of PR schedules in drug self-administration studies, see Stafford, LeSage, & Glowa, 1998). Under the PR schedule, a subject responds on a series of fixed-ratio (FR) schedules that are systematically increased until the subject fails to complete a ratio. The last ratio completed (termed the **breaking point**) is used as a measure of the reinforcing efficacy of the drug. The breaking point can be used to measure the relative ability of different drugs (or different doses of the same drug) to reinforce their administration. This measure tells us how hard a subject is willing to work for a certain drug or drug dose. In other words, the breaking point is an index of effort (Stafford et al., 1998).

A study by McLeod and Griffiths (1983) illustrates the use of a PR schedule to index the relative reinforcing value of various doses of a particular drug, specifically, the barbiturate pentobarbital. Subjects were men with extensive histories of drug (including barbiturate) use who resided in a residential research ward. They were allowed to work for pills containing placebo or one of three doses of pentobarbital (200, 400, or 600 mg). During training, subjects were given access to the four pills on separate days. Each pill was assigned a letter code, and subjects were told to try to remember the effects of each pill. During the performance phase of the experiment, one dose was available each day, and the doses were varied across days. To meet their response requirements, subjects had to either press two buttons in a specific sequence (i.e., complete a chain schedule) or ride a stationary bicycle for a certain period of time. When subjects completed the response requirements and received a pill, the response requirement for that dose increased for the next session (i.e., the activities became more effortful).

McLeod and Griffiths (1983) found that higher doses of pentobarbital maintained responding at larger PR values than did lower doses. For example, at the highest dose of pentobarbital (600 mg), one subject completed a PR value of 80,000 button-press response chains in a session that lasted almost 9 hours. These data indicate that higher doses of pentobarbital generally are more effective reinforcers than are lower doses, which is consistent with general findings with other drugs, in humans and nonhumans alike (e.g., Henningfield, Lucas, & Bigelow, 1986; Meisch & Lemaire, 1993; Young & Herling, 1986). As might be expected, higher doses of pentobarbital increased subjects' and staff's ratings of drug effect, and higher doses also were correlated with higher drug liking scores as assessed by a Likert scale. Although there are limitations to the use of PR schedules, the study by McLeod and Griffiths (1983) nicely demonstrates that such schedules provide valuable informa-

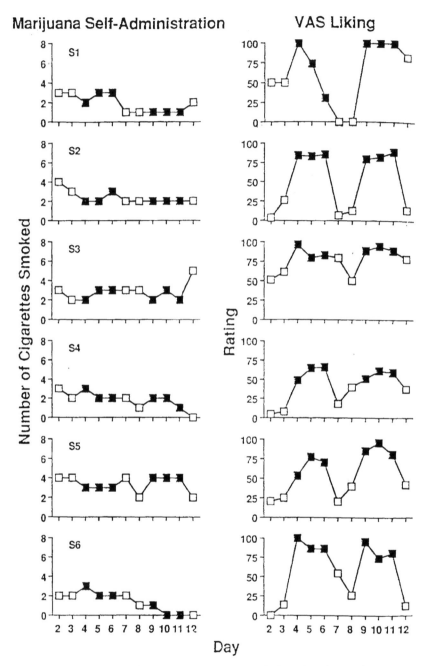

Figure 6-6. *Number of marijuana cigarettes smoked per day during the recreation period (left column) and visual-analogue ratings of drug "liking" (right column) for each subject. Symbol backgrounds represent dose conditions (open symbols: 0% THC; solid symbols: 2.3% THC). Data are from Kelly et al. (1994) and reproduced by permission.*

tion about the behavioral functions of drugs. It also illustrates the logic of single-access procedures for studying drug self-administration.

A study by Kelly, Foltin, Emurian, and Fischman (1994) is useful for contrasting a single-access procedure with a choice procedure. This study examined the reinforcing efficacy of various doses of delta-9-tetrahydrocannabinol (THC), the main active substance in cannabis (marijuana and its products). In one experiment, Kelly et al. used a single-access procedure in which male, cannabis-using volunteers lived in a residential research laboratory and could self-administer up to eight cannabis cigarettes per day. Cigarettes were obtained by responding on color-coded buttons, and the THC content did not change during any given day. THC contents of cigarettes were varied across days (0.0 or 2.3% w/w), and the reinforcing effectiveness of each THC dose was measured by the number of cigarettes that subjects smoked. Here, the assumption was that the more reinforcing THC concentration would lead to greater consumption.

As demonstrated in Figure 6-6, results indicated that THC level did not affect the number of cannabis cigarettes that subjects smoked (i.e., subjects smoked about the same number of active and placebo cigarettes). However, the higher THC level (2.3%) was correlated with higher visual-analogue scale (VAS) ratings of drug "liking." These data suggest that, although the higher dose of THC was "liked" more than the lower dose, the higher dose did not appear to function as a reinforcer. This finding emphasizes the difference between pleasurable and reinforcing events, and illustrates the importance of functionally determining, rather than inferring, a drug's behavioral actions.

In a second experiment, Kelly et al. (1994) combined the same single-access procedure used in the first experiment with a choice component. In this experiment, subjects were exposed to four 3-day blocks, each consisting of two "sample" days followed by a "choice" day. The experimental procedure on sample days was very similar to that used in the first experiment: only one concentration (and, therefore, dose) of THC (0.0, 2.0, or 3.5%) was available throughout each day and doses were varied across days. Unlike the first experiment, on sample days subjects were required to smoke at least one cigarette per day. On choice days within each block, subjects chose between the doses sampled on the previous two days (0.0, 2.0, or 3.5% THC). Thus, this second experiment used the single-access procedure of the first experiment on sample days and a discrete-trials choice procedure on choice days.

Results of the second experiment, shown in Figure 6-7, indicated that: a) as measured by the single-access procedure, the number of cigarettes that subjects smoked was not consistently related to THC dose (i.e., subjects smoked about the same number of cigarettes regardless of THC dose); b) as measured by the choice procedure, subjects preferred 3.5% THC cigarettes over the other two doses, and; c) in general, subjects reported similar VAS liking ratings for the two highest-dose cigarettes (i.e., 2.0 and 3.5% THC) and far lower VAS ratings for placebo (i.e., 0.0% THC) cigarettes. Taken together, the results of these two experiments demonstrate that whether or not the reinforcing effectiveness of THC differs as a function of concentration (and dose) depends on how reinforcing effectiveness is measured. In

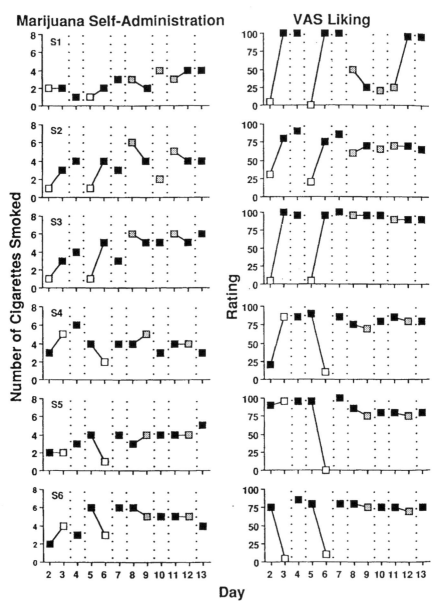

Figure 6-7. *Number of marijuana cigarettes smoked per day during the recreation period drug-availability interval (left column) and visual-analogue rating of drug "liking" (right column) for each subject. Symbol backgrounds represent dose conditions (open symbols: 0% THC; gray symbols: 2.0% THC; solid symbols: 3.5% THC). Unconnected points represent separate sessions in which subjects chose between doses sampled in the preceding two sessions. Data are from Kelly et al. (1994) and reproduced by permission.*

fact, from the results obtained under the single-access procedure alone, it would be reasonable to infer that THC was not a reinforcer, because the number of cigarettes smoked was not greater when THC was present than when it was absent. In contrast, however, findings under the choice procedure suggest that THC was a reinforcer, because cigarettes containing THC were consistently chosen relative to placebo cigarettes.

The findings reported by Kelly et al. (1994) show that the procedures used to index a drug's effects may influence obtained results. This point is further illustrated in a study demonstrating that the same dose of nicotine can serve as both a positive and a negative reinforcer (Henningfield & Goldberg, 1983). In this experiment, a person who self-administered 1.5 mg doses of nicotine intravenously at a very low, but nonzero, rate - indicating that the drug was a weak positive reinforcer - also worked to avoid receiving regularly-scheduled injections of the same nicotine dose. Specifically, in the avoidance study, 1.5 mg nicotine was administered every 15 minutes unless the person pressed a lever 10 times. Under this condition, substantial levels of responding occurred, and few nicotine injections were delivered. To be confident that nicotine itself was maintaining avoidance responding, Henningfield and Goldberg implemented a control condition in which saline solution was substituted for nicotine. If responding was maintained by avoidance of nicotine, then replacing the active drug with saline should have resulted in a decrease in avoidance responses. In fact, this is exactly what Henningfield and Goldberg found. Thus, for this person, nicotine served as a positive reinforcer under some conditions, but as a negative reinforcer under others.

One of the most important, and most often ignored, findings in behavioral pharmacology is that *the functional properties of a drug may depend critically on the procedures used to evaluate those properties.* Moreover, as discussed at length in Chapter 8, a drug's effects are not fixed, but vary depending upon a wide range of historical and current variables. For these reasons, it is wise to be cautious in interpreting the effects of individual experiments, and in making (or accepting) broad generalizations about any drug's behavioral effects. With extensive study, however, it is possible to make sense of a drug's effects and the variables that modulate them, and to summarize them meaningfully. A case in point concerns nicotine, which has been extensively studied in both humans and nonhumans (e.g., Henningfield et al., 1986). Much is known about the drug's effects, and it is now generally accepted that nicotine has substantial abuse potential. For example, in considering whether nicotine is "addictive," Stolerman and Jarvis (1995) conclude that:

> Patterns of use by smokers and the remarkable intractability of the smoking habit point to compulsive use as the norm. Studies in both animal and human subjects have shown that nicotine can function as a reinforcer, albeit under a more limited range of conditions than with some other drugs of abuse. In drug discrimination paradigms, there is some cross-generalization between nicotine on the one hand, and amphetamine and cocaine on the other. A well-defined withdrawal syndrome has been delineated which is alleviated by nicotine replacement. Nicotine replacement also enhances

outcomes in smoking cessation, roughly doubling success rates. In total, the evidence clearly identifies nicotine as a powerful drug of addiction, comparable to heroin, cocaine, and alcohol. (p. 8)

In this case, conclusions concerning the abuse potential of nicotine were supported by controlled experiments using self-administration and other proce-dures with humans and nonhumans, naturalistic observations of smokers in their everyday world, and treatment outcome studies. Few other drugs have been studied so carefully.

But what, you might ask, about the data showing that nicotine can serve as a negative reinforcer? Those data are valid; there are conditions under which nicotine serves as a negative reinforcer. But those conditions almost never occur in the everyday lives of human beings. Therefore, in understanding how the drug affects people who commonly use it - which is to say, how if affects tobacco users - nicotine's capacity to act as a negative reinforcer is of no practical importance. Other actions, however, are very important. Foremost among them is the drug's capacity to serve as a positive reinforcer, which it does under conditions commonly encountered by people.

Conditioned Reinforcement

Of course, the effectiveness of any drug as a positive reinforcer is not fixed, but instead depends on several different historical and current variables. Although the possibility has been essentially ignored in the nonhuman literature, conditioned reinforcement represents a potentially important mechanism through which the reinforcing effects of a given substance could be increased. This mechanism was explored in a recent study by Johanson, Mattox, and Schuster (1995; experiment 1), who used a choice procedure to assess whether a placebo capsule could come to function as a conditioned reinforcer due to a correlation with money, presumably a generalized conditioned reinforcer. In this study, volunteers were told they would receive two different drugs, which could be stimulants, sedatives, tranquilizing drugs, or placebo. On alternate days, participants were administered one of two differently colored placebo pills and were required to perform computer-generated tasks to earn money. Participants performed the tasks 15 minutes before and 30, 60, 90, and 120 minutes after placebo administration. One task consisted of a DMTS procedure, in which participants had to determine whether two patterns presented sequentially on the computer screen were the same or different. The second task required participants simultaneously to keep a cursor inside a moving box and a small circle inside a larger moving circle.

Although participants were told that they would be paid based on the accuracy of their performance on these computer tasks, payment actually was arranged by the computer independently of performance. After taking a capsule of one color (colors were counterbalanced across subjects), subjects "earned" more money at 30, 60, and 90 minutes after ingestion than they had earned prior to taking the capsule. In contrast, after taking a capsule of the other color, subjects "earned" less money at 30, 60, and 90 minutes after ingestion than they had earned prior to taking the capsule.

At 120 minutes after taking a capsule of either color, subjects "earned" the same amount of money as prior to taking it. Thus, conditions were arranged to simulate payoff conditions similar to those that would occur if a) capsules of one color increased accuracy and capsules of the other color decreased accuracy in a situation where, b) subjects actually were paid for the accuracy of their performances, and c) drug effects disappeared prior to the final test period.

Following exposure to the conditions just described, participants were allowed to self-administer the capsule of their choosing. Under this condition, most participants reliably chose the capsule correlated with higher earnings over the capsule correlated with lower earnings. These results suggest that correlating ingestion of capsules of a particular color with increased earnings established such capsules as conditioned reinforcers. Those conditioned reinforcers were sufficiently powerful to control choice behavior to a degree similar to that observed with unconditioned drug reinforcers (Johanson et al., 1995).

To assess the subjective effects associated with the different capsules and correlated payment conditions, participants completed three assays after each trial. The first assay was a version of the POMS. In this assay, participants indicated how they felt at the moment by allocating points on a 5-point scale (where 0 represented "not at all" and 5 represented "extremely") with respect to adjectives commonly used to describe mood states. The items used in the POMS were grouped into one of eight scales that describe the adjectives (Anger, Anxiety, Confusion, Depression, Elation, Fatigue, Friendliness, and Vigor). Johanson et al. (1995) used two additional scales, Arousal and Positive Mood, which were based on permutations of the original eight scales. The results of the POMS indicated that the higher-earnings condition significantly increased Elation, Positive Mood, and Vigor. It also decreased Confusion relative to the lower-earnings condition.

The second subjective assay involved a drug labeling exercise in which participants labeled the drug that they had received as either placebo, stimulant, sedative, or tranquilizer. In general, participants identified the capsules they had received as containing active drug significantly more often than they identified the capsules as placebo, but they identified them about equally often as a stimulant, sedative, and tranquilizer.

The final subjective assay used by Johanson et al. was a VAS that involved marking a point on a 100-mm line that corresponded to how much the participant liked the capsule. A point at one end corresponded to "disliked a lot," a point at 50 mm corresponded to "neutral," and a point at the other end corresponded to "like a lot." The location on the line where the point was marked did not differ significantly under the higher- and lower-earnings conditions.

The study by Johanson et al. (1995) provides clear evidence that what was assumed by subjects to be an active drug was established as a powerful conditioned reinforcer by being correlated with a nonpharmacological reinforcer, money. It is easy to envision how conditioned reinforcement contributes to drug use in humans' natural environment. As a case in point, most people on initial exposure find the smell and taste of cigars unpleasant. But, given a certain kind of history, some of those same people become cigar connoisseurs - for them, subtle characteristics in the taste and smell of fine cigars become conditioned reinforcers. Why? First, in a person who smokes cigars regularly, certain smells and tastes are reliably paired (i.e., correlated) with exposure to nicotine, which is an effective positive reinforcer. Such pairing probably is sufficient to establish general characteristics of cigar smoke as a conditioned reinforcer.

Subtle characteristics, however, probably acquire their conditioned reinforcing characteristics in large part due the actions of other cigar aficionados. Such individuals react positively to these characteristics, and reinforce similar reactions by novice smokers. In this way, a community of cigar smokers trains new members to discriminate subtle features of the taste and smell of cigar smoke, and also establishes those features as conditioned reinforcers.

Establishing Operations

The use of illicit as well as licit drugs often occurs within a social context in which social reinforcers such as approval and group membership may be made contingent upon drug use (Higgins, Hughes, & Bickel, 1989; Johanson et al., 1995). This process may establish drug-related stimuli as conditioned reinforcers, as well as engender drug use as operant behavior maintained by nonpharmacological consequences. That this is so calls attention to the fact that social reinforcement and drug effects can interact in complex, and often subtle, ways. The complexity of such interactions is further demonstrated in studies showing that drugs can actually make an individual more sensitive to social contingencies.

Such an effect was reported by Higgins et al. (1989), who used a discrete-trials choice procedure to assess the ability of d-amphetamine (0, 12.5, and 25 mg/70 kg) to increase the reinforcing effectiveness of social reinforcement relative to monetary reinforcement. Volunteers were studied in same-sex pairs of subject (who received drug) and partner (who did not receive drug), and each member of the pair wore a microphone to talk to the other. Each pair member was in a separate room during experimental sessions. Subjects were exposed to a discrete-trials procedure in which they could choose to talk to themselves for monetary reinforcement on a variable-interval 60-second schedule or to talk to their partner and receive no monetary reinforcement. During the monetary option, subjects were required to give speech monologues that consisted of naturalistic speech; humming, singing, or whistling was not reinforced. The major dependent variables were choice behavior, seconds of speech, and monetary earnings.

Subjective ratings in the form of VAS were taken immediately before, 30 minutes into, and at the end of the 60-minute sessions. Subjects completed 12 VAS that ranged from 0 ("not at all") at one end to 100 ("extremely") at the other end. The scales assessed drug effect, drug high, drug liking, good effects, bad effects, friendly, impaired, anxious, energetic, restless, sluggish, and elated.

Relative to placebo, d-amphetamine significantly increased choice for the social option, as well as speech rate and time spent speaking in that option. The drug-induced increase in choice for the social option necessarily resulted in a loss of earnings relative to the placebo condition. With respect to subjective ratings, *d*-amphetamine produced dose-dependent increases in drug effect, drug high, drug liking, friendly, elated, energetic, and good effects. All of these subjective ratings are consistent with increased sociability.

The data reported by Higgins et al. (1989) indicated that *d*-amphetamine can function as an establishing operation by increasing the relative reinforcing effectiveness of social reinforcement. If *d*-amphetamine is present when especially reinforcing social interaction occurs, this pairing may establish the drug as a conditioned reinforcer. This action could well combine with the drug's recognized action as an unconditioned reinforcer (McKim, 1997) to increase the likelihood of subsequent use. Here, of course, the direct effect of *d*-amphetamine is its action as an establishing operation. This effect, in turn, alters the stimulus function of the drug, making it a conditioned reinforcer. As is so often the case, the effects of the drug in this case are complex and situation-specific. Nonetheless, given adequate understanding of behavioral mechanisms of drug action, they are both orderly and understandable.

As discussed in Chapter 2 by definition an EO has two distinct effects: a) it momentarily increases or decreases the reinforcing effectiveness of some other environmental event (e.g., some object, stimulus, or activity); and b) it momentarily increases or decreases all behaviors that have previously resulted in obtaining or contacting that environmental event (Michael, 1993). In other words, humans and other animals will work to acquire certain objects, contact certain stimuli, and engage in certain activities because these events are valuable to them, and EOs are what make these events valuable. EOs are "motivational" variables, insofar as they influence the value of objects and events in an organism's life.

Construing motivation in terms of EOs has much to recommend it, in large part because EOs are quantifiable variables with specified functions. Therefore, they can be isolated and studied experimentally. Nonetheless, traditional conceptions of motivation, and of drug effects thereon, are not couched in terms of EOs. Probably the most well-known motivational drug effect is **amotivational syndrome**, which is said to be caused by self-administering cannabis. The amotivation hypothesis, as first proposed in the psychiatric literature, states that cannabis users exhibit apathy, unwillingness or inability to follow-through on long-term plans, introversion, and "regressive, childlike, magical thinking" (McGlothlin & West, 1968). More recent versions of the hypothesis describe the consequences of "heavy" or "chronic" cannabis use as a decrease in "ambition" or "drive" (Zimmer & Morgan, 1997). Evidence for amotivation usually comes in the form of inferences from behavior described as "lethargic," "apathetic," or "passive" (Foltin et al., 1990; Levinthal, 1996; McKim, 1997). The amotivational syndrome is then used to explain the behavior from which it is inferred. The result of this inferential process is a circular explanation, which is of no practical or explanatory value.

Another important problem with amotivation is that the variables that are responsible for it are never made explicit; for example, it is unclear what dose and pattern of use is sufficient to be termed "heavy." Moreover, terms like "lethargic," "passive," "ambition," and "drive" are ambiguous. One may legitimately ask, what is a "drive" and how does cannabis decrease it? In other words, we need to know how "drive" can be measured, and then determine the specific neuropharmacological or behavioral mechanisms through which cannabis affects it. Without some way to specify and quantify the variables involved in a hypothetical functional relation, such as the relation between cannabis and motivation that underlies the amotivational syndrome, that hypothesis is not a useful practical or explanatory device (Skinner, 1957).

Despite the imprecision of popular notions of amotivation, behavioral pharmacologists have attempted to examine cannabis's amotivational effects in several studies, reviewed by Foltin, Fischman, Brady, Bernstein, Capriotti, Nellis, and Kelly (1990). As they note, an objective, testable amotivation hypothesis can be stated this way: As doses of THC are increased, there will be a corresponding decrease in the frequency of some type of operant behavior emitted by subjects. If such an effect is observed under appropriately-controlled conditions, then THC is functioning as an EO to weaken the reinforcing efficacy of whatever reinforcer was maintaining that operant behavior. Therefore, it is producing "amotivation." If such an effect is evident with several different reinforcers, under a variety of maintenance conditions, then it might be justifiable to conclude that THC produces an "amotivational syndrome."

Studies using monetary reinforcement to examine the motivational effects of marijuana in human subjects have not provided convincing evidence of amotivation (e.g., Mello & Meldelson, 1985; Mendelson, Kuehnle, Greenberg, & Mello, 1976). Foltin et al. (1990) suggested that this inability to find amotivational effects may be due to the relative insensitivity of behavior maintained by money to motivational variables. They further suggested that requiring subjects to perform a less-preferred task (instrumental response) to earn access to a more-preferred task (contingent activity) might provide a more sensitive assay for determining the effects of cannabis on motivation. Support for the contingent-activity assay was provided in a previous study demonstrating that smoked cannabis reduced operant behavior maintained by contingent recreational activities. Foltin et al. (1990) extended the analysis of the motivational effects of smoked cannabis to repetitious "work" activities.

In this study, cannabis-experienced men, aged 19 to 30 years, lived in a residential laboratory for 15 consecutive days. Subjects smoked two 1-g cannabis cigarettes containing either 0.0% (placebo) or 2.7% THC each day under all experimental conditions. The duration of subjects' performance on four tasks was evaluated under three conditions: an initial baseline period, a contingent-activity period, and a second baseline period. During the initial baseline condition, subjects could engage in any of the four activities. Activity preferences were determined by assessing the length of time that subjects spent performing each activity; the task that a subject spent most of his time engaging in was deemed the "preferred" task, and all other tasks were termed "non-preferred." It was assumed that preferred tasks were "less effortful" for subjects to perform.

Following baseline, the contingent-activity condition began. In this condition, access to a preferred, or low-effort, activity depended upon the completion of a non-

Table 6-2. Summary of Studies Investigating Amotivational Syndrome

Study	Subjects	Doses/Regimen	Relevent Measures	Results
Carter & Doughty (1976)	82 Working-class Costa Rican males (41 users vs. 41 non-users matched for age, occupation, educational level, etc.).	Mean use approximately 40 mg. THC/day	Length and number of unemployment periods; preferred activity while intoxicated	Heaviest users had fewer and shorter periods of unemployment and higher incomes; most preferred to work while intoxicated
Mendelson, Kuehnle, Greenberg, & Mello (1976)	27 young adult American male volunteers residing on a hospital research ward (15 "heavy" users vs. 12 "casual" users).	Heavy users: 80-120 mg THC/day; Casual users: 40-60 mg THC/day	Number of points earned on a fixed-interval (FI) 1-s schedule (points could be used to purchase cannabis cigarettes or exchanged for cash); # of cannabis cigarettes purchased and smoked; # hours worked	Heavy users earned more points than casual users; heavy users purchased and smoked more cigarettes than casual users; periods of maximal work coincided with periods of maximal smoking
Mello & Mendelson (1985)	21 adult American female volunteers residing on a hospital research ward (5 "heavy" users vs. 7 "moderate" users vs. 9 "occasional" users).	Heavy users: 108 mg THC/day; Moderate users: 49 mg THC/day; Occasional users: 16 mg THC/day	Number of points earned on a second-order FI 1-s (FR 300) schedule, where completion of the response requirements resulted in one point (points could be used to purchase cannabis cigarettes or exchanged for cash); hours worked; money earned	No difference between groups in the number of points earned, hours worked, or money earned; periods of maximal work coincided with periods of maximal smoking

preferred, or high-effort, activity. Duration measures were again taken. Following placebo administration in the contingent-activity condition, a second baseline condition was implemented.

When the contingent-activity condition was in effect, subjects who had smoked active cannabis spent more time engaging in high-effort instrumental responses than subjects who had smoked placebo (Foltin et al., 1990). In other words, THC actually increased, rather than decreased, performance of high-effort activities. These data are consistent with cross-cultural studies in which frequent users of high-dose cannabis regularly engage in strenuous work after self-administering cannabis (Comitas, 1976; Zimmer & Morgan, 1997). In this study, it appears that THC may have made the high-effort activities less effortful, and researchers again failed to find any evidence of amotivation (see Table 6-2 for a summary of studies investigating amotivational syndrome). Furthermore, this study demonstrated the power of behavior-analytic techniques to test a common notion concerning drug action and to arrive at a more thorough understanding of a drug's many effects. Its results, and those of related studies, suggest that study of the motivational effects of drugs deserves continued attention by behavioral pharmacologists.

Drugs as Discriminative Stimuli

As discussed in Chapter 5, drug discrimination procedures are widely used in nonhuman research, primarily to examine correlations between neuropharmacological and behavioral effects of various compounds. Similar procedures also are used with humans. For example, Preston, Bigelow, Bickel, and Liebson (1987) attempted to develop sensitive, three-choice drug discrimination procedures with human subjects while simultaneously measuring subjective drug effects via traditional procedures. In this experiment, five adult, male, opioid-dependent volunteers residing on a research ward earned monetary reinforcement for correctly identifying the letter-coded drug that they received that day. Under double-blind conditions, subjects received one of three drugs: saline solution (placebo), hydromorphine, and naloxone. After discrimination training, generalization tests were conducted with various doses of the active training drugs. Among the dependent variables assessed by Preston et al. were three discrimination measures and four subjective measures.

To measure drug discrimination, each subject was exposed to three discrimination components: a) a discrete-choice component in which the subject identified which drug was administered by naming the appropriate letter code (A, B, or C); b) a component in which each subject distributed 50 points among the three drug alternatives, based on the certainty of his drug choice; and c) a free-operant component in which each subject responded under a FI 1-second schedule on computer keys labeled with the three drugs' letter codes. Responses on the correct button earned points that were exchangeable for money at the end of the session. In addition to these discrimination measures, Preston et al. employed the following subjective measures: VAS, a pharmacological class questionnaire, an adjective rating scale, and an abbreviated form of the ARCI.

Results indicated that subjects could easily discriminate among the three drugs. For example, naloxone at 0.15 mg was identified correctly on every trial in all three discrimination components. For all drugs, results were similar under all three components. The three drugs produced significant effects on the visual analog scales, the drug class identification questionnaire, the adjective rating scales, and the MBG (euphoria) scale from the ARCI. Hydromorphine produced significantly greater liking, good effects, high, and MBG scores relative to saline or naloxone. Naloxone produced higher bad effects, antagonist, and mixed agonist/antagonist scale scores than did saline or hydromorphine. Also, novel doses of each drug produced dose-related changes in drug-appropriate responses without any cross-generalization between hydromorphine and naloxone.

As have experiments involving nonhumans (see Chapter 5), this study demonstrated that three-choice discrimination procedures are viable. It also suggests that, in the case, of humans, three-choice procedures have several potential advantages, including: a) they are less time-consuming than two-choice procedures (e.g., Preston et al. trained discriminations after only two exposures to each of the three drugs); b) they show greater specificity of discriminations between similar drugs or different doses of the same drug, and; c) they can be integrated with subjective effects measures (e.g., visual analog scales) to provide a broader understanding of a drug's subjective effects.

As discussed in Chapter 5, drugs commonly are considered to be interoceptive stimuli. According to Catania (1992), an **interoceptive stimulus** is:

A stimulus inside the organism. The stimulus may be presented from outside, as when an experimenter passes electric current through an area of the brain, or it may be produced by the organism itself, as when responses produce proprioceptive stimulation on the basis of which the organism may discriminate among different movements. (p. 379)

An **exteroceptive stimulus**, in contrast, is "any stimulus presented at or outside of the organism's skin" (Catania, 1992, p. 374). Tones and lights, for instance, are exteroceptive stimuli. In essence, interoceptive stimuli are private events, whereas exteroceptive stimuli are public events. A light, for instance, may be seen by many people at the same time and affect their behavior in similar fashion. A drug taken by one person, however, can only directly affect his or her behavior. In both cases, however, reacting to the stimulus is mediated by events that occur within the organism, and there appears to be no fundamental difference in the behavioral functions of interoceptive and exteroceptive stimuli. In fact, interoceptive stimuli can belong to the same functional class as exteroceptive stimuli (Stolerman, 1993).

Such an outcome was demonstrated by DeGrandpre, Bickel and Higgins (1992), who used a matching-to-sample procedure to establish equivalance relations between interoceptive stimuli and exteroceptive stimuli. The interoceptive stimuli were produced by triazolam (0.32 mg/70 kg), a benzodiazepine, or placebo. Black symbols on white flash cards served as the exteroceptive stimuli. Subjects earned money for choosing the "correct" comparison stimulus (e.g., a sun symbol) in the presence of the appropriate interoceptive sample stimulus (e.g., triazolam).

As demonstrated in Figure 6-8, DeGrandpre et al. found that stimulus equivalence procedures engendered interoceptive-exteroceptive stimulus equivalance in human subjects. That is, subjects learned to choose the appropriate symbol based on how the drug made them feel. Furthermore, untrained interoceptive-exteroceptive stimulus relations emerged as a consequence of equivalence training. For example, when a new stimulus was presented on a nondrug day, subjects chose the visual comparison stimulus that was correlated with placebo, which produced an interoceptive stimulus similar to no drug. In other words, stimulus generalization

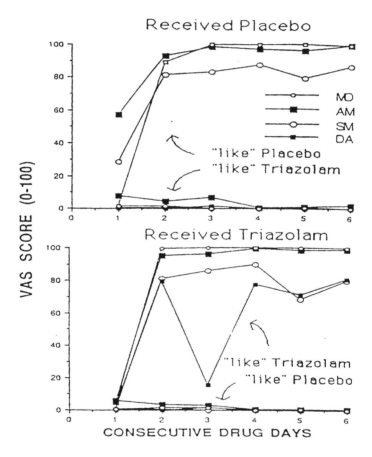

Figure 6-8. *Mean visual analogue scale (VAS) scores (range, 0-100) are shown for all 4 subjects for the "how much like Drug A?" and "how much like Drug B?" questions when placebo was administered (top panel) and when triazolam was administered (lower panel) as a function of consecutive placebo and triazolam days, respectively. If "Drug A" referred to placebo, then "Drug B" referred to triazolam, and vice versa. Data are from DeGrandpre et al. (1992) and reproduced by permission.*

occurred because of the physical similarity of two interoceptive stimuli (placebo and no drug).

Research of the type conducted by DeGrandpre et al. (1992) demonstrates that formerly neutral environmental stimuli can come to control drug-like responses without ever being paired with the drug itself (i.e., the stimuli become members of the same stimulus class) (Higgins et al., 1993). Such research also supports the results of drug discrimination and verbal report studies in demonstrating that people can readily detect, and report, drug-induced changes in their internal environment.

Concluding Comments

Basic research concerning drug effects in humans is necessary for two reasons. One is to allow researchers to determine whether results obtained with nonhumans, which are cheaper and easier to study, generalize to humans. In general, it appears that they do. The other is to allow researchers to investigate variables that cannot be studied in nonhuman subjects. One such variable is verbal behavior. A second is the presence of certain diseases or behavioral disorders. As discussed in other chapters of this book, both of these variables may influence drug effects, although they do not always do so.

As the experiments summarized in this chapter illustrate, behavioral pharmacologists have been innovative in devising procedures for determining behavioral loci and mechanisms of drug action in human subjects. Their findings illustrate that it is possible to conduct well-controlled basic research with a wide range of substances, including drugs of abuse. They also illustrate that procedures characteristic of the experimental analysis of behavior are useful for such studies. Finally, and importantly, they provide indubitable evidence that drug effects are fundamentally lawful, although they also are a function of many interrelated variables. Therefore, one should be cautious in interpreting experimental results, and in making or accepting simple statements about any drug's behavioral effects.

References

Baker, T. B., Morse, E., & Sherman, J. E. (1987). The motivation to use drugs: A psychobiological analysis of urges. In C. Rivers (Ed.), *The Nebraska symposium on motivation: Alcohol use and abuse* (pp. 257-323). Lincoln, NE: University of Nebraska Press.

Catania, A. C. (1992). *Learning*. Englewood Cliffs, NJ: Prentice Hall.

Comitas, L. (1976). Cannabis and work in Jamaica: A refutation of the amotivational syndrome. In: C. Dornbush, D. Freedman, & A. Fink (Eds.), *Chronic cannabis use* (pp. 24-32). New York: New York Academy of Sciences.

Davidson, M. C., & McCarthy, D. (1988). *The matching law: A research review*. Hillsdale, NJ: Erlbaum.

DeGrandpre, R. J., Bickel, W. K., & Higgins, S. T. (1992). Emergent equivalence relations between interoceptive (drug) and exteroceptive (visual) stimuli. *Journal of the Experimental Analysis of Behavior, 58*, 9-18.

de Villiers, P. (1977). Choice in concurrent schedules and a quantitative formulation of the law of effect. In W. K. Honig & J. E. R. Staddon (Eds.), *Handbook of operant behavior* (pp. 233-287). Englewood Cliffs, NJ: Prentice-Hall.

Dews, P. B., & Morse, W. H. (1958). Some observations on an operant in human subjects and its modification by dextro amphetamine. *Journal of the Experimental Analysis of Behavior, 1,* 359-364.

Ehrman, R. N., Robbins, S. J., Childress, A. R., & O'Brien, C. P. (1992). Conditioned responses to cocaine-related stimuli in cocaine abuse patients. *Psychopharmacology, 107,* 523-529.

Foltin, R. W., Fischman, M. W., Brady, J. V., Bernstein, D. J., Capriotti, R. M., Nellis, M. J., & Kelly, T. H. (1990). Motivational effects of smoked marijuana: Behavioral contingencies and low-probability activities. *Journal of the Experimental Analysis of Behavior, 53,* 5-19.

Grant, B. F., & Hartford, T. C. (1990). Concurrent and simultaneous use of alcohol with cocaine: Results of national survey. *Drug and Alcohol Dependence, 25,* 97-104.

Henningfield, J. E., & Goldberg, S. R. (1983). Control of behavior by intravenous nicotine injections. *Pharmacology Biochemistry and Behavior, 19,* 1021-1026.

Henningfield, J. E., Lucas, S. E., & Bigelow, G. E. (1986). Human studies of drugs as reinforcers. In S. R. Goldberg & I. P. Stolerman (Eds.), *Behavioral analysis of drug dependence* (pp. 69-112). Orlando, FL: Academic Press.

Higgins, S. T., Bickel, W. K., & Hughes, J. R. (1993). Methods in the human behavioral pharmacology of drug abuse. In F. van Haaren (Ed.), *Methods in behavioral pharmacology* (pp. 475-494). Amsterdam: Elsevier.

Higgins, S. T., Hughes, J. R., & Bickel, W. K. (1989). Effects of *d*-amphetamine on choice of social versus monetary reinforcement: A discrete-trial test. *Pharmacology Biochemistry and Behavior, 34,* 297-301.

Higgins, S. T., Rush, C. R., Hughes, J. R., Bickel, W. K., Lynn, M., & Capeless, M. A. (1992). Effects of cocaine and alcohol, alone and in combination, on human learning and performance. *Journal of the Experimental Analysis of Behavior, 58,* 87-105.

Johanson, C. E., Mattox, A., & Schuster, C. R. (1995). Conditioned reinforcing effects of capsules associated with high versus low monetary payoff. *Psychopharmacology, 120,* 42-48.

Kelly, T. H., Foltin, R. W., Emurian, C. S., & Fischman, M. W. (1994). Effects of D-9-THC on marijuana smoking, dose choice, and verbal report of drug liking. *Journal of the Experimental Analysis of Behavior, 61,* 203-211.

Levinthal, C. F. (1996). *Drugs, behavior, and modern society.* Needham Heights, MA: Allyn & Bacon.

McLeod, D. R. & Griffiths, R. R. (1983). Human progressive-ratio performance: Maintenance by pentobarbital. *Psychopharmacology, 79,* 4-9.

McGlothlin, W. H., & West, L. J. (1968). The marijuana problem: An overview. *American Journal of Psychiatry, 125,* 370-378.

McKim, W. (1997). *Drugs and behavior.* Upper Saddle River, NJ: Prentice-Hall.

Meisch, R. A. & Lemaire, G. A. (1993). Drug self-administration. In F. van Haaren (Ed.), *Methods in behavioral pharmacology* (pp. 257-293). Amsterdam: Elsevier.

Mello, N. K., & Mendelson, J. H. (1985). Operant acquisition of marihuana in women. *Journal of Pharmacology and Experimental Therapeutics, 235,* 162-171.

Mendelson, J. H., Kuehnle, J. C., Greenberg, I., & Mello, N. K. (1976). Operant acquisition of marihuana in man. *Journal of Pharmacology and Experimental Therapeutics, 198,* 42-53.

Michael, J. (1993). Establishing operations. *The Behavior Analyst, 16,* 191-206.

O'Brien, C. P., Ehrman, R. N., & Ternes, J. W. (1986). Classical conditioning in human opioid dependence. In S. R. Goldberg & I. P. Stolerman (Eds.), *Behavioral analysis of drug dependence* (pp. 329-356). Orlando, FL: Academic Press.

Preston, K. L., Bigelow, G. E., Bickel, W. K., & Liebson, I. A. (1987). Three-choice drug discrimination in opioid-dependent humans: Hydromorphine, naloxone and saline. *Journal of Pharmacology and Experimental Therapeutics, 243,* 1002-1009.

Robbins, S. J. & Ehrman, R. N. (1992). Designing studies of drug conditioning in humans. *Psychopharmacology, 106,* 143-153.

Sherman, J. E., Jorneby, M. S., & Baker, T. B. (1988). Classical conditioning with alcohol: Acquired preferences and aversions, tolerance and urges craving. In D. A. Wilkinson & D. Chaudron (Eds.), *Theories of alcoholism* (pp. 173-237). Toronto: Addiction Research Foundation.

Skinner, B. F. (1945). The operational analysis of psychological terms. *Psychological Review, 52,* 270-277.

Skinner, B. F. (1957). *Verbal behavior.* New York: Appleton-Century-Crofts.

Stafford, D., LeSage, M. G., & Glowa, J. R. (1998). Progressive-ratio schedules of drug delivery in the analysis of drug self-administration: A review. *Psychopharmacology, 139,* 169-184.

Stolerman, I. P. (1993). Drug discrimination. In F. van Haaren (Ed.), *Methods in behavioral pharmacology* (pp. 217-241). Amsterdam: Elsevier.

Stolerman, I. P., & Jarvis, M. J. (1995). The scientific case that nicotine is addictive. *Psychopharmacology, 117,* 2-10.

Wysocki, T., Fuqua, W., Davis, V., & Breuning, S. E. (1981). Effects of thioridazine (Mellaril) on titrating delayed matching-to-sample performance of mentally retarded adults. *American Journal of Mental Deficiency, 85,* 539-547.

Young, A. M., & Herling, S. (1986). Drugs as reinforcers: Studies in laboratory animals. In S. R. Goldberg & I. P. Stolerman (Eds.), *Behavioral analysis of drug dependence* (pp. 9-57). Orlando, FL: Academic Press.

Zimmer, L., & Morgan, J. P. (1997). *Marijuana myths, marijuana facts.* New York: The Lindesmith Center.

Chapter 7

Stimulus Properties of Drugs

Alan Poling[1], Thomas Byrne[2],
and Thomas Morgan[1]
[1]Western Michigan University
[2]Massachusetts College of Liberal Arts

As noted in Chapter 2, a **physical stimulus** is any object or event, whereas a **functional stimulus** is any object or event that affects behavior. Behavioral pharmacologists have long emphasized that drugs may affect behavior by acting as functional stimuli in the context of operant and respondent conditioning (e.g., Thompson & Pickens, 1971), and have proposed that this mechanism of drug action is relevant to understanding human drug abuse and the variability in drug effects that is commonly observed. The purpose of the present chapter is to summarize the potential stimulus properties of drugs and to consider how these properties can influence a person's reaction to a particular compound.

Drugs as Unconditional and Conditional Stimuli

As discussed in Chapter 2, an unconditional stimulus (US) elicits an unconditional response (UR) in organisms without special learning histories. Drugs frequently have such an action. For example, ipecac when taken orally reliably elicits vomiting in humans. Therefore, it is used therapeutically as an emetic in the treatment of oral drug overdoses and in certain cases of poisoning.

Even when a drug affects behavior by acting as a US, environmental variables may modulate observed effects. Such an outcome is evident in a study by Poling, Kesselring, Sewell, and Cleary (1983), who examined the lethality of combinations of pentazocine, a synthetic opioid with mixed agonist and antagonist properties, and tripelennamine (Talwin), an antihistaminic, in mice housed after injection either individually or in groups of 16. The combination, which has been used on the street as a substitute for heroin, killed more mice when they were housed together than when they were housed alone. This finding suggests that individuals suffering from an overdose of what users term "Ts and blues" (from the T on the Talwin pill, and the blue color of a common form of tripelennamine) should not be exposed to highly stimulating environments.

Greater toxicity in group-housed subjects relative to individually-housed ones has been demonstrated with other drugs, leading Green, Cross, and Goodwin (1995) to suggest that the crowded conditions common at raves (dance parties) may contribute to MDMA-related deaths (MDMA is known on the street as "ecstasy").

Be that as it may, there is clear evidence that most, if not all, of the effects of drugs, including their ability to cause death at certain doses, can be influenced by nonpharmacological variables.

Especially compelling evidence of the role of environmental variables in modulating the lethality of a drug is provided by a study conducted by Siegel, Hinson, Krank, and McCully (1982), who compared the lethality of a large dose (15 mg/kg) of heroin in three groups of rats. During the first part of the study, all rats in the two experimental groups received 15 injections of heroin over a 30-day period. Heroin was injected every other day, and the dose gradually was increased from 1 to 8 mg/kg. On days when heroin was not given, rats received an injection of dextrose (sugar solution). Heroin injections and dextrose injections were given in markedly different environments, specifically, the animals' colony or another room where loud white noise was present. Half of the rats received heroin in the colony area; the remainder were given drug in the room with white noise. On the final day of the study, rats in one of the experimental groups (Same) received 15 mg/kg heroin in the environment where they historically had received smaller doses, and rats in the other experimental group (Different) received 15 mg/kg heroin in the environment where dextrose had been given in the past. Control rats, previously given only dextrose, also received 15 mg/kg heroin. Half of these rats were given the drug in the colony room, whereas the remaining rats received heroin in the room with white noise.

The lethality of heron in the three groups of rats is shown in Figure 7-1. Although exposure to heroin alone produced some tolerance to the drug, as evidenced by the lower lethality (64%) in the Different group than in the Control group (96%), the environment in which the drug was administered strongly affected the degree of tolerance observed. In fact, mortality was twice as great in the group (Different) that received heroin in a novel environment (64%) as in the group (Same) that received the drug in the usual environment (32%). These findings cannot be explained in terms of heroin's pharmacological properties alone.

Siegel (e.g., 1989) has proposed that respondent conditioning may play a role in tolerance, and this analysis accounts nicely for the lethality data shown in Figure 7-1. Specifically, stimuli reliably correlated with drug administration are established as CSs that come to evoke CRs that are opposite in direction to the URs elicited by the drug US. These CRs compensate for (i.e., counteract) the URs elicited by the drug and, as the CRs increase in magnitude as a result of repeated CS-US pairings, reduce the magnitude of the observed response to the drug, for example, heroin-induced respiratory depression (which causes death). Diminution of an observed drug effect with repeated administrations of the drug is by definition tolerance.

Given the findings of Siegel et al. (1982) and other data suggesting that tolerance to opioids is situation-specific (e.g., Siegel, 1989), it is reasonable to propose that the likelihood of heroin abusers suffering problems with overdose would be greater if they took the drug under unusual circumstances. Although this proposition cannot be tested experimentally for obvious ethical reasons, some anecdotal evidence supports it. For instance, Siegel (1984) asked 10 heroin users who suffered serious

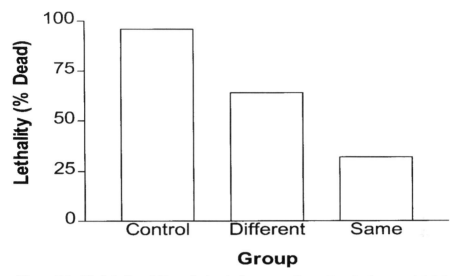

Figure 7-1. *The lethality of 15 mg/kg heroin in groups of rats. Rats in the group labeled Control had not previously been exposed to the drug. Groups labeled Same and Different had previously been exposed to lower doses of heroin under identical conditions, as explained in the text. These groups differed with respect to whether the 15 mg/kg dose was (Same) or was not (Different) administered in the environment in which prior drug injections occurred. Data are redrawn from Siegel et al. (1982).*

overdoses about the conditions where the problem occurred. Seven of them reported that the drug was taken in atypical circumstances when they overdosed.

Of course, as Pavlov's findings with respondently-conditioned salivation remind us, CRs do not always oppose URs in form. In fact, they can be nearly identical, and such an effect has been demonstrated with pharmacological USs. Pavlov himself reported such an outcome in dogs injected with apomorphine, which produces nausea, following tone presentations. After a few pairings, he found that the CS (tone) alone "sufficed to produce all the active symptoms of the drug, only in a lesser degree" (Pavlov, 1927, p. 35).

Conditioned withdrawal, evident in a study by Goldberg and Schuster (1970), provides another example of topographically similar CRs and URs. Goldberg and Schuster studied monkeys that were self-administering morphine and were physically dependent on the drug. Eventually, a red light was paired with injections of nalorphine, an opioid antagonist. Nalorphine precipitated withdrawal and, after a number of pairings, the red light did so as well. That is, when the light came on the monkeys salivated and vomited, just as they did when nalorphine was administered. Interestingly, the red light continued to elicit such effects for up to 120 days after morphine was no longer administered. Conditioned withdrawal has been demonstrated in humans (e.g., O'Brien, Testa, O'Brien, Brady, & Wells, 1977) and may have implications for drug abuse and its treatment.

Conditioned immunosuppression provides a third example of CRs resembling drug-induced URs. For example, Adler, Cohen, and Bovbjerg (1982) conducted a study in which rats in the Experimental group first drank a novel solution containing saccharin (CS), and then were injected with a drug (cyclophosphamide) (US) that impairs immune function (UR). Rats in the Control group did not drink the solution before being injected with the drug. Days later, the level of antibody production induced by exposure to a foreign substance (sheep's blood) was measured in rats that did or did not consume saccharine shortly before testing. Antibody production was reduced (CR) by exposure to saccharine (CS) in animals for which it had previously been paired with cyclophosphamide (i.e., those in the Experimental group), but not for animals exposed to saccharine without such pairing (i.e., those in the Control group). Here, both the drug and the stimulus respondently paired with it inhibited the immune response.[1]

Conditioned nausea in patients receiving chemotherapy provides a fourth example of respondent conditioning in which CRs and drug-elicited URs are similar. The chemotherapeutic agents used to treat cancer cause nausea, and patients who receive such treatment frequently become sick to their stomach upon approaching the clinic where treatment is administered. This phenomenon involves respondent conditioning: The stimuli that constitute the clinic are reliably paired with treatment, which elicits nausea, and these stimuli eventually elicit a similar response. For example, approaching the clinic, smelling the clinic, and seeing the nurses and doctors may all elicit nausea similar to that initially elicited only by the chemotherapy. In fact, just thinking about going to the clinic may cause patients to feel sick.

If, perchance, a patient eats before receiving chemotherapy, he or she may develop an aversion to the taste and smell of the food. This effect is evident in a study by Bernstein (1978). Bernstein's study involved three groups of children who were undergoing chemotherapy for cancer. Children in one group were given a novel-flavored ice cream before their treatment, children in a second group were not given ice cream before their treatment, and children in the third group were given ice cream without chemotherapy. Several weeks later the children were given a choice between eating ice cream and playing a game. Although 73% of the children who had ice cream but no therapy chose ice cream, only 21% of the children who had the ice cream before chemotherapy did so. In this case, a single respondent pairing was sufficient to reduce the reinforcing capacity of ice cream.

---

[1] It is noteworthy that in the studies by Goldberg and Schuster (1979) and Adler et al. (1982), drugs were used primarily as tools to study important learning phenomena. That is, the effects of nalorphine and cyclophosphamide were not of interest. Instead, the well known effects of those agents were used to examine important behavioral phenomena, conditioned withdrawal and conditioned immunosuppression. Although this aspect of behavioral pharmacology is not emphasized in this text, drugs can be useful tools for examining behavioral processes.

An opposite effect –one in which the reinforcing efficacy of stimuli is increased by being respondently paired with a drug–is evident in the "needle freak" phenomenon (Levine, 1974). **"Needle freaks"** are people with extensive histories of intravenous drug self-administration who, unlike most of us, report that drug injection is pleasurable and engage in such behavior even when it does not lead directly to drug injection. For instance, after injecting a drug bolus, they may continue to move the plunger in and out, thereby withdrawing and injecting their own blood. Such behavior is reinforcing, it appears, only by virtue of a history in which it reliably precedes delivery of a reinforcing stimulus, the drug. Absent such a history, people characteristically fear and avoid needles.

As the examples discussed in this section clearly illustrate, if a drug has US properties, then a previously neutral stimulus that reliably precedes the drug's administration may come through respondent conditioning to evoke a CR. As those examples further illustrate, stimuli predictive of drugs sometimes produce effects that are comparable to those produced by the drug. In other cases, however, pre-drug stimuli appear to control "compensatory" responses, that is, effects opposite to those produced by the drug. That this is the case is of theoretical interest. Although it is not presently possible to predict accurately when CRs will resemble drug-elicited URs, Eikelboom and Steward (1982) have proposed that this will be the case when the drug produces its effects by initially stimulating receptors that initiate activity in the central nervous system, which leads in turn to effector action. In contrast, when the drug directly stimulates the effector system, CRs will be compensatory. As Siegel (1989) explains, ". . . the CR will be in the same direction as the drug effect if the drug has an afferent site of action, and the CR will be opposite in direction to the drug effect if the drug has an efferent site of action" (p. 121). Whether this analysis will prove adequate to account for the effects of previously neutral stimuli respondently paired with behaviorally-active drugs remains to be determined. In any case, the fact that some such explanation is needed underscores the fact that a drug's behavioral effects are far from simple, even when the drug is acting as a US.

Perhaps because it is difficult to control when their detectable effects appear and disappear, drugs have rarely been studied as conditional stimuli. Nonetheless, researchers have demonstrated that a drug can acquire CS properties if a) the organism receiving it can detect its presence, and b) its presence reliably precedes exposure to a US. For instance, Bormann and Overton (1993) demonstrated that morphine could act as a CS in rats. They did so by pairing morphine injections with electric shock. The shock alone reduced drinking. Morphine did likewise when its presence historically was paired with shock presentation, but not otherwise.

One can readily imagine how CS effects of a drug might be of importance in determining its effects in the natural environment of humans. Consider a young man who has a history of masturbating after drinking alcohol. The way this history came about isn't especially important–perhaps our man regularly drinks in bars frequented by sexually appealing (but inaccessible) people. He comes home from the bars aroused and uninhibited, and plays with himself, something that he rarely does on other occasions. If this pattern occurs repeatedly, it may well be that drinking alcohol will produce some degree of arousal, for the detectable effects of the drug have been correlated predictably with stimuli that produce arousal. This effect might, in turn, increase the reinforcing effect of alcohol. It might also increase the probability that the person would engage in sexual activity while drinking, because the arousal elicited by the drug could serve as an establishing operation for sexual stimulation. Such effects are not, of course, intrinsic to alcohol, but occur only in individuals with particular histories. Although hypothetical, this example, like the real examples discussed previously, should serve to indicate that even such seemingly simple learning processes as respondent conditioning can dramatically alter a drug's effects.

Drugs as Discriminative Stimuli

Given the momentary effectiveness of some form of reinforcement, a particular behavior occurs more often in the presence of a **discriminative stimulus** (S^D) than in its absence because, historically, the behavior has been more successful in producing that form of reinforcement in the presence of the discriminative stimulus than in its absence. Two conditions must be met for a drug to be established as a discriminative stimulus: 1) the drug must produce effects that can be detected by the organism receiving it, and 2) that organism must have a history of differential reinforcement in the presence and absence of the drug.

The discriminative stimulus properties of drugs have been studied for over three decades. Thousands of studies using drug discrimination procedures have been published, and their results indicate that there is a strong correlation between the subjective effects of drugs and the neurochemical events that mediate these effects (e.g., Colpaert & Balster, 1988; Glennon & Young, 1987; Stolerman, 1993). Drug discrimination studies have been conducted with both human (Chapter 6) and nonhuman (Chapter 5) subjects, and results have been similar across species (Kamien, Bickel, Hughes, & Higgins, 1993). In essence, speaking nontechnically, drug discrimination studies allow researchers to ask subjects how drugs "make them feel," even if the subjects are nonverbal.

In a typical **drug discrimination procedure**, one response (e.g., depressing the leftmost of two levers) is reinforced when drug is given and another response (e.g., depressing the other lever) is reinforced following either vehicle control administration, administration of another drug, or administration of a different dose of the training drug. Stimulus-appropriate responses usually are reinforced under an intermittent schedule, for example, a fixed-ratio (FR) 20. In this case, only responses that occurred prior to the emission of 20 responses on one or the other lever would be used in assessing whether the drug was serving as an S^D. Subsequent responses would be excluded from this determination to prevent confusing control of behavior by an antecedent stimulus (the drug) with control of behavior by its consequences. If, for instance, right-lever responses were reinforced and left-lever responses extinguished during a test session, it would hardly be surprising if a subject emitted the vast majority of its total responses on the former lever. Such differential responding is **schedule-controlled**, not **stimulus-controlled**, and can occur in the presence as well as the absence of a putative discriminative stimulus.

After subjects reliably discriminate between the training stimuli, novel drugs can be introduced to determine whether their subjective effects are similar to those of the training stimuli. Also, putative antagonists can be administered to determine whether they block the detectable effects of the training drug(s). Generalization testing (i.e., testing involving novel compounds) characteristically is conducted during extinction, to ensure that the novel drugs are not themselves established as discriminative stimuli. For the same reason, extinction also is characteristically arranged during testing with putative antagonists.

In general, substantial **stimulus generalization** is obtained when drugs with similar neurochemical actions are substituted for the training drug. When stimulus generalization occurs, the novel drugs engender primarily training-drug-appropriate responding. For example, if a pigeon is trained to peck the leftmost of two keys following injections of morphine and the rightmost key following injections of saline solution (the morphine vehicle), it will primarily respond on the left key when tested with other mu opioid agonists, such as heroin. Drugs from other classes (e.g., amphetamine, ethanol, LSD), however, will engender primarily right-key responding. Such results are easily interpreted: In lay terms, the pigeon "feels as though it has received morphine" after injections of heroin, but not after injections of amphetamine, ethanol, or LSD.

Harder to interpret are results indicative of partial generalization, which occurs when a test compound engenders some, but not close to exclusive, training-drug-appropriate responding. For example, a pigeon trained to discriminate 5.6 mg/kg morphine from vehicle may emit 60% of its responses on the morphine-appropriate operandum when tested with 5.6 mg/kg of the experimental drug U50,488H. How should these data be interpreted? One possibility is that the subjective effects of the two drugs are similar, but they differ in potency. Animals can detect quantitative as well as qualitative differences in the effects of drugs, as illustrated when other doses of the training drug are substituted for the training dose. When this occurs, a generalization gradient like the one illustrated in Figure 7-2 characteristically is obtained.

If U50,488H produces detectable effects that are equivalent to those of morphine, but the former drug is less potent, then giving a dose larger than the 5.6 mg/kg dose that produced 60% morphine-appropriate responding in our hypothetical example should engender stronger generalization, and a sufficiently high dose of U50,488H should generate nearly exclusive morphine-appropriate responding.

[2]The latter term if misleading is one assumes that discriminative stimulus properties are fixed properties of a drug. In fact, discriminative stimulus properties are learned, and therefore variable across time and individuals. For example, 5.6 mg/kg morphine may or may not serve as a discriminative stimulus, depending on the organism's history. If the drug does have discriminative stimulus properties, the behavior it controls also depends on operant history. Therefore, referring to the "discriminative stimulus properties of morphine," is meaningful only with respect to a particular context.

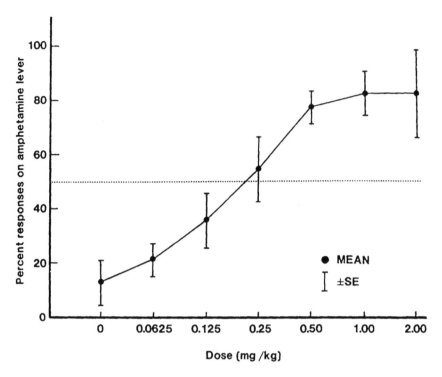

Figure 7-2. *Generalization gradient obtained when novel doses of* d-*amphetamine were tested in rats trained to discriminate 1.0 mg/kg* d-*amphetamine from vehicle. Each point represents mean performance across 12 test sessions (±1 standard error). Data are from Kuhn, Appel, and Greenburg (1974) and reproduced by permission.*

Researchers recognize that there are both qualitative and quantitative aspects of a drug's detectable effects, which are often referred to as the "cue state" or the "discriminative stimulus properties of the drug."[2] Therefore, they evaluate a range of doses in generalization tests.

Assume that several doses of U50,488H were evaluated in our morphine-trained pigeon, from a low dose that had no effect on behavior (as indexed by response rate) to a high dose that strongly reduced responding. Assume in addition that no dose of U50,488H engendered greater than 60% morphine-appropriate responding. The fact that a full range of U50,488H doses were tested rules out the possibility that U50,488H and morphine produce equivalent subjective effects, but differ in potency. How, then, should such results be interpreted? In truth, there is no agreement among researchers. Some have dismissed such results as indicative of disorganized responding, which cannot be interpreted. From their perspective, our hypothetical results would provide no useful information about the subjective effects of U50,488 and morphine. Other researchers use arbitrary criteria to dichotomize responding as either indicative of generalization, or not. For example, if a test drug engenders at least 80% training-drug-appropriate responding, then the two are assumed to produce similar subjective effects. All lower values are taken to be indicative of an absence of shared properties. From this perspective, our hypothetical results indicate that the subjective effects of U50,488H are unlike those of morphine. A third group argues that partial generalization is as meaningful in tests with novel compounds as in tests with various doses of the training compound, and should be interpreted in similar fashion. They would analyze our results as indicating that there are some common features in the subjective effects of the two drugs, but there are differences as well.

These differences, which can be to some extent be quantified via verbal report in studies with humans, probably reflect the fact that the two drugs share some neurochemical actions, but not others. For example, it may be that morphine only affects mu opioid receptors, whereas U50,488H affects both mu and kappa receptors. Therefore, U50,488H would produce some effects not associated with morphine. Humans might, for instance, report that both drugs made them feel euphoric and sedated, but only U50,488H made them urinate frequently and think bizarre thoughts. Pigeons, of course, could not describe verbally any differences in the drug states, and might not experience them in exactly the same way as humans, but nonetheless would respond differently to them, as indicated by their key-pecking behavior. Although such an analysis is perfectly reasonable, it is problematic in one respect: As discussed in Chapter 5, the results of drug discrimination studies are affected, in part, by procedural details.

You will perhaps recall from that chapter the results of a study by Makhay, Young, and Poling (1998), who used a three-response procedure to establish morphine, U50,488H, and vehicle as discriminative stimuli. They found no cross-generalization between U50,488H and morphine. This result is in contrast to results obtained in subjects trained and tested in two-response arrangements (i.e., morphine-vehicle or U50,488H-vehicle discriminations), which frequently behave much like our hypothetical pigeon. Although drug discrimination procedures are widely used and simple in concept, the results that they yield often are influenced by procedural details. Moreover, regardless of the exact procedure used, their results are not necessarily easy to interpret. These characteristics have not prevented drug discrimination procedures from playing a valuable role as a tools for neuropharmacologists. Like all tools, however, they must be well understood and used with care to yield optimal results.

With respect to analyzing drug effects in the everyday environment, it is important to recognize that there is almost infinite latitude in the range of behaviors that a drug can control by serving as an S^D, and this helps to explain how a given drug can produce very different behavioral effects across individuals. Consider the behavior of different people who have drunk roughly equivalent quantities of ethanol (beverage alcohol). There are violent drunks, amorous drunks, gross drunks, and playful drunks. Why? The reasons undoubtedly involve the actions of multiple and interactive variables, historical as well as current. One factor likely to be of considerable importance is an individual's reinforcement history while drinking. Consider two 21-year-old college students.

One plays shortstop on a local softball team and eventually begins to stop after games to sink a few beers with fellow players. For reasons that need not concern us, those individuals favor a bawdy good time and positively reinforce crude language, risqué jokes, and the not-too-subtle double entendre. The initiate is shaped into emitting such behavior, which is heavily reinforced when it occurs. After a few drinking bouts, the foulness of the shortstop's mouth might well do Chris Rock proud.

Our second student is first exposed to ethanol in the company of self-proclaimed intellectuals who sniff brandy while pondering intellectual issues. These academics reinforce fine language and reference to the classics; "deposition of fecal boli" is their term for what dogs do on the lawn. The student whose drinking history is with this company is likely to behave rather differently when imbibing than the softball player considered earlier. That this is so has nothing to do with the direct effects of ethanol, which should be very similar in both students, but rather reflects unlike conditioning histories during drug exposure.

Note, however, that in the examples given above the drinking of ethanol and the sensory consequences affected thereby are but part of a complex of stimuli that are uniquely correlated with particular reinforcement contingencies. The likelihood that the softball player will play the rowdy during future drinking bouts depends upon the extent to which these bouts occur in situations that resemble in their totality the after-games milieu. In addition, if reinforcement contingencies change, discriminative stimuli eventually fail to control behavior. Should the shortstop's friends undergo a religious conversion and hence come to punish coarse language, the player's behavior while drinking in their company—assuming that they did not turn away from beer in turning to god—eventually would change. If fact, should the group arrange sufficiently powerful contingencies of reinforcement and punishment, soon enough the shortstop would while drinking disparage filthy language and praise the lord with equal zeal. Unlikely though it is, this scenario emphasizes that the discriminative stimulus properties of a drug, and consequently its behavioral effects, can vary over time in the same individual, as well as across different people.

A study by Poling and Appel (1978), using rats as subjects, provides clear evidence that both qualitative and quantitative aspects of a drug's behavioral effects can be modified by changing its discriminative stimulus properties. In the first phase of this investigation, six rats were exposed to a fixed-interval (FI) 60-second schedule of food delivery. d-Amphetamine, street "speed," at the relatively low dose of 0.5 mg/kg increased response rates of all subjects under this schedule (see Figure 7-3).

In the second phase of the study, all animals were exposed to conditions in which an FR 20 schedule was in effect during some sessions and an FI 60-sec schedule was in effect during others. These conditions were arranged over a total of 63 sessions. For three subjects, the FR 20 schedule was in effect during 21 sessions, each preceded by an injection of 0.5 mg/kg d-amphetamine, and the FI 60-sec schedule was in effect for 42 sessions, each preceded by saline injection; drug (FR 20) and

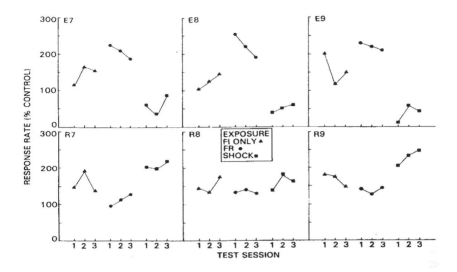

Figure 7-3. *Individual rat's response rates under an FI 60-second schedule of food delivery during sessions in which they received 0.5 mg/kg* d-*amphetamine. Each data point represents a single drug injection, expressed as a percentage of the mean control rate maintained in 12 baseline sessions under that training phase (the 4 sessions that preceded each of the 3 drug injections in that phase). Conditions are labeled according to whether an FR 20 schedule or punishment was arranged during the training sessions preceding drug testing. For rats E7, E8, and E9, the FR schedule and punishment were explicitly correlated with* d-*amphetamine injections; for the other rats, drug injections were random with respect to the FR schedule or punishment. Data are from Poling and Appel (1978).*

saline (FI 60-sec) sessions occurred in an irregular temporal sequence. The remaining subjects also were exposed to the FR 20 schedule for 21 sessions and received *d*-amphetamine (0.5 mg/kg) prior to 21 of the 63 sessions. For these animals, however, drug injections did not reliably precede either FR 20 or FI 60-sec sessions. That is, the FR 20 schedule followed 7 of the 21 injections of d-amphetamine (33%) and 14 of the 42 saline sessions (33%). At the end of this phase, 0.5 mg/kg *d*-amphetamine increased the response rates of all animals under the FI 60-sec schedule. As shown in Figure 7-3, the magnitude of the rate increase was much larger for those animals in which drug injection had been perfectly correlated with the FR 20 schedule than for those for which the relation was random.

In the third 63-day phase, all animals were exposed to sessions during which responding under the FI 60-second schedule sometimes was punished by electric shocks delivered under a variable-interval (VI) 5-minute schedule. For three subjects, each of the 21 punishment sessions was preceded by a 0.5 mg/kg injection of *d*-amphetamine; for the others, punishment sessions followed 7 drug injections and no punishment followed 14 drug injections. Thus, as in phase two, *d*-amphetamine was uniquely correlated with a change in environmental contingencies for three rats only. Therefore, *d*-amphetamine was discriminative for punishment in some of the rats, but not for others. That is, for the former animals but not for the latter, the probability of a response producing shock historically was greater in the presence of *d*-amphetamine. At the end of this phase, 0.5 mg/kg *d*-amphetamine substantially increased rates of responding under the FI 60-second schedule when given to subjects for which drug injections and shock sessions were random with respect to one another. In contrast, the drug reduced rates of FI responding when administered to rats for which *d*-amphetamine and shock sessions had been perfectly correlated (Figure 7-3).

In this study, *d*-amphetamine was not simply discriminative for the presence or absence of reinforcer availability. Instead, for some rats, the drug was first discriminative for the availability of reinforcers (food) under an FR 20 schedule. Later, again for only some animals, it was discriminative for scheduled punishment (electric shock delivery under a VI 5-minute schedule). Relative to the FI 60-second schedule, the FR 20 engendered higher response rates. So, too, did *d*-amphetamine when it was correlated with the FR 20. Response-dependent electric shocks reduced response rates under the FI 60-second schedule of food delivery, as did *d*-amphetamine when it was correlated with the punishment schedule. These results indicate that *d*-amphetamine, the prototype of stimulant drugs, could either increase or decrease the response rate of an individual animal under the same fixed-interval schedule, depending on the environmental contingencies with which the drug had been correlated and hence its discriminative stimulus properties. This result emphasizes that the behavioral effects of drugs, like those of other stimuli, may depend on the behavioral history of the organism as well as the current environment and the physical (e.g., pharmacological) properties of the stimulus.

Distinguishing between Discriminative and Motivational Effects

In some cases, changes in behavior produced by a drug may appear to involve its actions as an S^D, but in actuality a different mechanism of action is involved. Consider a group of experienced middle-class American marijuana smokers. While smoking, they are quite likely to engage in verbal (and other) behavior indicative of hunger—"the munchies" in user slang. It is possible that this may reflect the actions of the drug as an S^D, in which case users would have to have a history in which food-related responses were more successful (in gaining food or some other reinforcer, such as verbal support from peers) in the presence of drug than in its absence. If such a history is lacking, the drug must be producing its effects in some other manner. One way in which this might come about is if the drug acted as a motivation-altering variable, or **establishing operation** (EO) (see Chapter 2). That drugs can act as EOs is clear if one considers how amphetamines reduce food-seeking responses in humans, or the manner in which polyethylene glycol (which reduces extracellular fluid volume) increases fluid-maintained operant responses. Other examples of this mechanism of drug action are provided in Chapter 8.

Although the control of behavior exercised by an EO can resemble that associated with an S^D, it is important to distinguish the two functions. As Michael

(1982) points out, "In everyday language we can and often do distinguish changing people's behavior by changing what they want and changing their behavior by changing their chances of getting something that they already want" (p. 154). Drugs can do both, but in the former case they are serving as an EO, and in the later as an S^D .Whether a drug is acting as an establishing operation or as a discriminative stimulus cannot be determined without knowledge of the operant history of the person in question. In many cases, knowledge of past as well as current circumstances are required to determine a drug's behavioral mechanism of action.

State-dependent Learning

As usually defined, **state-dependent learning** occurs when behavior acquired in the presence of a particular drug is performed better on subsequent occasions when that drug is present than when it is absent. Conversely, similar behavior acquired in the absence of drug is performed less well on subsequent occasions when that drug is present than when it is absent (Overton, 1978; Weingartner, 1978). In the past 30 years, state-dependent learning has been demonstrated with a variety of drugs, including stimulants, sedatives, opioids, and hallucinogens, and with a range of species, among them dogs, goldfish, mice, rats, cats, and humans. Several different experimental tasks have been used in studies of state-dependent learning and it is evident that the behavioral procedure employed, as well as pharmacological variables (e.g., the kind and dose of drug employed), determine whether or not the phenomenon occurs (Poling & Cross, 1993).

State-dependent learning is evident in a study by Hill, Schwin, Powell, and Goodwin (1973). They studied 32 experienced marijuana smokers in a two-day experiment. The subjects were randomly assigned to one of four groups, each comprising eight subjects. Two conditions were examined: Marijuana was smoked during the D condition and a placebo was smoked during the N condition. For different groups, conditions were arranged in the order D-D, N-N, N-D, and D-N. All subjects were exposed to a visual avoidance task, a word association recall task, a verbal learning task measuring memory for sets of words, and a task requiring recall of ordered objects. Only the last task will be considered here. As Hill et al. (1973) described it:

> [On day 1 in] the object recall test subjects were shown seven plastic objects.
> . . . They were asked to name each so that subsequent deficits in recall
> presumably would reflect memory loss rather than inattention. The sub-
> jects were then asked to order the objects from left to right. On day 2
> subjects were asked to recall the seven objects and then arrange them in the
> same order as on day 1. (p. 242)

Mean errors per subject in each of the four groups are shown in Figure 7-4. These results indicate good performance in the state-unchanged groups (i.e., subjects in the N-N and D-D groups made few errors) and relatively poor performance in the state-changed groups (i.e., subjects in the N-D and D-N groups made several errors). Moreover, the decrement in performance was roughly symmetrical across the two changes in state (i.e., subjects in the N-D and D-N groups made a similar number

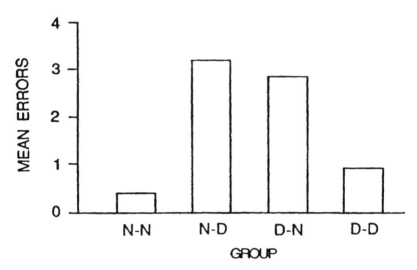

Figure 7-4. *Mean number of errors made by men performing an ordered object recall task. Data are from day 2, on which the subjects smoked marijuana (drug, D, or placebo, N). The task was learned on day 1, on which the subjects smoked marijuana (D) or placebo (no drug, N). Procedural details are described in text. Data are redrawn with permission from Hill, Schwin, Powell, and Goodwin (1973).*

of errors). There is, however, some evidence that smoking marijuana interfered with performance regardless of whether or not a state change occurred. This evidence involves the greater number of errors made by subjects in the D-D and N-D groups relative to the D-N and N-N groups, respectively.

How can these results be explained? One possibility is that the diminution of performance in subjects trained with drug present and tested with drug absent reflects altered stimulus control. Similarly, performance in subjects trained with drug absent and tested with drug present could reflect a stimulus change decrement: By virtue of the subject receiving drug in it, the test environment differs from the training environment, hence the test environment does not control behavior in the same way or to the same degree as the training environment. These possibilities are consistent with a behavioral analysis of state-dependent learning and some researchers have suggested that state-dependent learning and control of behavior by pharmacological discriminative stimuli are essentially equivalent (e.g., Schuster & Balster, 1977; Overton, 1983). Others disagree (e.g., Colpaert Niemegeers, & Janssen, 1976; Nielson, DeWitt, & Gill, 1978).

Disagreement over the mechanisms responsible for state-dependent learning underscores an important point: State-dependent learning is a descriptive, not explanatory, construct and the mechanisms responsible for it cannot be specified with confidence. Perhaps for this reason, contemporary behavioral pharmacologists rarely study the phenomenon, preferring instead to examine uncontaminated discriminative stimulus control of behavior. Nonetheless, drugs habitually used by humans, including caffeine, nicotine, marijuana, and ethanol (Lowe, 1988), can produce the changes in behavior known collectively as state-dependent learning: Under certain conditions, behaviors acquired in the presence of these drugs are not performed well in the absence of drug and vice versa. As Heistad (1957) pointed out over 40 years ago, such effects could create obvious difficulties for humans who use drugs. Given this, further studies of state-dependent learning appear to be justified.

Drugs as Positively Reinforcing Stimuli

All reinforcers are stimuli that strengthen behaviors which closely precede them in time. Positive reinforcers involve adding something to the environment; negative reinforcers involve taking something away. As discussed in Chapter 2, what functions as a reinforcer for a particular person at a given time and place depends upon the individual's prior experiences and current circumstances. Consider cigarette smoking. Early exposures to cigarettes typically are not in themselves positively reinforcing but may be repeated due to nonpharmacological reinforcers (e.g., peer praise) associated with the experience. With continued exposure, however, tolerance develops to the unpleasant effects of cigarette smoke (e.g., nausea), and cigarette smoke eventually becomes positively reinforcing due to the nicotine it contains. In this example, the reinforcing properties of smoking emerge gradually, through a process that involves interaction between the behavior of an individual (i.e., repeated administration) and the direct effects of a drug (nicotine). Behavioral actions of drugs which develop in this manner are frequently termed **functional** (as opposed to direct).

As noted in Chapters 5 and 6, drugs as positive reinforcers have been studied in laboratory experiments with both nonhuman and humans subjects. Over 100 compounds have been tested for whether they serve as positive reinforcers in nonhumans. In general, there is good correspondence between those drugs that serve as positive reinforcers in nonhumans and those that serve as positive rein-forces—and are used recreationally and abused—by humans (e.g., Griffiths, Bigelow, & Henningfield, 1980; Meisch & Lemaire, 1993; Young & Herling, 1986). The primary exception are hallucinogenic compounds, such as LSD, mescaline, and psilicybin. No data indicate that nonhumans will behave in ways leading to the delivery of these drugs; instead, behavior that prevents their delivery is strengthened (as discussed in the next section). Of course, these relations may not obtain in all circumstances: LSD might well serve as a positive reinforcer for nonhumans given special, and as yet unspecifiable, training. It has, however, been suggested that social variables, primarily the way in which a group reacts to drug taking by its members, are uniquely important in controlling humans' self-administration of hallucinogens.

A wide range of opiates, sedative-hypnotics, stimulants, and other drugs maintain the drug taking of nonhumans in environments devoid of obvious predisposing factors. That is, rats and monkeys will take certain drugs without being stressed, food-deprived, provided with nondrug reinforcement, or treated in any unusual manner to learn drug self-administration. All that is required is exposure to a situation in which a response leads to drug delivery. Given this exposure, the behavior leading to drug delivery occurs often, and high levels of intake result. For example, drug-naive monkeys allowed to press a bar producing intravenous injections of morphine self-administer enough of the drug to produce physical dependence (Thompson & Schuster, 1964). Moreover, unless protective contingen-

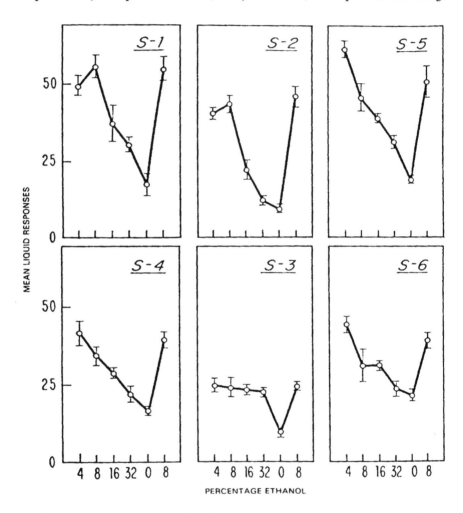

Figure 7-5. *Mean number of liquid-reinforced responses (lever presses) emitted by six individual rats (±1 standard error) during one-hour sessions in which food was not concurrently available. During each condition, liquid was available under an FR 1 schedule during seven consecutive sessions. Ethanol concentration was varied across conditions in the order listed, and prior to the sessions shown all subjects were exposed to an intermittent (i.e., FI 26-s) food delivery schedule with ethanol concurrently available. Data are from Poling and Thompson (1977).*

cies that limit drug intake are arranged, monkeys under some conditions will self-administer enough morphine or *d*-amphetamine to kill themselves (Johanson, Balster, & Bonese, 1976). Such findings indicate that some drugs are powerful unconditioned reinforcers.

Special histories are required to establish other drugs as reinforcers in nonhumans. For example, ethanol (beverage alcohol) administered via the oral route does not reliably serve as a positive reinforcer for most strains of rats and monkeys. If, however, these animals are induced to drink substantial quantities of the drug, either by making it available while they are eating their daily food, or by concurrently exposing them to an intermittent schedule of dry food delivery, it will subsequently serve as a reinforcer (e.g., Meisch, 1975; Meisch & Lemaire, 1993). Such an outcome is evident in Figure 7-5, which shows the number of lever-presses maintained by 0, 4, 8, 16, and 32% ethanol solutions in rats previously exposed to an FI 26-second schedule of food delivery while 8% ethanol was available. After this exposure, all of the ethanol solutions engendered substantially more responding than did water alone.

Of course, when food is used to induce drinking, animals characteristically are food deprived. That was the case for the rats that generated the data shown in Figure 7-5. In such animals, ethanol might serve as a reinforcer because of its caloric value, not because of its pharmacological effects. Apparent support for this contention stems from the observation that absolute levels of ethanol intake characteristically decrease when food deprivation is reduced. Findings with other drugs, however, indicate that food deprivation generally increases intake of a wide variety of drugs that are not a source of calories (Carroll & Meisch, 1984), and Kliner and Meisch (1989) propose that the behavioral mechanism of action of food deprivation is an increase in the reinforcing effects of drugs. In any case, ethanol and many other drugs clearly serve as effective positive reinforcers in a range of species, regardless of whether food deprivation is arranged.

In general, it appears that the procedures used to establish drugs as reinforcers do not appreciably influence subsequent patterns of self-administration. As Young and Herling (1986) indicate, "Once contingent drug delivery has gained control of a behavioral repertoire, the development and maintenance of future behavior appear controlled primarily by prevailing access conditions rather than by the conditions important in initially establishing the drug as a reinforcer" (p.16). Researchers have examined many variables that influence drug self-administration by nonhumans, and their findings indicate that *behavior maintained by drugs is similar to behavior maintained by other kinds of positive reinforcers in terms of its sensitivity to environmental variables*. Therefore, drug-maintained behavior is influenced in lawful fashion by the amount and delay of reinforcement, the schedule under which drug is available, the consequences of alternative behavior, and the establishing operations in effect. Given an appropriate history, antecedent stimuli can also be a powerful determinant of drug self-administration.

Under comparable maintenance conditions, drugs may generate similar patterns of self-administration in humans and nonhumans. Such an effect is evident

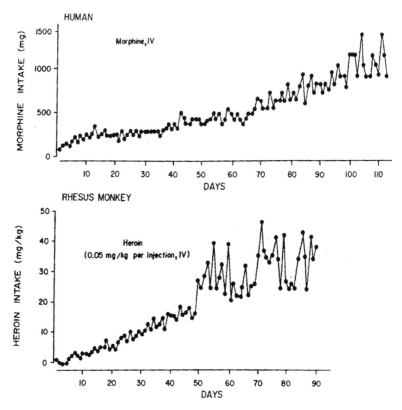

Figure 7-6. *Similar patterns of opioid intake in a human and a rhesus monkey under conditions of continuous drug availability. Each graph shows the amount of drug taken over successive days. The human data are replotted from an experiment in which a volunteer with a history of drug abuse was permitted was permitted to regulate his intravenous morphine intake (Wikler, 1952). The monkey data are from an unpublished study in which lever-press responses by rhesus monkeys produced intravenous injections of heroin. From Griffiths, Bigelow, and Henningfield (1980) and reproduced by permission.*

in Figure 7-6, which shows across consecutive days the amount of morphine self-administered by a human and the amount of heroin self-administered by a rhesus monkey. Although the dependent variable in this figure is total drug intake per day, in most laboratory studies, number of responses (usually expressed as response rate) and number of drug deliveries are the primary dependent variables (Meisch & Lemaire, 1993). Response rate under a given schedule is sometimes taken as a direct index of reinforcing effectiveness, the notion being that more effective reinforcers engender higher rates. Because drugs can directly affect response rates, including rates of the behaviors that lead to their delivery, care must be taken in using rate as a measure of the effectiveness of reinforcement. Other procedures, including progressive-ratio schedules, concurrent schedules, and ratio schedules that allow demand curves to be generated (see Chapters 2, 5, and 8) are useful for quantifying the reinforcing properties of drugs.

The **conditioned place preference** procedure is also used to study drugs as positive reinforcers. This procedure, which involves placing an animal on one side (e.g., the left, which is painted white) of an alley after drug injection, then determining whether the animal subsequently prefers that side in the absence of drug, essentially determines whether stimuli correlated with the drug are established as conditioned reinforcers. It is useful as a rapid but rough-and-ready screen for reinforcing effectiveness, but does not allow for the kind of fine-grained quantification provided by free-operant assays. Bozarth (1987) provides full coverage of procedures used to assess drugs as positive reinforcers.

Given the magnitude of the drug abuse problem in the United States and elsewhere, it is not surprising that self-administrations procedures—which involve using drugs as positive reinforcers—have been used in many published studies. Studies of drug self-administration are important for three reasons. First, they indicate that drugs can exercise powerful control over behavior in the absence of any obvious psychopathology. Second, by extrapolation, they provide information about the variables that control human drug use and abuse. Third, they allow for the examination of pharmacological and behavioral treatments that may reduce or eliminate established drug intake. For example, pre-treatment with opioid antagonists such as naloxone and nalorphine essentially eliminates the reinforcing effects of heroin and morphine. Unfortunately, both naloxone and nalorphine have undesirable properties that limit their value as treatments for treating opioid abuse. But the fact that they do block the positively reinforcing effects of mu opioid agonists has galvanized a search for long-lasting, orally effective antagonists that produce no serious adverse effects. When and if such an agent is found, it will undoubtedly be a valuable tool in treating heroin and morphine abuse.

Studies of drugs as positive reinforcers in humans yield similar information to that produced in animal studies (see Chapter 6). As Henningfield, Lucas, and Bigelow (1986) point out, studies with humans also allow researchers to determine whether characteristic patterns of self-administration differ in people with different demographic characteristics (e.g., postoperative pain treatment patients, recreational drug users, addicts), and to evaluate the extent to which subject-reported drug effects correlate with other measures of behavior.

Drugs as Negatively Reinforcing Stimuli

A drug is serving as a negatively reinforcing stimulus if an organism will respond to escape or avoid it. For example, mice will respond to escape from exposure to ozone and ammonia vapors (Tepper & Wood, 1985; Wood, 1979), and monkeys will behave so as to avoid exposure to LSD (Hoffmeister, 1975). In both cases, the drug is negatively reinforcing. Humans, too, regularly avoid contact with certain drugs, including prescribed medications. A child with diabetes, for instance, may avoid painful premeal insulin injections by staying outdoors, safely away from the parent waiting to give the injection, or a person with schizophrenia may avoid exposure to a neuroleptic by vomiting soon after the medication is administered. In these cases, the result is failure to administer a drug, and to comply with the intended treatment program.

Negative Reinforcement and Patient Noncompliance

Patient noncompliance is certainly a major medical problem (Benet, 1996; Haynes, Taylor, & Sackett, 1979). According to Sackett and Snow (1979), on average 38% of patients fail to comply with short-term medication regimens, and 46% fail to comply with long-term treatments. More recently, Kass, Gordon, Morley, Meltzer, and Goldberg (1987) reported similar results, in that 40% of their subjects made major errors in self-medicating during long-term treatment. It is tempting to speculate that negative reinforcement contributes to the high incidence of noncompliance reported in these and other studies. But the fact that patients frequently fail to take medications as intended by their physicians does not, in itself, indicate that these medications are serving as negative reinforcers. Remember that negative reinforcers strengthen behaviors that prevent or terminate exposure to them. A patient's failure to self-administer a medication may indicate simply that the drug is not positively reinforcing. Such a drug may have no functional stimulus properties whatever and surely need not function as a negative reinforcer.

Regardless of whether patient noncompliance results from a drug's negatively reinforcing properties or the absence of positively reinforcing properties, principles of behavioral psychology can be used to increase the likelihood of compliance. Research in this area is carefully reviewed by Masek (1982) and Epstein and Cluss (1982). A number of specific procedures have proven useful in increasing patient compliance. One involves careful monitoring of drug intake, a difficult but not impossible task, coupled with systematic reinforcement of appropriate drug taking and punishment of inappropriate self-administration. For example, a hypertensive patient and spouse might draw up a behavioral contract such that the patient gives the spouse $70 at the beginning of each week. Each day that the spouse actually sees the patient ingest scheduled medication, $10 is returned; any time medication is not taken in the approved fashion, $10 is sent to an organization despised by the patient. Here, short-term consequences are being arranged so as to support a behavior, adherence to a medication regiment, the assumed long-term consequences of which, good health, are too delayed and uncertain to control behavior.

Providing appropriate rules for administering medications may also help to increase the odds of compliance. As emphasized throughout this book, human behavior can be rule-governed as well as contingency-shaped, and it appears that much health-related behavior, including complying with doctors' orders, is of the former sort. A significant goal for researchers in behavioral medicine is to discern the conditions under which the likelihood of patients' rule following is maximized.

Determinants of Negative Reinforcement

Whether a given drug and dosage serve as a negative reinforcer depends upon prior and current conditions. The narcotic antagonist naloxone, for instance, at low doses typically does not serve as a negative reinforcer in subjects that are not physically dependent on opioids but will maintain avoidance behavior if physical dependence is presence (e.g., Downs & Woods, 1975; Goldberg, Hoffmeister, Schlichting, & Wuttke, 1971; Tang & Morse, 1975). In addition to the presence or absence of physical dependence, the schedule under which an opioid antagonist is administered can determine its stimulus function. For example, Downs and Woods (1975) initially exposed physically-dependent monkeys to conditions in which every 30th response terminated a stimulus associated with injections of naloxone. Responding was well maintained under this schedule. Responding also was well maintained for as many as 15 days in a subsequent condition in which responding produced naloxone injections (under a second-order schedule). Although responding eventually declined, these results indicate that, depending on current and prior circumstances, naloxone can serve as a positive or a negative reinforcer in the same subject.

As discussed in Chapter 2, a common misconception among individuals only minimally conversant with behavioral principles is the notion that a drug is serving as a negative reinforcer if it is self-administered by a person undergoing withdrawal symptoms, which are alleviated by the drug. The logic behind this analysis, albeit faulty, is as follows: Drug administration is an escape response which serves to terminate the aversive state of withdrawal, ergo the drug must be a negative reinforcer. Although it may be intuitively appealing, this analysis violates the convention of classifying reinforcers as positive or negative according to their *physical* characteristics, not their effects on some real or posited internal state of the subject.

If a drug serves as a negative reinforcer, stimuli that reliably precede exposure to it may come to serve as conditioned negative reinforcers. Conversely, a drug can acquire through conditioning negatively reinforcing properties if its administration predictable precedes exposure to an established negative reinforcer. Finally, drugs that serve as negative reinforcers also frequently serve as positive punishers, that is, as stimuli that reduce the future probability of occurrence of behaviors that lead to their administration. A series of experiments by Goldberg and associates provides clear evidence that the stimulus properties of a given drug are not fixed, but depend critically on history and current context. Initially, they demonstrated that monkeys would respond reliably under FI schedules to self-administer certain doses of nicotine (e.g., Goldberg & Spealman, 1982; Goldberg, Spealman, & Goldberg, 1981). Therefore, the drug served as a positive reinforcer. Under other conditions, however, nicotine was a positive punisher (Goldberg & Spealman, 1983). This effect was demonstrated under a multiple FR FR schedule of food delivery, where the first response in each ratio also produced a nicotine injection under one of the two components. Response-dependent nicotine injections reduced response rate by over

70% in that component, therefore, the drug was a positive punisher. Although perhaps counterintuitive, as Young and Herling (1986) point out:

> Such disparate effects are not unique to nicotine. It is well established that electric shock may function to reinforce behaviors leading to its presentation or to punish behaviors maintained by other reinforcers, depending on the exact conditions of its presentation an the behavioral history of the subject (see review by Morse & Kelleher, 1977). Furthermore, the range of drugs reported to produce the suppression of food or fluid intake called conditioned taste aversion includes drugs that function effectively as reinforcers (i.e., White, Sklar, & Amit, 1977; Wise, Yokel, & de Wit, 1976). . . . Such experiments emphasize the multiple functions that drugs can serve. Demonstration that a drug serves as a reinforcer or punisher under one set of conditions does not rule out the possibility that the same drug, at the same doses, can serve other, even opposite behavioral functions under other conditions. (p. 43)

Concluding Comments

The fact that drugs may acquire functional stimulus properties through conditioning, as well as have the ability to affect behavior in the absence of conditioning, has two important implications for understanding drug effects in humans. The first is that the behavioral actions of a given drug may differ dramatically across individuals, depending upon their conditioning histories with respect to it. One person may dance while intoxicated at a party because that response was richly reinforced in similar circumstances in the past; another may sing for the same reason. In both cases, ethanol would be affecting behavior as a discriminative, as well as an unconditional, stimulus.

The second implication is that a drug's behavioral actions within an individual may vary over time. Ethanol, for instance, possesses aversive taste properties and typically does not serve as a positive reinforcer upon initial exposure. With repeated exposure to the drug's pharmacological properties, however, it frequently comes to serve as a powerful positive reinforcer. As noted earlier, behavioral actions that develop through such an interaction of behavioral and pharmacological variables are termed functional, as opposed to direct, effects. Any attempt to account for the behavioral actions of drugs across individuals, or within an individual over time, is unlikely to succeed unless it considers functional as well as direct actions. Behaviorally active drugs are not magic bullets that selectively and inevitably change behavior in particular ways. They are, rather, stimuli, and as such produce effects that may differ as a function of the conditions under which they are, and have been, administered (Branch, 1991).

References

Adler, R., Cohen, N., & Bovjberg, D. (1982). Conditioned suppression of humoral immunity in the rat. *Journal of Comparative and Physiological Psychology, 96,* 517-520.

Benet, L. Z. (1996). Principles of prescription order writing and patient compliance instructions. In J. G. Hardman, L. E. Limbard, P. B. Molinoff, R. W. Ruddon, & A. G. Gilman (Eds.), *The pharmacological basis of therapeutics* (pp. 1697-1706). New York: McGraw-Hill.

Bernstein, I. L. (1978). Learned taste aversions in children receiving chemotherapy. *Science, 200*, 1302-1303.

Bormann, N. M., & Overton, D. A. (1993). Morphine as a conditioned stimulus in a conditioned emotional response paradigm. *Psychopharmacology, 112*, 277-284.

Bozarth, M. A. (1987). *Methods for assessing the reinforcing properties of abused drugs.* New York: Springer-Verlag.

Branch, M. (1991). Behavioral pharmacology. In I. H. Iversen & K. A. Lattal (Eds.), *Experimental analysis of behavior* (Part 2, pp. 21-77). Amsterdam: Elsevier.

Carroll, M. E., & Meisch, R. A. (1984). Increased drug-reinforced behavior due to food deprivation. In T. Thompson, P. B. Dews, & J. E. Barrett (Eds.), *Advances in behavioral pharmacology* (Vol. 4, pp. 47-88). New York: Academic Press.

Colpaert, F. C., & Balster, R. L. (1988). *Transduction mechanisms of drug stimuli.* Berlin: Springer.

Colpaert, F. C., Niemegeers, C. J., & Janssen, P. A. (1976). Theoretical and methodological considerations on drug discrimination learning. *Psychopharmacologia, 46*, 169-177.

Downs, D. A., & Woods, J. H. (1975). Naloxone as a negative reinforcer in rhesus monkeys: Effects of dose, schedule, and narcotic regimen. *Pharmacology Reviews, 27*, 397-406.

Eikelboom, R., & Stewart, J. (1982). Conditioning of drug-induced physiological responses. *Psychological Review, 89*, 507-527.

Epstein, L. H., & Cluss, P. A. (1982). A behavioral medicine perspective on adherence to long-term medical regimens. *Journal of Consulting and Clinical Psychology, 50*, 950-971.

Glennon, R. A., & Young, R. (1987). The study of structure-activity relationships using drug discrimination methodology. In M. A. Bozarth (Ed.), *Methods of assessing the reinforcing properties of abused drugs* (pp. 373-390). Berlin: Springer.

Goldberg, S. R., & Schuster, C. R. (1970). Conditioned nalorphine-induced abstinence changes: Persistence in post morphine-dependent monkeys. *Journal of the Experimental Analysis of Behavior, 14*, 33-46.

Goldberg, S. R., & Spealman, R. D. (1982). Maintenance and suppression of behavior by intravenous nicotine injections in squirrel monkeys. *Federation Proceedings, 41*, 216-220.

Goldberg, S. R., & Spealman, R. D. (1983). Suppression of behavior by intravenous injections of nicotine or by electric shocks in squirrel monkeys: Effects of chlordiazepoxide and mecamylamine. *Journal of Pharmacology and Experimental Therapeutics, 224*, 334-340.

Goldberg, S. R., Hoffmeister, F., Schlichting, U. U., & Wuttke, W. (1971). Aversive properties of nalorphine and naloxone in morpine-dependent rhesus monkeys. *Journal of Pharmacology and Experimental Therapeutics, 179*, 267-276.

Goldberg, S. R., Spealman, R. D., & Goldberg, D. M. (1981). Persistent behavior at high rates maintained by intravenous self-administration of nicotine. *Science, 214,* 573-575.

Goldberg, S. R., Spealman, R. D., & Shannon, H. E. (1982). Aversive properties of nalorphine and naloxone in morphine-dependent rhesus monkeys. *Journal of pharmacology and Experimental Therapeutics, 179,* 267-276.

Green, A. R., Cross, A. J., & Goodwin, G. M. (1995). Review of the pharmacology and clinical pharmacology of 3,4-methylenedioxymenthamphetamine (MDMA or "Ecstacy"). *Psychopharmacology, 119,* 247-260.

Griffiths, R. R., Bigelow, G. E., & Henningfield, J. E. (1980). Similarities in animal and human drug-taking behavior. In N. Mello (Ed.), *Advances in substance abuse* (Vol. 1, pp. 1-90). Greenwich, CT: JAI Press.

Haynes, R. B., Taylor, D. W., & Sackett, D. L. (1979). *Compliance in health care.* Baltimore: Johns Hopkins Press.

Heistad, G. T. (1957). A bio-psychological approach to somatic treatments in psychiatry. *American Journal of Psychiatry, 114,* 540-545.

Henningfield, J. E., Lucas, S. E., & Bigelow, G. E. (1986). Human studies of drugs as reinforcers. In S. R. Goldberg & I. P. Stollerman (Eds.), *Behavioral analysis of drug dependence* (pp. 69-122). Orlando, FL: Academic Press.

Hill, S. Y., Schwin, R., Powell, B., & Goodwin, D. W. (1973). State-dependent effects of marijuana on human memory. *Nature, 243,* 241-242.

Hoffmeister, F. (1975). Negatively reinforcing properties of some psychotropic drugs in drug-naive rhesus monkeys. *Journal of Pharmacology and Experimental Therapeutics, 192,* 467-477.

Johanson, C. E., Balster, R., & Bonese, S. (1976). Self-administration of psychomotor stimulant drugs: The effects of unlimited access. *Pharmacology Biochemistry and Behavior, 4,* 45-51.

Kamien, J. B., Bickel, W. K., Hughes, J. R., & Higgens, S. T. (1993). Drug discrimination by humans compared to nonhumans: Current status and future directions. *Psychopharmacology, 111,* 259-270.

Kass, M. A., Gordon, M., Morley, R. E., Meltzer, D. W., & Goldberg, J. J. (1987). Compliance with topical timolol treatment. *American Journal of Opthamology, 103,* 187-193.

Kliner, D. J., & Meisch, R. A. (1989). Oral pentobarbital intake in rhesus monkeys: Effects of drug concentration under conditions of food deprivation and satiation. *Pharmacology Biochemistry and Behavior, 32,* 347-354.

Kuhn, D. M., Appel, J. B., & Greenberg, I. (1974). An analysis of some discriminative properties of *d*-amphetamine. *Psychopharmacologia, 15,* 347-356.

Levine, D. G. (1974). Needle freaks: Compulsive self-injections by drug users. *American Journal of Psychiatry, 131,* 297-300.

Lowe, G. (1988). State-dependent retrieval effects with social drugs. *British Journal of Addiction, 32,* 143-158.

Makhay, M., Young, A. M., & Poling, A. (1998). Establishing morphine and U50,488H as discriminative stimuli in a three-choice assay with pigeons. *Experimental and Clinical Psychopharmacology, 6,* 3-9.

Masek, B. J. (1982). Compliance and medicine. In D. M. Doleys, R. L. Meredith, & A. R. Ciminero (Eds.), *Behavioral medicine: Assessment and treatment strategies* (pp. 527-536). New York: Plenum Press.

Meisch, R. A. (1975). The function of schedule-induced polydipsia in establishing ethanol as a positive reinforcer. *Pharmacological Review, 27,* 465-473.

Meisch, R. A., & Lemaire, G. A. (1993). Drug self-administration. In F. van Haaren (Ed.), *Methods in behavioral pharmacology* (pp. 257-300). Amsterdam: Elsevier.

Michael, J. L. (1982). Distinguishing between discriminative and motivational functions of stimuli. *Journal of the Experimental Analysis of Behavior, 37,* 149-155.

Morse, W. H., & Kelleher, R. T. (1977). Determinants of reinforcement and punishment. In W. K. Honig & J. E. R. Staddon (Eds.), *Handbook of operant behavior* (pp. 174-200). Englewood Cliffs, NJ: Prentice Hall.

Nielson, H. C., DeWitt, J. R., & Gill, J. H. (1978). Some failures of the drug discrimination hypothesis of state-dependent learning. In F. C. Colpaert & J. A. Rosecrans (Eds.), *Stimulus properties of drugs: Ten years of progress* (pp. 423-443). Amsterdam: Elsevier.

O'Brien, C. P., Testa, T., O'Brien, T. J., Brady, J. P., & Wells, B. (1977). Conditioned narcotic withdrawal in humans. *Science, 195,* 1000-1002.

Overton, D. A. (1978). Major theories of state-dependent learning. In B. T. Ho, D. W. Richards, III, & D. L. Chute (Eds.), *Drug discrimination and state-dependent learning* (pp. 283-318). New York: Academic Press.

Overton, D. A. (1983). State-dependent learning and drug discrimination. In L. L. Iverson, S. D. Iverson, & S. H. Snyder (Eds.), *Handbook of psychopharmacology* (Vol. 18, pp. 59-128). New York: Plenum Press.

Pavlov, I. P. (1927). *Conditioned reflexes.* (G. V. Anrep, Trans.). Oxford, England: Clarendon.

Poling, A., & Appel, J. B. (1978). *d*-Amphetamine and fixed-interval performance: Effects of establishing the drug as a discriminative stimulus. *Pharmacology Biochemistry and Behavior, 9,* 473-476.

Poling, A., & Cross, J. (1993). State-dependent learning. In F. van Haaren (Ed.), *Methods in behavioral pharmacology* (pp. 245-256). Amsterdam: Elsevier.

Poling, A., & Thompson, T. (1977). Suppression of ethanol-maintained lever pressing by delaying food availability. *Journal of the Experimental Analysis of Behavior, 28,* 271-283.

Poling, A., Kesselring, J., Sewell, R. G., Jr., & Cleary, J. (1983). Lethality of pentazocine and tripellenamine combinations in mice housed individually and in groups. *Pharmacology Biochemistry and Behavior, 18,* 103-105.

Sackett, E. L., & Snow, J. C. (1979). *The magnitude of compliance and noncompliance.* Baltimore: Johns Hopkins Press.

Schuster, C. R., & Balster, R. (1977). The discriminative stimulus properties of drugs. In T. Thompson & P. B. Dews (Eds.), *Advances in behavioral pharmacology* (Vol. 1, pp. 85-138). New York: Academic Press.

Siegel, S. (1984). Pavlovian conditioning and heroin overdose: Reports by overdose victims. *Bulletin of the Psychonomic Society, 22,* 427-430.

Siegel, S. (1989). Pharmacological conditioning and drug effects. In A. J. Goudie & M. W. Emmett-Oglesby (Eds.), *Psychoactive drugs: Tolerance and sensitization* (pp. 115-180). Clifton, NJ: Humana Press.

Siegel, S., Hinson, R. E., Krank, M. D., & McCully, J. (1982). Heroin "overdose" death: Contribution of drug-associated environmental cues. *Science, 216,* 436-437.

Stolerman, I. P. (1993). Drug discrimination. In F. van Haaren (Ed.), *Methods in behavioral pharmacology* (pp. 217-244). Amsterdam: Elsevier.

Tang, A. H., & Morse, W. H. (1975). Termination of a schedule complex associated with intravenous injections of nalorphine in morphine-dependent monkeys. *Pharmacology Reviews, 27,* 407-417.

Tepper, J. W., & Wood, R. W. (1985). Behavioral evaluation of the annoying properties of ozone. *Toxicology and Applied Pharmacology, 78,* 404-411.

Thompson, T., & Pickens, R. (1971). *Stimulus properties of drugs.* New York: Appleton-Century-Crofts.

Thompson, T., & Schuster, C. R. (1964). Morphine self-administration, food-reinforced and avoidance behaviors in rhesus monkeys. *Psychopharmacologia, 5,* 87-94.

Young, A. M., & Herling, S. (1986). Drugs as reinforcers: Studies in laboratory animals. In S. R. Goldberg & I. P. Stolerman (Eds.), *Behavioral analysis of drug dependence* (pp. 9-67). Orlando, FL: Academic Press.

Weingartner, H. (1978). Human state-dependent learning. In B. T. Ho, D. W. Richards, III, & D. L. Chute (Eds.), *Drug discrimination and state-dependent learning* (pp. 361-382). New York: Academic Press

White, N., Sklar, L., & Amit, Z. (1977). The reinforcing action of morphine and its paradoxical side effect. *Psychopharmacology, 52,* 63-66.

Wikler, A. (1952). A psychodynamic study of a patient during experimental self-regulated re-addiction to morphine. *Psychiatry Quarterly, 26,* 270-293.

Wise, R. A., Yokel, R. A., & DeWit, H. (1976). Both positive reinforcement and conditioned aversion from amphetamine and from apomorphine in rats. *Science, 191,* 1273-1275.

Wood, R. W. (1979). Behavioral evaluation of sensory irritation evoked by ammonia. *Toxicology and Applied Pharmacology, 50,* 157-162.

Chapter 8

Variables that Influence Drug Action

Alan Poling
Western Michigan University

The primary objective of any science is to account for variability in its subject matter. Therefore, the primary task for behavioral pharmacologists is explaining the variations in drug effects that are observed across people, or in the same person across time or conditions. Previous chapters have described a number of mechanisms through which drugs produce their behavioral effects, and several variables that modulate those effects. The purpose of this chapter is to consider further the variables that influence drug action.

Pharmacological and Physiological Variables

It is impossible to make sense of the effects of drugs without understanding such fundamental pharmacological concepts as dose dependence, pharmacokinetics, tolerance, cross-tolerance, accumulation, physical dependence, and drug interaction. Chapter 3 summarized these and other pharmacological concepts, and in so doing introduced a number of variables that influence the behavioral effects of drugs. Table 8-1 lists four of the most important pharmacological variables that influence drug effects. Because these variables were discussed at some length in Chapter 3, they will not be covered further here.

Table 8-1. Pharmacological Variables that May Influence　　Drug Effects

- Drug dose, physical form, and route of administration
- Time of drug administration relative to when effects are assessed
- Historical exposure to the drug in question and to other substances
- Simultaneous exposure to other drugs

As also discussed in Chapter 3, the **fate of a drug**—its absorption, distribution, biotransformation, and excretion—depends, in part, on the physical characteristics of the individual in whom it occurs. So, too, does the neurochemical initiation of its behavioral effects, as outlined in Chapter 4. Table 8-2 lists several physical characteristics of individuals that may influence the behavioral effects of drugs.

Table 8-2. Physical Characteristics of Individuals that May Influence Drug Effects

- Species
- Genotype
- Age
- Gender
- Body composition (e.g., blood volume, muscle mass, body fat)
- Presence of disease
- Blood flow
- pH of blood, urine, and other body fluids

Of course, not all of the variables listed in Table 8-2 influence the effects of every drug. Nor does a given variable necessarily influence the action of different drugs in the same way. For instance, as described in Chapter 3, the disease cirrhosis is likely to increase the magnitude and duration of the behavioral effects of drugs that are inactivated by the liver, decrease the effects of drugs that are activated by the liver, and do nothing to the actions of drugs that are not metabolized by the liver. Understanding how the variables listed in Tables 8-1 and 8-2 influence drug action is essential for the individualization of drug therapy for behavioral and other disorders, and for making sense of the effects of any drug. Every good pharmacology book (e.g., Hardman, Limbird, Molinoff, Ruddon, & Gilman, 1996) covers these variables in detail, and anyone trained in pharmacology will be conversant with them. In fact, the influence of several of these variables, such as dose and history of exposure, is so strong and pervasive that laypeople are well aware of their importance. Fewer people, however, are aware of how learning can influence drug effects, and the manner in which drug-environment interactions can contribute to a drug's behavioral effects. These are topics of paramount importance to behavioral pharmacologists, and they are the focus of the balance of this chapter.

Characteristics of Stimuli and Responses that Influence Drug Effects

Many of the interesting actions of humans and other animals involve stimulus-controlled operant or respondent behavior (see Chapter 2). In such cases, drugs can influence behavior by altering sensory or response capabilities. They can also influence behavior by altering the momentary reinforcing (or punishing) effectiveness of the historical consequences of the response. Although these three mechanisms of drug action are different, in each case the control of behavior by an antecedent stimulus is diminished. It is, however, possible to distinguish these effects, and behavioral pharmacologists have developed strategies for doing so (e.g., Heise & Milar, 1984; Picker & Negus, 1993). For our purposes, it is sufficient to discuss how these mechanisms of drug action contribute to differential drug effects across people and situations.

Antecedent Stimuli and Drug Effects

Behavior is under **stimulus control** "when a change in a particular property of a stimulus produces a change in some response characteristic, as in the rate or probability with which a response occurs" (Rilling, 1977, p. 432). It is recognized widely that drugs are capable of altering stimulus control, and studies of drug effects on **stimulus-controlled responding**—or, to use an older phrase, on discrimination and perception—are common in behavioral pharmacology (e.g., Appel & Dykstra, 1977; Picker & Negus, 1993; Thompson, 1978).

As Picker and Negus (1993) point out, "A wide variety of stimuli have been used in experiments examining the effects of drugs on stimulus control, and this work has revealed that the characteristics of the stimuli employed in a stimulus control experiment can have a profound influence on a drug's ability to alter stimulus control" (p. 136). It is probably obvious that if a drug influences behavior by altering a particular sensory modality, then the effects of that drug should be limited to behaviors controlled through that modality. For example, some aminoglycoside antimicrobials, such as neomycin and kanamycin, can damage sensory cells in the inner ear, and thereby reduce auditory acuity (Chambers & Sande, 1996). At high doses, such drugs disrupt behaviors that require auditory pitch discrimination (Stebbins & Coombs, 1975), but not similar behaviors controlled by, for example, visual stimuli. Therefore, whether or not these drugs disrupt behavior depends on the nature of the antecedent stimuli controlling behavior. In contrast, high doses of depressants such as ethanol (beverage alcohol) impair sensory acuity and stimulus control, regardless of the stimulus modality. That is, their disruption of stimulus control is far less selective than that of the aminoglycoside antibiotics.

A study examining the effects of morphine on rats' ability to detect electric shock (Poling, Simmons, & Appel, 1978) provides an example of a drug affecting an organism's ability to detect one stimulus, but not another. In this study, rats learned to detect electric shocks of low (0.05mA) and moderate (0.20 mA) intensity in a discrete-trials two-choice discrimination procedure. In brief, subjects were trained with food reinforcement to pull a chain, initiating a trial in which lights above two response levers were illuminated. On half of the trials, selected at random, electric shock was also presented. Following trials in which shock occurred, a response on a specified lever (left for two rats, right for the other two) was followed by trial termination and food delivery. A response on the other lever was followed by trial termination and an 8-second period during which the chamber was darkened and chain-pulls failed to initiate trials. Conditions were identical during non-shock trials, except the locations of the correct-response and incorrect-response levers were reversed relative to shock trials. Animals had an unlimited time in which to make a lever press after initiation of a trial, and all daily sessions lasted until 200 trials were completed. For two rats, shock intensity was initially set at 0.05 mA; for the other two, a 0.20 mA intensity was initially used. When responding stabilized at these intensities, a probe design was used to evaluate the effects of several doses of morphine (2.5-20 mg/kg). Following completion of dose-response testing, subjects initially exposed to 0.20 mA shocks were exposed to 0.05 mA shocks and vice-versa, and a second dose-response determination occurred.

Results are summarized in Figure 8-1 The mean percentage of correct responses during vehicle control sessions did not differ appreciably during shock and non-shock trials at either shock intensity; percent correct responding during shock and non-shock trials was substantially higher at the 0.20 mA intensity than at the 0.05 mA intensity. Morphine produced dose-dependent decreases in percent correct responses during shock trials at the 0.05 mA intensity. The drug did not affect percent correct responses during non-shock trials at this intensity, nor during shock or non-shock trials at the 0.20 mA intensity. Thus, it appears that morphine selectively decreased the ability of rats to detect low-intensity electric shocks, with the magnitude of the effect produced directly related to the dose administered. Similar results have been reported in other studies with both rats and monkeys (e.g., Dykstra, 1979, 1980).

The observant reader may recognize that the data presented in Figure 8-1 are consistent with the notion that, *in general, drugs affect behavior under strong discriminative stimulus control less than they affect similar behavior under weaker stimulus control.* This principle of drug action was illustrated in Chapter 5 through a comparison of drug

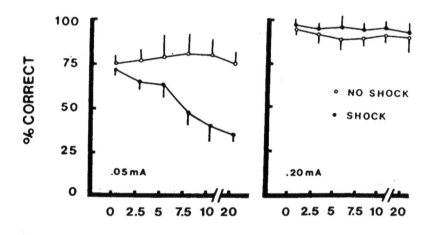

MORPHINE DOSE[MG/KG]

Figure 8-1. *Mean percent correct responses during shock and non-shock trials as a function of shock intensity and morphine dose. For the group of four rats, each control (0 mg/kg) data point represents the three vehicle control sessions that immediately preceded each of the five drug sessions, while each drug data point represents a single session. Vertical lines indicate one standard error. Data are from Poling, Simmons, and Appel (1978) and reproduced by permission.*

effects under two versions of a fixed-consecutive-number (FCN) schedule, the FCN and the FCN-S^D. Both schedules require the subject to respond a specified number of times on a work operandum, then a single time on a reinforcement operandum. Under the FCN-S^D schedule, but not the FCN schedule, an exteroceptive stimulus change is correlated with completion of the response requirement on the work operandum. Accuracy is higher (i.e., stimulus control is stronger), and drug-induced accuracy reductions generally are smaller (e.g., Laties, 1972; Picker & Negus, 1993), under the former variant. These findings were interpreted in Chapter 5 as indicating that differences in the degree of stimulus control in the absence of drug (i.e., baseline accuracy) modulated drug effects.

There is, however, an alternative explanation. Under the FCN-S^D schedule, switching from the work operandum to the reinforcement operandum is controlled by an exteroceptive stimulus, that is, by a change in the external environment. In contrast, switching under the FCN schedule is controlled by interoceptive stimuli–that is, by events occurring within the organism that are not the result of exposure to an external discriminative stimulus. It may be that behaviors controlled by interoceptive and exteroceptive stimuli are differentially sensitive to drug effects, as Laties (1972) suggested several years ago. But to demonstrate convincingly that this is the case, one must show differential drug effects under conditions where comparable baseline performances are evident when behavior is controlled by interoceptive and exteroceptive stimuli. This has rarely been attempted, and it appears that in most cases the differential drug effects that have been demonstrated under conditions of interoceptive and exteroceptive stimulus control can be subsumed under the general principle of degree of stimulus control modulating drug action.

Certainly there is good support for this principle, which also accounts for the fact that *drugs often disrupt learning to a greater extent than performance of already learned behavior*. Such an effect is readily demonstrated under repeated acquisition procedures (Chapter 5) that comprise learning and performance components. Under the former component, a new sequence of responses is learned each session. Under the latter, the same sequence of responses is emitted each session. Relatively few errors occur under the performance component (i.e., stimulus control is strong) relative to the learning component (where stimulus control is weaker), and drugs that increase errors under the latter component characteristically have little or no effect on accuracy under the former component (Thompson & Moerschbaecher, 1979; Picker & Negus, 1993).

If learning is especially sensitive to drug-induced disruption, then it is unsurprising that drinking alcohol while driving–risky behavior regardless of who engages in it–may be especially likely to result in an accident when done by inexperienced drivers. For such persons, the complex stimulus control that is required to drive safely is weakly established, hence, it is readily disrupted by alcohol. Moreover, many beginning drivers have little experience with drinking, and therefore are not tolerant to alcohol's disruptive effects. Even those with drinking histories will have done little driving while drinking, and performing the response in question in the drug state is necessary for behavioral tolerance to develop. Behavioral tolerance is an interesting phenomenon that merits attention.

Behavioral Tolerance

Behavioral tolerance (also termed contingent tolerance) is evident when the development of tolerance depends on performing the response in question in the drug state. That is, exposure to the drug alone is not sufficient to produce tolerance. This phenomenon is clearly evident with ethanol (beverage alcohol) in a study by Chen (1968). In this investigation, 12 rats were trained in a maze-running task. Once performance stabilized in the absence of drug, they were divided at random into two groups of six. Subsequently, rats in the Behavioral Group received 1.2 g/kg alcohol 20 minutes before each of four daily maze-running sessions. Rats in the Physiological Group also received four exposures to 1.2 g/kg alcohol. For them, however, the drug was administered 1 minute after the maze-running session on the first three days, and 20 minutes before the fourth session.

Relative to their performance in the absence of drug, rats in the Behavioral Group did very poorly during their first exposure to alcohol. With repeated exposure to alcohol, however, they developed tolerance to the drug's effects. By the fourth test session, they completed about the same number of runs as occurred prior to their exposure to alcohol. Rats in the Physiological Group were only tested in the drug state on day four, at which time their performance was very similar to that of the Behavioral Group when it was first exposed to alcohol. That is, the drug was highly disruptive.

In Chen's experiment, exposure to alcohol alone was not sufficient to produce tolerance, insofar as the two groups had equivalent drug histories, but only the Behavioral Group was unaffected by alcohol following three prior exposures to the drug. Clearly, performing the behavior of interest in the drug state was necessary for tolerance to develop. Procedures similar to those used by Chen have been used to demonstrate behavioral tolerance with drugs from many different classes (Branch, 1993). In some cases, of course, exposure to a drug *per se* is sufficient to induce tolerance. Nonetheless, tolerance may develop more rapidly or to a greater degree in subjects who regularly perform the response of interest in the presence of drug. Behavioral tolerance can occur in conjunction with cellular or kinetic tolerance. Interestingly, when tolerance develops under one maintenance condition, tolerance may not be evident under other maintenance conditions, even when the form of the behavior is the same. This effect is evident in a study by Smith (1990a). In this study, rats were exposed to three different environments (test chambers), each associated with a different schedule of reinforcement. In a black-walled chamber, subjects could avoid electric shocks (otherwise delivered every 5 seconds) by poking their noses into a hole. In a commercial test chamber, they could earn food by lever pressing under a fixed-interval (FI) 5-minute schedule. In a plastic chamber, they could earn food by lever pressing under a fixed-ratio (FR) 40 schedule. Subjects were exposed to each test condition once each day. When administered acutely, cocaine (3-17 mg/kg) produced dose-dependent increases in avoidance responding and dose-dependent decreases in food-maintained responding under both schedules.

After initial dose-response determinations, Smith administered 13 mg/kg cocaine each day. For the first four weeks, the drug was administered just after all behavioral testing ended. Then, in blocks of four weeks, the drug was administered shortly before testing under the FR, FI, and avoidance schedules, respectively.

Substantial tolerance developed under the FR schedule when drug was administered just before the FR session. Responding under the other schedules was not affected during this phase of the study. Even though tolerance had developed under the FR, cocaine initially reduced responding under the FI. Tolerance subsequently developed to this effect. In the final phase of the study, cocaine increased responding under the avoidance schedule, as it had initially. Again, tolerance was situation-specific. Interestingly, tolerance did not develop to the rate-increasing effects of cocaine under the avoidance schedule.

Smith's results indicate that the specific conditions under which behavior is maintained can powerfully influence whether or not tolerance is observed. Even though lever-press responding under the FR schedule had returned to baseline levels following chronic cocaine administration, the drug disrupted lever-press responding under the FI schedule. Here, a history of lever pressing in the presence of cocaine was not adequate to produce tolerance under the FI. Instead, what was required was a history of lever pressing under the FI schedule in the presence of cocaine. Tolerance established for FR lever pressing did not generalize to FI lever pressing.

Smith's (1990a) data provide a compelling demonstration of the specificity of tolerance. They also provide some support for the **reinforcement-loss hypothesis,** which has long been popular in behavioral pharmacology. It was first advanced over 30 years ago by Schuster, Dockens, and Woods (1966) as an attempt at predicting when tolerance would and would not develop to a drug's effects on operant behavior. They proposed that:

> Behavioral tolerance will develop in those aspects of the organism's behavioral repertoire where the action of the drug is such that it disrupts the organism's behavior in meeting the environmental requirements for reinforcement. Conversely, where the actions of the drug enhance, or do not affect, the organism's behavior in meeting reinforcement requirements, we do not expect the development of behavioral tolerance. (p. 181)

Smith's (1990a) findings are consistent with this analysis in two respects. First, the rate reductions produced by cocaine under the FR and FI schedules were associated with a reduction in reinforcement rates compared to control levels, and tolerance occurred under these schedules. Second, the rate increases produced by cocaine under the avoidance schedule were associated with an increase in reinforcement rates compared to control levels, and tolerance failed to occur under this schedule.[1] Both of these results are as predicted by the reinforcement-loss model of tolerance. So, too, are the results of a number of other studies. Nonetheless, and

[1] The reader may recognize that these results can be interpreted in another way: Tolerance may develop to the rate-reducing effects of cocaine, but not to its rate-increasing effects, regardless of how these effects influence rates of reinforcement. Other studies have shown that this is not the case.

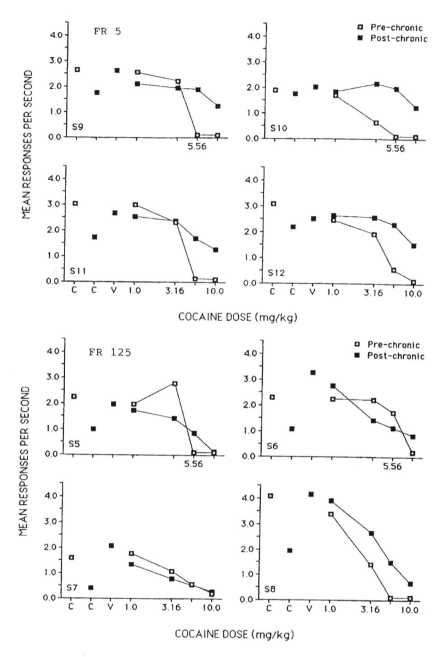

Figure 8-2. *Effects of cocaine before and after chronic exposure to daily injections of 5.6 mg/kg in pigeons exposed to simple FR 5 (upper frames) and FR 125 (lower frames) schedules of food delivery. Data are from Nickel, Alling, Kleiner, and Poling (1993) and reproduced by permission.*

despite its elegant simplicity, the reinforcement-loss hypothesis is not consistently supported by experimental findings (Corfield-Sumner & Stolerman, 1978; Wolgin, 1989).

For example, tolerance to the rate-reducing effects of cocaine and several other drugs develops readily under short FR schedules (e.g., FR 5), but develops less readily, if at all, under long FR schedules (e.g., FR 125), although drug-induced reinforcement loss occurs regardless of FR size (e.g., Genovese, Elsmore, & Witkin, 1988; Hoffman, Branch, & Sizemore, 1987; Hughes & Branch, 1991; Smith, 1986b, 1990b). This effect is evident in Figure 8-2, which shows that in pigeons tolerance developed to the effects of cocaine under an FR 5 schedule of food delivery, but not under an FR 125 schedule.

The reinforcement-loss hypothesis as proposed by Schuster et al. (1966) cannot account for the effects of FR size on tolerance. As Branch and his colleagues have emphasized (Hoffman et al., 1987; Hughes & Branch, 1991), reinforcement loss may be a necessary but not sufficient condition for the development of tolerance under FR schedules.

In a significant extension of the reinforcement-loss model, Smith (1986a) suggested that the development of tolerance may be influenced by relative, as well as absolute, reinforcement loss. In his study, which used rats as subjects, tolerance to the rate-increasing and reinforcement-decreasing effects of 1.0 mg/kg d-amphetamine under an interresponse-time-greater-than-t (IRT>t) schedule of food delivery failed to develop when a multiple IRT>t random-ratio (RR) schedule was arranged. Tolerance developed (i.e.,. rates decreased) rapidly when the RR component was terminated. Reinstatement of the RR component produced increases in responding under the IRT > t component.

A possible interpretation of these results is in terms of the costliness of drug-induced reinforcement decreases under the IRT > t schedule relative to the total reinforcement received each session. As Smith (1986a) put it,

> Pharmacological tolerance is thought to sometimes be influenced by a behavioral process such as "response cost," so that more "costly" drug effects result in more rapid tolerance development than do less "costly" drug effects. The relative "costliness" of drug-related lost reinforcers is clearly not the same under all conditions, however. When all, or even most, of the total available reinforcers come from a single schedule, then responding under that schedule may be greatly influenced by those lost reinforcers and behavioral tolerance may develop rapidly. (pp. 298-299)

Results of Smith's (1986a) study demonstrate unequivocally that the context in which a drug's effects are evaluated can play an important role in determining whether or not tolerance is observed. These results, and those of other studies summarized in this section and in prior discussions of Siegel's respondent conditioning model of tolerance (Chapters 2 and 7), make it clear that environmental variables, including drug-behavior interactions, modulate not just the initial effects of a drug, but also the extent to which behavior adapts to those effects. This is a point of fundamental importance, and we have digressed from considering stimulus and response characteristics in order to make it. We now return to those variables.

Response Characteristics and Drug Effects

Perhaps because convenience and precedent dictate that they study simple repetitive movements, such as key pecks by pigeons and lever presses by rats and monkeys (Chapter 5), behavioral pharmacologists have largely ignored the topography (physical form) of operant behavior as a potential determinant of drug action. There is, for example, no mention of this variable in a recent text devoted to methods in behavioral pharmacology (van Haaren, 1993). Some researchers have, however, shown that response characteristics influence drug effects, as when substances that produce tremors or muscular weakness selectively disrupt operants defined by force requirements (e.g., Fowler, 1992).

In some cases, drugs simply disrupt motor activity. For example, curare prevents muscular contractions, making it impossible to emit most operant responses. Other drugs produce more specific incapacitation. Ethanol, for instance, at sufficiently high doses makes it impossible for men to produce and sustain erections, although they may be able to emit other responses. Sildenafil citrate (Viagra), in contrast, works in the opposite direction. It allows many men with erectile dysfunction to produce erections in erotic situations.

As the example of ethanol illustrates, drugs can produce changes in behavior that are incompatible with the performance of some operant responses, but not others. For example, extrapyramidal side effects (Parkinsonian reactions and tardive dyskinesias), which encompass a variety of uncontrollable movements, frequently occur in people treated with neuroleptic drugs (e.g., Poling, Gadow, & Cleary, 1991). Whether these side effects are serious for a given patient depends, in part, on the specific movements involved and on the behaviors that are especially important for the patient. For instance, drug-induced tongue thrusting and chewing movements might interfere with a person's ability to sing, and would be especially dire for a person who made a living by singing. Drug-induced tremors of the hands probably would be less significant with respect to that person's livelihood. In contrast, for a surgeon, tremors, but not tongue-thrusts, would be professionally debilitating.

In addition to the physical form of the behavior, the conditions under which it is maintained play an important role in determining drug effects. For this reason, as pointed out in Chapter 5, it is almost always impossible to describe in a meaningful way how a drug affects broad categories of behavior, such as "aggression," "locomotion," or "sleep." As a case in point, predatory attack, intermale attack, and infanticide are often considered as "aggressive" behaviors in rodents, and assays involving these behaviors are used frequently to examine drug effects on "aggression" (Kemble, Blanchard, & Blanchard, 1993). In mice, however, fluprazine does not alter predation on insect larvae, but it does reduce intermale attact and infanticide (Parmigiani & Palanza, 1991). Thus, the drug's effect on "aggressive" behavior varies.

Even if "aggression" is broken into subcategories, drug effects may depend on the specifics of the response in question and the maintenance conditions. For instance, as with the predation of mice on insect larvae, fluprazine does not alter rats' predation on earthworms. The drug does, however, disrupt rats' predation on leopard frogs (Schultz & Kemble, 1986). Here, the characteristics of the prey species –which influences, in part, the form of the predatory behavior-modulated drug effects. Clearly, no simple statement regarding the effects of fluprazine on "aggression" is possible. The same typically is true regarding the effects of other drugs on similarly large and ill-defined response categories.

Consequences of Operant Behavior and Drug Effects

In some cases, drugs act as establishing operations, which (as discussed in Chapters 2 and 7) alter the reinforcing (or punishing) effectiveness of other stimuli. When this occurs, drug effects are **consequence-dependent**. That is, the action of the drug on operant behavior depends on the kinds of events that control the response in question. A noteworthy example of a consequence-dependent drug effect involves the ability of certain sedative-hypnotic drugs selectively to increase punished responding.

This effect was first demonstrated by Geller and Seifter (1960), who initially exposed rats to a multiple FR 1 variable-interval (VI) 2-minute schedule of food delivery. A tone was present during the FR 1 component, but not during the VI 2-minute component. After responding stabilized, conditions were changed so that responses during the tone produced a brief electric shock (delivered to the rat's feet), as well as food. This procedure was punishing, insofar as response rates in the presence of the tone decreased relative to pre-shock levels. Geller and Seifter reported that three sedative-hypnotic drugs with marked anxiolytic properties, phenobarbital, pentobarbital, and meprobamate, increased punished responding. In contrast, a stimulant (d-amphetamine) and a neuroleptic (promazine) decreased punished responding. Geller and Seifter proposed that their procedure assessed "conflict," and variations of it have frequently been used by researchers interested in conflict behaviors as animal models for the study of anxiety (Commissaris, 1993). Those researchers have reported that these animals models have good predictive validity for, as Commissaris (1993) notes, with the exception of propranolol and yohimbine, "there is a strong concordance between the effects of drugs in the clinical management of anxiety and the effects of drugs on conflict behavior" (p. 465). In most cases, drugs that have selective antipunishment effects also produce anxiolytic (anxiety-reducing) effects in humans.

Of course, when rates are much different in the presence and absence of punishment, it may be the case that what appear to be punishment-specific drug effects actually are rate-dependent effects (which were introduced in Chapter 5 and are discussed further in the following section). This possibility has been evaluated and generally rejected. For example, Cook and Catania (1964) exposed monkeys to a concurrent VI 6-minute VI 2-minute schedule of food delivery. A VI 2-minute schedule of shock delivery was also in effect during the VI 2-minute food schedule.

By adjusting shock intensity, Cook and Catania produced comparable response rates during the two food schedules. After this occurred, they examined the effects of meprobamate.

As shown in Figure 8-3, meprobamate produced dose-dependent increases in punished responding, but not in unpunished responding. This occurred even though rates were roughly equal in the absence of drug, which shows that the effects of meprobamate were punishment-selective, not rate-dependent. Similar effects have been demonstrated for several other sedative-hypnotic drugs. In fact, many drugs said to have "disinhibitory" properties (e.g., ethanol, various barbiturates and benzodiazepines) attenuate the effects of punishment, and this may be a major aspect of their behavioral mechanism of action.

Even with such drugs, however, antipunishment effects are not always observed. For instance, McKearney (1976) examined the effects of d-amphetamine and pentobarbital under FI 5-minute schedules of food delivery and stimulus-shock termination. After responding stabilized, a punishment contingency was added such that every thirtieth response produced a brief shock. After responding stabilized, drug effects were evaluated.

As usually occurs, under the food-reinforcement schedule d-amphetamine reduced the rate of punished responding and pentobarbital increased it. Results were reversed, however, under the shock-postponement schedule, where d-amphetamine

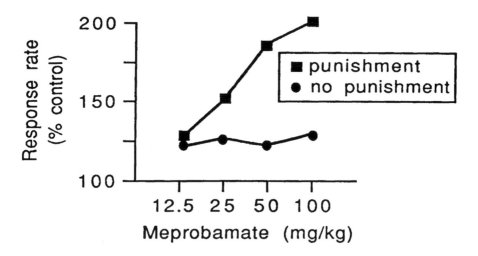

Figure 8-3. *Response rates of a squirrel monkey under a concurrent VI 6-min VI 2-min schedule of food delivery as a function of meprobamate dose. Drug effects were examined under conditions where electric shock punishment was arranged under the VI 2-min component and rates were comparable in the two components. Data are redrawn from Cook and Catania (1964) and reproduced by permission.*

increased punished responding and pentobarbital decreased it. As Branch (1993) emphasizes:

> These results illustrate an important fact; one must be careful not to oversimplify the description of a drug's effects on behavior. Before the advent of Behavioral Pharmacology, effects of drugs on "behavior" were discussed, giving rise to terms like "stimulant" and "depressant." Such terms, however, quickly became far too general. Subsequently, descriptions about drug effect on avoidance behavior, punished behavior, positively reinforced behavior, etc., gained popularity. Data such as those of McKearney, however, indicate that even these "refinements" in descriptions of drug action may be incorrect. Behavioral Pharmacology has shown that drug effects depend critically on the specifics of the variables responsible for the behavior being examined. Seemingly minor characteristics of stimulus circumstances, scheduling of consequences, and other variables all can contribute to a drug's action on behavior. One of the major goals of Behavioral Pharmacology is to be able to offer meaningful, relatively general statements about drug-behavior interactions. These general statements, however, will have to be of a form that explains the complexity that already has been shown to exist. (pp. 48-49)

Put differently, *descriptions of the behavioral effects of drugs and the variables that modulate drug effects should be as simple as possible, but no simpler.* Although not all of these variables are operative in every situation, it is clear that the consequences of behavior, as well it's antecedents, its form, the specific relations among stimuli and responses that maintain behavior, and the context in which those relations are arranged are important determinants of drug action. So, too, it appears, is the rate of behavior in the absence of drug, as discussed in the following section.

Rate-Dependent Drug Effects

As described in Chapter 5, in one of the first influential studies in behavioral pharmacology Dews (1955) reported that pentobarbital's behavioral effects were strongly influenced by the ongoing rate of behavior in the absence of drug, that is, they were **rate dependent**. Subsequent studies reported rate-dependent effects for drugs from many different classes. Of course, as noted previously, not all drugs with rate-dependent effects mimic pentobarbital's ability to increase high-rate responding at doses that reduce low-rate responding. For example, at low-to-moderate doses, amphetamines increase low-rate operant responding but reduce high-rate operant responding (Dews & Wenger, 1977).[2]

---

[2]According to Kelleher and Morse (1969), low-rate operants are separated in time by more than one second; shorter interresponse times are indicative of high-rate responding. This standard has not been universally applied. One criticism of rate dependency as an explanatory construct is that high and low rates are some times defined after the fact, e.g., rates increased by a moderate dose of amphetamine are "low," whereas those reduced by the same dose are "high." This criticism loses force if rate dependency is envisioned as purely descriptive.

One common technique for studying rate-dependent drug effects involves giving drugs to subjects exposed to schedules that engender very different response rates, for example, short FR and long FI schedules of food delivery. Another common technique involves a detailed analysis of drug effects on responding under FI schedules. Animals exposed to such schedules typically emit few responses early in the interval but respond much more rapidly as the interval progresses. Hence, if each fixed interval is divided temporally into a number of sequential segments (e.g., 10), a range of baseline rates will be evident.

In most studies concerned with rate-dependent drug effects, data are plotted as shown in Figure 8-4. Here, drug-induced proportional changes in response rates (i.e., drug rates expressed as a percentage of control rates) are graphed as a function of control rates. Drug rates are scaled linearly and control rates are scaled logarithmically and data are interpreted as showing rate dependency if the data fall along a straight line with a slope other than zero.

When data concerning the effects of d-amphetamine on schedule-controlled responding are graphed as just described, the regression line that best fits the data frequently has a slope of about -1 (Gonzales & Byrd, 1977a, b). In such cases, as illustrated in Table 8-3, response rate in the presence of drug is constant regardless of control rate, and control and drug rates are independent of one another. Nonetheless, when drug rates are expressed as a percentage of control rates, it appears

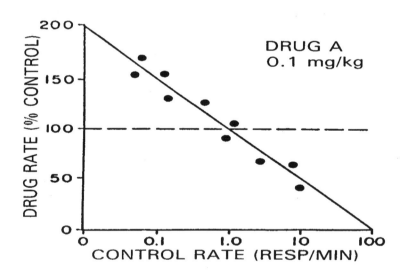

Figure 8-4. *Data showing what commonly are considered as rate-dependent effects for a hypothetical drug. Each data point represents the effects of administering the drug on a single occasion under a condition associated with a particular response rate in the absence of drug. Note that the magnitude and direction of the change in responding induced by the drug are dependent on the rate of behavior in the absence of drug.*

Table 8-3. Hypothetical Data Showing Rate Constancy

Absolute Control Rate	Absolute Drug Rate	Drug Rate as a Percentage of Control
0.10 responses/minute	10.00 responses/minute	10,000
1.00 responses/minute	10.00 responses/minute	1,000
10.00 responses/minute	10.00 responses/minute	100
100.00 responses/minute	10.00 responses/minute	10

that the effects of the drug depend upon the rate of behavior in the absence of drug. In view of this, Gonzales and Byrd (1977a) have proposed rate constancy as an alternative to the rate-dependency "hypothesis." Byrd (1981) describes **rate constancy** as follows:

> According to rate constancy, a drug reduces the variability in the rate at which the behavior occurs, and responding approaches a more constant rate. The higher the drug dose, within limits, the more constant and uniform the rate. (p. 85)

Advocates of the rate constancy analysis recommend that data be plotted with absolute drug rate along the y-axis and absolute control rate (both plotted in logarithmic coordinates) along the x-axis (Byrd, 1981). This suggestion has rarely been followed.

To date, research concerning rate-dependent drug effects has almost exclusively involved nonhuman subjects. While there is no good reason to believe that rate-dependent drug effects cannot be observed with humans in their usual environment, those who hope to extend the rate-dependency analysis of drug effects to human behavior should recognize that rate dependency is an explanatory construct only in that it describes a relation between two variables: the relative change in response rate following drug administration and the nondrug response rate. As McKearney and Barrett (1978) contend:

> It is important to note that neither in its initial statement nor in its later elaboration by Dews or his colleagues was this [the rate-dependency analysis] any more than a description of the effects of certain drugs, and as a factor that might predict drug effects in certain situations. It did not, and indeed does not, directly "explain" the effects of drugs. It is still a descriptive statement, not a "theory" or "hypothesis," and its generality and biological significance, rather than truth or falsity, are what should be elaborated experimentally. (p. 26)

Nevertheless, several early studies provided evidence that the rate and temporal patterning of responding was a much more powerful and general determinant of drug effect than the consequences that were maintaining behavior. This was demonstrated in early studies of nonhumans (e.g., Cook & Catania, 1964; Kelleher & Morse, 1964) in which roughly comparable rates of responding were maintained under schedules of food delivery, escape from electric shock, or termination of a stimulus associated with forthcoming shock. In the Cook and Catania study, only FI schedules were examined, whereas Kelleher and Morse used both FI and FR schedules. In both studies, the effects of several drugs (chlordiazepoxide, chlorpromazine, d-amphetamine, and imipramine) did not depend on the consequences that maintained behavior. In the Kelleher and Morse investigation, the effects of both chlorpromazine and d-amphetamine differed under the FR and FI schedules. The former evoked considerably higher response rates than did the latter, thus these findings are consistent with the notion that the effects of certain drugs are rate-dependent, irrespective of the consequences maintaining behavior.

More recent investigations, however, "provide overwhelming evidence that the type of event controlling behavior can be an important aspect of the environment contributing to the behavioral effects of a number of drugs" (Barrett, 1981, p. 175). This is evident in the results of a study by Barrett (1976), who found that pentobarbital, ethanol, and chlordiazepoxide increased monkeys' responding maintained by food delivery but decreased similar rates of responding engendered by shock presentation. Cocaine, in contrast, similarly affected responding maintained by the two events. Other examples of drugs producing consequence-dependent effects were provided earlier in this chapter.

Although rate-dependent analyses of drug effects were once a cornerstone of behavioral pharmacology, it has become clear that such analyses are limited in scope and explanatory value. Nonetheless, it also is clear that baseline response rates do influence, in part, the observed effects of many drugs. Given this, it is important that researchers distinguish between rate-altering and other effects of the substances that they study.

A case in point is a study by Dykstra and Appel (1972), which was designed to examine the effects of LSD on auditory discrimination in rats. In this study, rats initially were trained through differential reinforcement to discriminate between 600 and 1,000 hertz tones. After extended training, response rates were high in the presence of the tone during which food was available (S^D), and much lower in the presence of the tone during which extinction was arranged (S^{delta}). That is, the rats' behavior appeared to be stimulus controlled. After this occurred, Dykstra and Appel exposed the rats to tones of other frequencies in the presence and absence of 0.08 and 0.16 mg/kg doses of LSD, thereby establishing generalization gradients.

In the absence of drug, response rates declined progressively as the difference between the frequency of the test stimulus and the S^D increased. Dykstra and Appel (1972) reasoned that, if LSD interfered with rats' ability to discriminate among auditory stimuli, then generalization gradients should be flatter in the presence of the drug than in its absence. That is, responses rates during presentation of stimuli that differed from the S^D should be higher during the drug condition than during baseline. Such an effect was observed when absolute response rates were considered, suggesting that LSD altered stimulus control. But when absolute rates were considered, it was apparent that "these effects can be attributed to drug-induced changes in the animal's rate of responding; thus, the drug is not affecting sensitivity but is, rather, affecting the animal's response output" (Dykstra & Appel, 1972, p. 722).

This study illustrates the importance of disentangling a drug's effects on sensory function from its effects on the behavior used to index sensory function. Doing so is as important in studies of humans as in studies of laboratory animals. As Appel and Dykstra (1977) note:

> While the effects which humans report following LSD or morphine might indeed reflect drug-induced changes in acuity, threshold, or other index of ability to detect the presence or absence of visual or painful stimuli, we cannot objectively study such changes except by measuring some corre-lated change in behavior which is assumed to indicate the subject's "capacity to discriminate." But such behavior may also be altered by these same drugs; thus, it becomes difficult, if not impossible, to separate the effect of the drug on discriminatory processes (sensitivity) from its effect on the subject's behavior or response criterion (bias) in the presence of the discrimination situation. (p. 141)

Signal detection theory (Green & Swets, 1966) was devised to separate the effects of nonpharmacological variables on sensitivity (response accuracy) as op-posed to response bias (a tendency to select one of the response alternatives) and has been employed occasionally to study drug-behavior interactions (e.g., Appel & Dykstra, 1977; Pontecorvo & Clissold, 1993). The assumptions and methods of signal detection theory are too complex to be covered here. For our purposes, it is sufficient to emphasize that a drug is apt to have many different behavioral effects, and it is all too easy to confuse one with another. If, for instance, Dykstra and Appel (1972) had not recognized the possibility that LSD's effects were rate dependent in their study and looked at their data with this in mind, they would have erroneously concluded that the drug disrupted auditory discrimination. Such mistakes can best be avoided by, first, being fully cognizant of the variables that influence drug action and, second, not holding strongly to preconceived notions about a drug's behavioral effects. LSD, for example, is the prototype of hallucinogenic drugs, and the most notable effect of such drugs is perceptual. Thus, most people probably assume that the drug disrupts visual and other discriminations. Nonetheless, LSD characteristi-cally does not do so (e.g, Dykstra & Appel, 1974; Appel, Poling, & Kuhn, 1982). Sometimes, scientific findings are inconsistent with widely held beliefs.

Learning and Drug Effects

As emphasized throughout this book, behavioral pharmacology is unique in emphasizing that drugs can be construed as stimuli that affect behavior in the context of operant and respondent conditioning. Many of the functional stimulus properties of drugs are not innate characteristics of the compounds, but are instead acquired as the result of a particular history. Put differently, they are learned. Given this, drug effects are not fixed across people, but rather vary to some degree as a function of differences in learning histories and the variables that those histories comprise. The extent to which learning influences drug action varies as a function of the drug and effect being considered but, as emphasized in Chapters 2, 5, 6, 7 and 10, its importance can be considerable. To emphasize this point further, we now consider three studies by Hughes and his associates that demonstrate how drug effects can be modulated by rules. Rules, that is, what people say to themselves and to others about the effects of drugs, can be construed as cognitive factors and are the "set" in the "set and setting" traditionally proposed to modulate drug effects. "Setting," of course, is the actual environment in which drug effects are assessed.

A study by Hughes, Pickens, Spring, and Keenan (1985) provides clear evidence of verbal mediation of drug effects. In that study, cigarette smokers were given concurrent access to nicotine and placebo gums during a period of abstinence from smoking. In the first experiment, subjects were told that they would receive either nicotine or placebo gum. Under these conditions, they consistently administered nicotine but not placebo gum, which suggests that nicotine was serving as a reinforcer. Two subsequent experiments examined the possibility that subjects self-administered nicotine at a greater rate than placebo gum because they believed that the gum with more side effects (nicotine gum) was the active gum, not because the nicotine gum was more reinforcing. In the second study, subjects were told they would receive either a marketed nicotine gum or a different nicotine gum (actually placebo) that was as effective but had fewer side effects. In the third study, subjects were told that the placebo gum had more side effects than the nicotine gum. In both studies, subjects did not self-administer nicotine gum at a rate greater than placebo gum, indicating that instructions altered the reinforcing effectiveness of nicotine. In a similar study, Hughes, Strickler, King, Higgins, Fenwick, Gulliver, and Mireault (1989b) gave two groups of cigarette smokers concurrent access to placebo and nicotine gums. One group, but not the other, was explicitly told that nicotine was available. Subjects who were informed of nicotine availability self-administered nicotine at a greater rate than placebo, but the uninformed subjects did not. As in the Hughes et al. (1985) study, it appears that instructions altered the reinforcing effectiveness of nicotine.

A third study by Hughes and his associates (Hughes, Gulliver, Amori, Mireault, & Fenwick, 1989a) found that, when cigarette smokers tried to stop smoking, both receiving nicotine gum and receiving a placebo described as nicotine gum increased the number of days abstinent and decreased the number of cigarettes smoked. This outcome suggest that instructions alone had therapeutic effects. Several other dependent variables were examined in this study, which used a three (instructed that gum was placebo, nicotine gum, or unspecified) by two (placebo gum or nicotine gum) factorial design. Some interactions between the treatment variables occurred and the overall results indicated that "the effects of instructions and nicotine (1) are not mutually exclusive, (2) vary across independent variables, and (3) can interact such that instructions modify the therapeutic and subjective effects of nicotine" (Hughes et al., 1989a, p. 486).

Although the authors of a major review article (Hull & Bond, 1986) suggested that instructions rarely influence drug action, at least when alcohol is the drug in question, the findings of Hughes et al. (1989a) call this conclusion into question. In their study, instructions influenced whether nicotine produced any therapeutic, reinforcing, or subjective effects, not just the magnitude of these effects. Here, both the pharmacological effects of nicotine and instructions were important determinants of behavior. Rules (instructions) apparently altered the behavioral functions of the subjective effects of the drug. As Hughes et al. (1989a) noted in discussing gum self-administration, "when subjects are told they are receiving nicotine gum, the stimulus effects are probably labeled as indicators of therapeutic efficacy [which renders these effects positively reinforcing] whereas when they were told they received placebo, the same stimulus effects are labeled as side-effects [which renders them aversive]" (p. 490).

The findings of Hughes and his coworkers clearly demonstrate that what people are told about nicotine influences the drug's behavioral effects. Similar effects have been demonstrated with other drugs, including marijuana and cocaine, and with placebo substances (Poling & LeSage, 1992). In fact, it appears that in general instructions indicating that subjects will receive active drug increase the magnitude of placebo effects and the amount of placebo medication self-administered.

The studies considered here and elsewhere in this book demonstrate that rules can significantly influence both the quantitative and qualitative effects of active drugs and placebos. Certainly the rules, or instructions, that people are given concerning various substances can substantially alter the behavioral effects of those substances. Self-generated rules appear to be capable of doing the same. Consider an athlete who begins using anabolic steroids. It is probable that drug self-administration is preceded by the person covertly verbalizing something to the effect that "taking this will make me stronger." This rule describes a behavior (taking the steroid) and a desired outcome (getting stronger). Following the rule leads to the initiation and maintenance of such behavior. That this process works is evident by the fact that anabolic steroids (drugs that resemble testosterone in their effects) have recently been classified as controlled - they have abuse potential. But this potential does not appear to reside in their immediate subjective effects. Unlike most drugs of abuse, they do not make people "feel good" soon after they are taken. Also unlike most such drugs, they probably do not function as positive reinforcers in the absence of verbal mediation. That this is so does not, however, in any way reduce the dangers associated with them, or make them fundamentally unlike other drugs of abuse. Verbal mediation—which is learned behavior—often plays a role in determining the effects of abused substances (see Chapter 10), and of many other drugs as well.

Concluding Comments

It should by now be apparent to the reader that many variables, not all intuitively obvious, interact to determine a drug's behavioral effects. As emphasized in this chapter, these factors include response rate in the absence of drug, the consequences that maintain (or suppress) behavior, and the degree to which responding is stimulus-controlled. The topography of the behavior in question may also influence a drug's effects, as when a compound that induces tremor disrupts performance of an operant response that requires fine-motor skill but has no such effect when only gross responses are demanded. A drug's stimulus properties also dictate its behavioral effects, as do pharmacological variables such as dosage and schedule of administration.

Because drug effects depend upon a wide range of factors, both currently operative and historical, it stands to reason that a given drug can produce dramatically different behavioral actions in different people, or in the same individual at different times and places. Consider two adolescents with mental retardation who engage in self-injurious biting, for which each is treated with the same dose of a neuroleptic drug. Self-injury allows one adolescent to terminate aversive encounters with staff but enables the second to prevent such encounters. Here, biting would be maintained as an escape response for the first client and as an avoidance response for the second. It would not be surprising if the drug's effects on self-biting differed in these individuals, for neuroleptics often interfere with avoidance responding at doses that have no effect on escape responding. If this held true in the present example, Client 1's self-biting would be unaffected by doses of a neuroleptic that suppressed the response in Client 2. This is perfectly lawful and comprehensible if the role of behavioral and environmental variables in determining drug effects is acknowledged, but a mystery if they are ignored. A drug's behavioral effects are rarely simple, but they are always lawful. Making this point clear and isolating the factors that contribute to a drug's behavioral actions are two major contributions to the understanding of drug effects in humans that have arisen from the efforts of behavioral pharmacologists.

References

Appel, J. B., & Dykstra, L. A. (1977). Drugs, discrimination, and signal detection theory. In T. Thompson & P. B. Dews (Eds.), *Advances in behavioral pharmacology* (Vol. 1, pp. 140-166). New York: Academic Press.

Appel, J. B., Poling, A., & Kuhn, D. (1982). The behavioral pharmacology of psychotomimetics. In F. Hoffmeister & G. Stille (Eds.), *Handbook of experimental pharmacology* (Vol. 55, pp. 45-56). New York: Springer-Verlag.

Barrette, J. E. (1976). Effects of alcohol, chlordiazepoxide, cocaine, and pentobarbital on responding maintained under fixed-interval schedules of food or shock presentation. *Journal of Pharmacology and Experimental Therapeutics, 196*, 605-615.

Barrette, J. E. (1981). Differential drug effects as a functional of the controlling consequences. In T. Thompson & C. Johanson (Eds.), *Behavioral pharmacology of human drug dependence* (pp. 159-181). Washington, DC: US Government Printing Office.

Branch, M. N. (1993). Behavioral factors in drug tolerance. In F. van Haaren (Ed.), *Methods in behavioral pharmacology* (pp. 329-347). Amsterdam: Elsevier.

Chambers, H. F., & Sande, M. A. (1996). The aminoglycosides. In J. Hardman, L. E. Bimbird, P. B. Molinoff, R. W. Ruddon & A. G. Gilman (Eds.), *The pharmacological basis of therapeutics* (pp. 1103-1121). New York: McGraw-Hill.

Chen, C. S. (1968). A study of the alcohol-tolerance effect and an introduction of a new behavioral technique. *Psychopharmacologia 12*, 433-440.

Commissaris, R. L. (1993). Conflict behaviors as animal models for the study of anxiety. In F. van Haaren (Ed.), *Methods in behavioral pharmacology* (pp. 443-474). Amsterdam: Elsevier.

Cook, L., & Catania, A. C. (1964). Effects of drugs on avoidance and escape behavior. *Federation Proceedings, 23*, 818-835.

Dews, P. B., & Wenger, G. R. (1977). Rate dependency of the behavioral effects of amphetamine. In T. Thompson & P. B. Dews (Eds.), *Advances in behavioral pharmacology* (Vol. 1, pp. 167-227). New York: Academic Press.

Dykstra, L. A. (1979). Effects of morphine, diazepam and chlorpromazine on discrimination of electric shock. *Journal of Pharmacology and Experimental Therapeutics, 209*, 297-303.

Dykstra, L. A. (1980). Discrimination of electric shock: Effects of some opioid and nonopioid drugs. *Journal of Pharmacology and Experimental Therapeutics, 213*, 234-240.

Dykstra, L. A., & Appel, J. B. (1972). Lysergic acid diethylamide and stimulus generalization: Rate-dependent effects. *Science, 177*, 720-722.

Dykstra, L. A., & Appel, J. B. (1974). Effects of LSD on auditory perception: A signal detection analysis. *Psychopharmacologia, 34*, 289-307.

Fowler, S. C. (1992). Force and duration of operant responses as dependent variables in behavioral pharmacology. In T. Thompson, P. B. Dews & J. E. Barrett (Eds.), *Neurobehavioral pharmacology* (pp. 83-128). Hillsdale, NJ: Erlbaum.

Geller, I., & Seifter, J. (1960). The effects of meprobamate, barbiturates, *d*-amphetamine and promazine on experimentally-induced conflict in the rat. *Psychopharmacologia, 1*, 482-492.

Genovese, R. F., Elsmore, T. F., & Witkin, J. M. (1988). Environmental influences on the development of tolerance to the effects of physostigmine on schedule-controlled behavior. *Psychopharmacology, 96*, 462-467.

Gonzales, F. A., & Byrd, L. D. (1977a). Mathematics underlying the rate-dependency hypothesis. *Science, 195*, 546-550.

Gonzales, F. A., & Byrd, L. D. (1977b). Rate-dependency hypothesis. *Science, 198*, 1977.

Green, D. M., & Swets, J. A. (1966). *Signal detection theory and psychophysics*. New York: Wiley.

Hardman, J. G., Limbird, L. E., Molinoff, P. B., Ruddon, R. W., & Gilman, A. G. (1996). *The pharmacological basis of therapeutics*. New York: McGraw-Hill.

Heise, G. A., & Milar, K. S. (1984). Drugs and stimulus control. In L. L. Iversen, S. D. Iversen & S. J. Snyder (Eds.), *Handbook of psychopharmacology* (Vol. 18, pp. 129-190). New York: Plenum Press.

Hoffman, S. H., Branch, M. N., & Sizemore, G. M. (1987). Cocaine tolerance: Acute versus chronic effects as dependent upon fixed-ratio size. *Journal of the Experimental Analysis of Behavior, 47*, 363-376.

Hughes, C. E., & Branch, M. N. (1991). Tolerance to and residual effects of cocaine in squirrel monkeys depend on reinforcement-schedule parameter. *Journal of the Experimental Analysis of Behavior, 56,* 345-360.

Hughes, J. R., Gulliver, S. B., Amori, G., Mireault, G., & Fenwick, J. E. (1989a). Effects of instructions and nicotine on smoking cessation, withdrawal symptoms and self-administration of nicotine gum. *Psychopharmacology, 99,* 486-491.

Hughes, J. R., Pickens, R. W., Spring, W., & Keenan, R. M. (1985). Instructions control whether nicotine will serve as a reinforcer. *Journal of Pharmacology and Experimental Therapeutics, 235,* 106-112.

Hughes, J. R., Strickler, G., King, D., Higgins, S. T., Fenwick, J. W., Gulliver, S. B., & Mireault, G. (1989b). Smoking history, instructions and the effects of nicotine: Two pilot studies. *Pharmacology Biochemistry and Behavior, 34,* 149-155.

Hull, J. G., & Bond, C. F. (1986). Social and behavioral consequences of alcohol consumption and expectancy: A meta-analysis. *Psychological Bulletin, 99,* 347-360.

Kelleher, R. T., & Morse, W. H. (1964). Escape behavior and punished behavior. *Federation Proceedings, 23,* 808-817.

Kelleher, R. T., & Morse, W. H. (1969). Determinants of the behavioral effects of drugs. In D. H. Tedeschi & R. E. Tedeschi (Eds.), *Importance of fundamental principles in drug evaluation* (pp. 1-60). New York: Appleton-Century-Crofts.

Kemble, E. D., Blanchard, D. C., & Blanchard, R. J. (1993). Methods in behavioral pharmacology: Measurement of aggression. In F. van Haaren (Ed.), *Methods in behavioral pharmacology* (pp. 539-559). Amsterdam: Elsevier.

Laties, V. G. (1972). The modification of drug effects on behavior by external discriminative stimuli. *Journal of Pharmacology and Experimental Therapeutics, 183,* 1-13.

McKearney, J. W. (1976). Punishment of responding under schedules of stimulus-shock termination: Effects of *d*-amphetamine and pentobarbital. *Journal of the Experimental Analysis of Behavior, 26,* 281-287.

McKearney, J. W., & Barrett, J. E. (1978). Schedule-controlled behavior and the effects of drugs. In D. E. Blackman & D. J. Sanger (Eds.), *Contemporary research in behavioral pharmacology* (pp. 1-68). New York: Plenum Press.

Nickel, M., Alling, K., Kleiner, M., & Poling, A. (1993). Fixed-ratio size as a determinant of tolerance to cocaine: Is relative or absolute size important? *Behavioural Pharmacology, 4,* 471-478.

Parmigiani, S., & Palanza, P. (1991). Fluprazine inhibits intermale attack and infanticide, but not predation, in male mice. *Neuroscience and Biobehavioral Research, 15,* 511-513.

Picker, M., & Negus, S. (1993). Drugs and stimulus control: Generalization, discrimination and threshold procedures. In F. van Haaren (Ed.), *Methods in behavioral pharmacology* (pp. 117-145).

Poling, A., & LeSage, M. (1992). Rule-governed behavior and human behavioral pharmacology: A brief comment on an important topic. *Analysis of Verbal Behavior, 10,* 37-44.

Poling, A., Gadow, K., & Cleary, J. (1991). *Drug therapy for behavior disorders: An introduction.* New York: Pergamon Press.

Poling, A., Simmon, M., & Appel, J. B. (1978). Morphine and shock detection: Effects of shock intensity. *Psychopharmacological Communications, 2,* 333-336.

Pontecorvo, M. J., & Clissold, D. B. (1993). Complex and delayed discriminations: automated repeated measures techniques. In F. van Haaren (Ed.), *Methods in behavioral pharmacology* (pp.147-193). Amsterdam: Elsevier.

Rilling, M. (1977). Stimulus control and inhibitory processes. In W. K. Honig & J. E. R. Staddon (Eds.), *Handbook of operant behavior* (pp. 432-480). Englewood Cliffs, NJ: Prentice-Hall.

Schultz, L. A., & Kemble, E. D. (1986). Prey-dependent effects of fluprazine hydrochloride on predatory aggression northern grasshopper mice (*Onychomys leucogaster*) and rats (*Rattus norvegicus*). *Aggression and Behavior, 12,* 267-275.

Schuster, C. R., Dockens, W. S., & Woods, J. H. (1966). Behavioral variables affecting the development of amphetamine tolerance. *Psychopharmacologia, 9,* 170-182.

Smith, J. B. (1986a). Effects of chronically administered *d*-amphetamine on spaced responding maintained under multiple and single-component schedules. *Psychopharmacology, 88,* 296-300.

Smith, J. B. (1986b). Effects of fixed-ratio length on the development of tolerance to decreased responding by *l*-nantradol. *Psychopharmacology, 90,* 259-262.

Smith, J. B. (1990a). Situational specificity of tolerance to decreased operant responding by cocaine. *Pharmacology Biochemistry and Behavior, 36,* 993-995.

Smith, J. B. (1990b). Effects of fixed-ratio requirement on observed tolerance to decreased responding by clonidine. *Pharmacology Biochemistry and Behavior, 36,* 993-995.

Stebbins, W. C., & Coombs, S. (1975). Behavioral assessment of ototoxicity in nonhuman primates. In B. Weiss & V. G. Laties (Eds.), *Behavioral toxicology* (pp. 401-428). New York: Plenum Press.

Thompson, D. M. (1978). Stimulus control and drug effects. In D. E. Blackman & D. J. Sanger (Eds), *Contemporary research in behavioral pharmacology* (pp. 159-208). New York: Plenum Press.

Thompson, D. M., & Moerschbaecher, J. M. (1979). Drug effects on repeated acquisition. In T. Thompson & P. B. Dews (Eds.), *Advances in behavioral pharmacology* (Vol. 2, pp. 229-260). New York: Academic Press.

van Haaren, F. (1993). *Methods in behavioral pharmacology.* Amsterdam: Elsevier.

Chapter 9

Clinical Drug Assessment

Scott H. Kollins, Kristal Ehrhardt, and Alan Poling
Western Michigan University

Ever since the first effective antipsychotic drug, chlorpromazine (Thorazine), was introduced in the early 1950s, medications have played a major role in the treatment of people with behavior disorders, especially those diagnosed as "mentally ill." Today, dozens of different psychotropic medications are available, and they collectively account for roughly 10-15% of all prescriptions written in the United States (Baldessarini, 1996).

There is no shortage of studies examining the safety and efficacy of psychotropic medications. By law, a series of clinical trials must be conducted before any new medication is marketed, and studies continue long after a medication is introduced. In fact, hundreds of studies have examined the effects of certain popular behavior-change medications, such as methylphenidate (Ritalin) and chlorpromazine. As discussed in Chapter 1, behavioral pharmacologists have long argued that within-subject experimental designs, direct and repeated measures of behavior, and visual data analysis provide the best general approach for determining how drugs affect behavior. Several authors have claimed that this approach is as useful for clinical drug evaluation as for applied research in other areas (e.g., DuPaul & Barkley, 1993; Kennedy & Meyer, 1998; Poling & Cleary, 1986a, b; Singh & Beale, 1986; Wysocki & Fuqua, 1982), and this claim is repeated in the present chapter. Finally, the possibility of meaningfully relating behavioral mechanisms of drug action to clinical effects is considered.

Differences in Evaluating Behavior-Change and Other Medications

When drugs are prescribed in any clinical setting, the goal is to alter some aspect of the client's functioning so as to improve health and to increase comfort. There is an important conceptual difference, however, in the domains of functioning that are altered by psychotropic drugs and other medications. Consider two hypothetical examples. In one, following several days of an increasingly sore throat, a woman goes to her family physician who, after conducting a throat culture, determines that she has a large colony of *Streptococcus pyogenes bacteria living in her mouth and throat*. To treat this condition, the doctor prescribes an antibiotic, amoxicillin, that specifically targets those bacteria. The woman's symptoms (complaints of a sore throat) are directly related to the bacteria living in her throat and the drug prescribed selectively acts on those bacteria. On a return visit one week later, the physician can determine the extent to which the drug has been effective not only by asking the client how her throat feels, but also by conducing a second throat culture. In this case, there is a clear and accessible biological cause (bacteria) of the behavioral symptoms (verbal reports of discomfort).

Now consider another scenario. Following several weeks of feeling sad and depressed, the same woman become so distraught that she considers ending her own life. Once these thoughts become prominent, she realizes that she needs professional help and visits her psychiatrist. Upon examination, which includes the woman describing her emotional state and her thoughts of suicide, the psychiatrist determines that she is experiencing a major depressive episode and prescribes a selective serotonin-reuptake inhibitor, paroxetine (Paxil). After three weeks, the client again visits her psychiatrist. This time, she reports that she is feeling better and is no longer considering harming herself. In this case, although there are biochemical models of mental illness, the behavioral symptoms (verbal reports of depression and suicidal ideation) can *not* be attributed with certitude to a biological cause, and there is no practical means of ascertaining the effects of the drug at that level of analysis.

In the case of strep throat, the disease process is well understood and consistent across individuals. So, too, is the mechanism through which amoxicillin alters that process and thereby alleviates behavioral symptoms. Like other penicillins, amoxicillin disrupts cell wall synthesis in gram-negative bacteria, including *streptococci*, causing cell walls to leak and bacteria to die. By killing the bacteria that cause a sore throat, amoxicillin alleviates the symptoms of the disease. The manner in which the bacteria cause symptoms can be described in detail – they release toxins and initiate an immune response – and the mechanism of therapeutic action is well understood and can be measured. Moreover, these processes are generally invariant across individuals with strep throat, and, consequently, most people with the disorder respond favorably to amoxicillin.

In the case of depression, however, the relation between the pharmacological mechanism of action of paroxetine and the symptoms of depression, which themselves vary considerably across individuals, is more tenuous. Although the drug is known to interfere with the reuptake of serotonin, the manner in which this neurochemical change leads to client-reported changes in affect and ideation cannot be specified. Put differently, the details of the disease process responsible for depression (if such there be) and the manner in which paroxetine interferes with that process to alleviate symptoms are a matter of speculation. Furthermore, although serotonin-specific reuptake inhibitors have been demonstrated to alleviate symptoms of depression in large group trials, effects are not uniform across treated individuals and it is impossible to predict *a priori* who will respond favorably to the drug.

Clinical Research and Everyday Drug Evaluation

The example of paroxetine illustrated that psychotropic drugs are unique insofar as they are used to deal with problems that are defined by, measured in terms of, and best understood at the level of, overt behavior. The effects of these drugs on the biological processes responsible for the behavioral symptoms are not clearly understood, and clinical effectiveness cannot be evaluated at this level of analysis. Therefore, clinical evaluations of psychotropic drugs must assess whether medication (the independent variable) significantly improves some targeted aspect(s) of the participant's behavior (the dependent variable) without producing intolerable adverse reactions (side effects). To determine whether a pharmacological intervention is successful in treating a behavior disorder, three questions must be answered: (a) What were the desired effects of the medication? (b) Were those effects obtained? (c) Were there any significant adverse reactions? These are easy questions to ask, but they are not so easy to answer, whether in the context of formal research or in practical everyday drug evaluations.

As Sprague and Werry (1971) pointed out, every prescription of a psychotropic medication is in essence an experiment in which the physician and other care providers hypothesize that administering a specific drug will produce a desired change in one or more aspects of a client's behavior. In the context of controlled research, the essential four features of a sound drug evaluation are that: (a) treatment effects must be adequately measured; (b) medication must be administered according to the experimental regimen; (c) experimental conditions and their sequencing must allow observed changes in behavior to be attributed with confidence to the drug, and; (d) data analysis must be adequate for detecting clinically important changes in client behavior. If these conditions are met, the evaluation is, in principle, sound. These same characteristics are important in the practical evaluation of medication, although assessment procedures employed outside research settings rarely meet the rigorous standards advocated by scientists. When a child diagnosed with Attention Deficit Hyperactivity Disorder (ADHD) receives methylphenidate for the first time, the child's parents and physician are not interested in conducting a study worthy of presentation to the scientific community, but only in determining whether the drug is an appropriate treatment. They must, however, consider treatment goals and outcomes with the same care as do researchers. If they do not, there is no way for them to know whether the child is helped, hurt, or not affected by the drug.

When competent adults contract for treatment by a physician, the evaluation process is relatively simple: The client and physician agree on treatment goals and a medication, and the treatment is successful if the client deems it so and the physician detects no serious adverse effects. Evaluation is complicated, however, when the client by virtue of age or disability is not able to decide whether to initiate or continue drug treatment. As Thomas Greiner (1958) pointed out four decades ago:

> Sensible adult patients will usually balk when a drug is causing symptoms, but the very young and the very old are forced to take drugs, can't complain or stop on toxic symptoms, may not even connect them with the drug. The mentally deficient of any size or age cannot protect themselves either, and they also merit special care to avoid toxic doses. (p. 349)

Poling (1994) proposed that the appropriate drug use with populations requiring special protections (e.g., people with mental retardation, children) is defined by three characteristics:

1). *The goals of treatment are clear and in the patient's best interests.* A persistent problem in everyday clinical practice is the use of psychotropic drugs to treat vague and ill-defined disorders. The problem has three aspects. One is that failure to specify precisely what signs and symptoms a drug is to improve makes it difficult to pick an appropriate medication. A second is that it is impossible to know whether a drug produced the desired effect unless one knows precisely what the desired effect entails. A third is that it is unclear whether the goals of treatment are in the patient's best interest unless those goals are specified in terms of precise changes in behavior.

2). *Treatment decisions are made on the basis of real drug effects.* Too often, decisions about the effectiveness of medication are made on the basis of subjective evaluations of questionable validity and reliability. For example, DuPaul, Barkley, and McMurray (1991) indicated that "...a large percentage of physicians prescribing stimulant medications [for children with a diagnosis of ADHD] do not collect objective data to establish treatment efficacy, optimal dose, or the need for a change in dosage" (p. 211). In the absence of such data, decisions about the value of stimulant medication for a particular client may well reflect factors other than changes in the client's behavioral and physiological status.

Other authors provide guidelines for monitoring medication effects in special populations, including school children (e.g., DuPaul et al., 1991; Rapport, 1987) and people with mental retardation (e.g., Kalachnik, 1988; Poling, 1994). They point out the non-medical personnel, such as behavior analysts and school psychologists, are by virtue of training and access to clients in an especially favorable position for collecting data that accurately reflect a client's response to medication. Such data, which obviously should be collected with due regard to ethical and legal standards (see DeMers, 1994), are required if treatment decisions are to be made on the basis of real drug effects.

3). *Drug therapy is flexible and integrated with nonpharmacological interventions.* Drug treatment alone will not meet the needs of many people with behavior disorders. Relative to other behavior-change interventions, psychotropic medications are cheap and easy to administer. Moreover, should they fail to produce desired changes in behavior, responsibility for the failure does not obviously rest with direct care staff. Finally, even when they do not produce the desired therapeutic effect, they may make troublesome clients easier to manage (e.g., through sedation). For these reasons, there is a temptation to offer pharmacological interventions as a substitute for a comprehensive and individualized treatment program. This practice fails to maximize quality of life for the client, benefits only caregivers, and cannot be justified. There is no substitute for comprehensive planning and programming to maximize the capacity of people with special needs to function in, and derive pleasure from, their worlds.

Of course, neither the people nor the worlds in which they function are static. Although it is foolish to try repeatedly to reduce medication in a person who is responding favorably when drug is present and has consistently deteriorated when drug was withdrawn in the past, it is equally foolish to assume that a person's need for, and response to, medication will not change over time. Appropriate use of medication requires constant monitoring and evaluation; there is no status quo in psychopharmacology. The strategies and tactics that are appropriate for such monitoring are very similar to those that are appropriate for actual research, which are discussed in the balance of this chapter.

Strategies and Tactics of Clinical Drug Research

Psychotropic drugs have some special characteristics (e.g., slow onset of effects) that must be considered in their evaluation. In addition, there are established conventions for clinical drug studies, such as the use of placebo-controlled and double-blind conditions, and determination of dose-response relations (see Gadow & Poling, 1986). Nonetheless, their efficacy can be determined via the same general tactics and strategies that are used to evaluate other behavior-change interventions. There is no mystery to designing a clinical drug study: One determines whether any independent variable (including medication) affects behaviors of interest by comparing levels of behavior (the dependent variable) when the independent variable is and is not operative, or is operative at different levels. Factors other than the independent variable that might affect the dependent variable (extraneous variables) are held constant across conditions or rendered inoperative. If levels of the dependent variable differ when treatment is and is not present (or is present at different levels), it is logical to assume that behavior changed as a function of treatment, which is therefore deemed active.

Of course, there are many specific experimental designs that may be used in clinical drug evaluations. There is no one best way to conduct a drug evaluation, no panacean design that succeeds where others fail. The manner in which a researcher evaluates medications will depend on several factors. One factor, and not the least important, is a scientist's training and theoretical persuasion. A psychiatrist well versed in group designs and statistical analyses is unlikely to favor the same designs as a behavior analyst. A second factor is the research question that the study is attempting to answer. An investigator concerned with whether fluoxetine (Prozac) interacts with cognitive-behavior therapy in alleviating depression is obliged to use a different design than a researcher who is asking whether naloxone reduces self-injury in children with mental retardation. All research designs are limited with regard to the kinds of information that they can provide; matching research design to research question, therefore, is of no small consequence. A third factor that influences experimental design is the availability of resources – personnel, time, money, equipment, and subjects. Practicality guides the successful treatment evaluator.

Experiments can be considered along a number of dimensions; three of particular significance are depicted in Figure 9-1. This figure emphasizes that experiments can differ with respect to whether: (1) demonstration of a treatment effect depends primarily upon a comparison of (a) the behavior of the same subject(s) under different conditions or (b) the behavior of different subjects under different conditions; (2) a subject's behavior is observed (a) occasionally or (b) repeatedly; and (3) data are analyzed through (a) inferential statistics or (b) visual inspection.

Discussions of experimental designs frequently do not clearly differentiate these three dimensions. Instead, group and single-case designs are generically contrasted. Group designs are presented as involving single (or occasional) observations of each subject's performance and statistical data analysis, whereas repeated observations and visual (graphic) data analysis are represented as features of single-case designs. Indirect and direct measures of behavior also are commonly considered as features of group and single-case designs, respectively.

Each of the cells in Figure 9-1 represents a potentially viable experiment. As explained in Chapter 1, there is good reason to distinguish two general approaches to research, with the single-case approach (represented by the lower right front cell of Figure 9-1) viewed as characteristic of behavior analysis and the group approach (represented by the upper left front cell) viewed as characteristic of traditional psychology. The latter approach also is characteristic of much of mainstream medicine, including psychiatry and clinical drug evaluations. Traditional and behavior analytic approaches to clinical drug evaluation are not discrete categories,

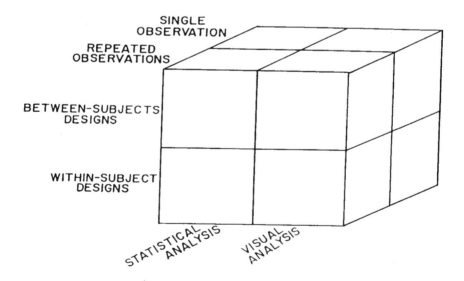

Figure 9-1. *Classification of experimental strategies along three significant dimensions.*

but they favor different tactics and strategies, and provide fundamentally different kinds of information about drug effects. Differences in the methodology character-istic of the two approaches, and in the kinds of information that they provide, are clearly evident in a comparison of studies.

Behavior-Analytic Drug Evaluations: An Early Example with Chlorpromazine

Withdrawal designs, multiple-baseline designs, and alternating-treatments de-signs are among the named experimental configurations commonly used in applied behavior analysis that can be readily adapted to clinical drug evaluation (see Poling, 1986, Poling & Cleary, 1986a, b). In a **withdrawal (or reversal) design**, conditions alternate (e.g., between drug and placebo) and each condition is arranged until performance stabilizes. In a **multiple-baseline design**, two or more dependent variables (e.g., problem behaviors in different subjects) are measured. Treatment is introduced for the different behaviors in a temporally-staggered fashion, for example, first to treat the target behavior of Subject A, then, after Subject A's behavior stabilizes, to treat the target behavior of Subject B. (This design can also begin with the treatment of all target behaviors, after which treatment is withdrawn in a sequence that is temporally staggered across target behaviors). In a **multielement** (or **alternating-treatments**) design, behavior is measured repeatedly under rapidly alternating values of the independent variable. Figure 9-2 illustrates these designs.

A study conducted two decades ago by Marholin, Touchette, and Steward (1979) provides a good example of a withdrawal design, and of the use of behavior-analytic strategies in clinical drug evaluation. This study examined how chlorprom-azine affected four adults with mental retardation. All of these people had been receiving the drug for many months, for unclear reasons and with unknown effects. (A fifth person also was studied under a similar but more complex withdrawal design; for simplicity, this subject will not be considered here). To ascertain the effects of the drug, several important behaviors were carefully measured by direct observation in workshop and ward settings. Among the dependent measures were compliance to verbal requests, accuracy and rate of performance of workshop tasks, time on task, eye contact, talking to self, talking to others, standing, walking, being within three feet of others, being in bed, approaching others, and touching others. During the first 19 days of recording, chlorpromazine was administered in the same manner as in preceding months. This was followed by a 23-day drug-free (placebo) phase, and a 25-day period in which drug treatment was reinstated. Momentary time-sampling procedures, in which the percentage of intervals in which target behaviors occurred were recorded, were used to quantify dependent variables under all conditions.

Some of the data collected by Marholin et al. are shown in Figure 9-3. The effects of withdrawing chlorpromazine differed appreciably across subjects, but some desirable behaviors did emerge in all of them when the drug was withdrawn. Certainly the medication was not producing consistently beneficial effects: "Changes in the behavior of these severely retarded adults which we attributed to chlorprom-

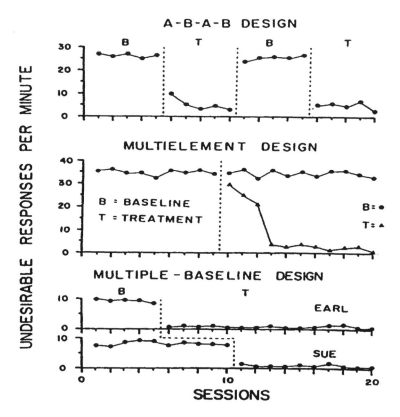

Figure 9-2. *Hypothetical data from experiments using withdrawal (A-B-A-B),*
multielement, and multiple-baseline (across subjects) designs. Each set of data suggests that
the treatment was effective in reducing undesired behavior.

azine were diverse and generally of no clear relevance to the clients' well being,
access to the environment, or physical or psychological comfort" (Marholin et al.,
1979, p. 169). Because Marholin et al. provided a quantitative analysis of a range
of behaviors under controlled conditions involving the alternate presence and
absence of drug, they were able to make such an assertion with relative confidence.
Given their findings, further use of chlorpromazine with any of the clients could not
be justified on ethical or practical grounds.

For many years, it was widely believed that antipsychotic drugs were useful in
dealing with a wide range of problems in people with mental retardation. In addition,
such drugs were thought to be generally safe. More recently, studies like the one
conducted by Marholin et al. (1979) have shown that most people with mental
retardation do not respond favorably to antipsychotic medications, although some
clients (especially those with a dual diagnosis of schizophrenia and mental retarda-

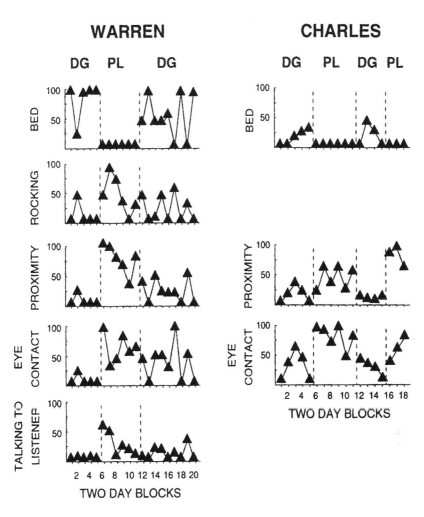

Figure 9-3. *Percentage of intervals during which a number of social behaviors occurred during drug (D) and placebo (P) conditions. Taken from Marholin et al. (1979) and reproduced by permission.*

tion) do derive significant benefit from them (for review see Baumeister, Sevin, & King, 1998). Other studies have demonstrated that these drugs produce a range of vexing side effects, including tardive dyskinesia (uncontrollable movements of the lips, tongue, face, trunk, or limbs) (e.g., Guiltieri, Schroeder, Hicks, & Quade, 1986). It is now generally acknowledged that antipsychotic medications historically have been overprescribed for people with mental retardation, and that such medications are relatively restrictive interventions that should be used with due caution.

Early reports of efficacy in most people with mental retardation reflected, in many cases, nonselective drug-induced reductions in behavior, including disruptive responses that were targeted for deceleration (Gadow & Poling, 1988). Studies that carefully quantified drug effects on desirable as well as undesirable behaviors – which is to say, studies like the one conducted by Marholin et al. (1979) – were required to profile drug effects adequately. Unfortunately for the many people with mental retardation who have been inappropriately medicated with antipsychotic drugs, such studies did not appear in the early clinical literature. In fact, to this day, thorough analyses of the behavioral effects of psychotropic drugs in people with mental retardation are rare. This is due, in part, to the practical and ethical difficulties associated with conducting controlled research with special, protected populations.

Behavior-Analytic Drug Evaluations: Two Examples with Methylphenidate

Mental retardation is the most common developmental disability, observed in approximately 1% of the population, but ADHD is even more common. The prevalence of ADHD, which is characterized by developmentally inappropriate levels of inattention, impulsivity, and hyperactivity, is estimated to be 3-5% in school-aged children (American Psychiatric Association, 1994). Stimulant medication, most notably methylphenidate (Ritalin), is the most common treatment for children diagnosed with ADHD. Approximately 750,000 school children receive stimulant medication each year (DuPaul et al., 1991).

As Stoner, Carey, Ikeda, and Shinn (1994) pointed out, a critical issue in determining the effects of methylphenidate, or any other psychotropic drug, is selecting appropriate outcome measures. As they indicate,

Basic principles of behavioral assessment, as outlined in a variety of sources (e.g., Barlow, Hayes, & Nelson, 1984; DuPaul & Barkley, 1993; Shapiro & Kratochwill, 1988) provide clear guidelines for choosing or developing outcome measures. Briefly, these principles suggest that to assess changes in behavior, measures should (a) use rate of responding as a primary dependent measure; (b) be socially valid; (c) be accurate (i.e., demonstrate sound psychometric properties); (d) be capable of repeated administration prior to, during, and following treatment; (e) provide standardized counts of behavior; and (f) demonstrate sensitivity with respect to precise measurement of critical effects. (p. 102)

Stoner et al. (1994) proposed that curriculum-based measurement (CBM) may have these characteristics. The major purpose of their study was to examine the feasibility of using CBM to evaluate the short-term effects of methylphenidate on academic performance. In essence, CBM involves collecting brief samples of a student's fluency in performing activities sampled directly from her or his curriculum. For example, Stoner et al. evaluated two boys' math skills by determining each student's speed and accuracy in solving problems based on the computation skills covered by his math curriculum. Performance was evaluated during 2-minute probes that were arranged repeatedly across the course of the experiment. Reading skills were evaluated by having students read 1-minute passages that were randomly selected from their reading texts. The number of words read correctly and the number of errors that occurred during these probes were recorded.

Drug effects also were indexed through the use of two standardized behavior rating scales, the Academic Performance Rating Scale (APRS) and the Child Attention Problems Scale (CAP), which were completed by the students' primary classroom teachers. Both students, their teachers, and one of the student's parents also completed the Stimulant Drug Side Effects Rating Scale.

Stoner et al. examined the effects of 5, 10, and 15 mg doses of methylphenidate on these measures in two boys with a diagnosis of ADHD. The experiment was conducted as two case studies, but the ordering of conditions was reversed across the two subjects, so that some features of a crossover design were evident.

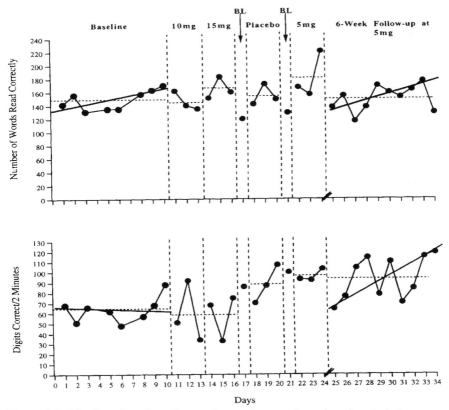

Figure 9-4. *Number of words read correctly per minute and number of math digits correct per 2 minutes by a boy diagnosed with ADHD under the indicated conditions. Dosages refer to the amount of methylphenidate administered each day. Taken from Stoner, Carey, Ikeda, and Shinn (1994) and reproduced by permission.*

CBM data for one of the subjects, Bill, appear in Figure 9-4. These data suggest that his academic performance was best at 5 mg methylphenidate. Bill's best score on the CAP occurred during the placebo phase; his APRS scores were similarly high during the placebo, 5 mg, and 15 mg phases. Adverse side effects were reported only at 10 mg.

The other subject, Dan, in contrast, did best in both math and reading at the highest (15 mg/kg) dose of methylphenidate. He received the best APRS rating at this dose, and the second-best CAP rating (the best rating came at 10 mg/kg). Adverse but tolerable side-effects were reported at 10 and 15 mg/kg doses; they decreased in severity over time.

The results obtained by Stoner et al. (1994) indicate that there were individual differences in the effects of a given drug dose and the effects of a given dose in a particular subject depended, in part, on the aspect of performance that was measured. These findings are consistent with the results of many other studies. In fact, Stoner et al. (1994, p. 102) pointed out that, "For any child, the same dose of methylphenidate may produce positive, negative, or no change in performance, depending on the evaluation task (Rapport, 1987)." Because drug effects are influenced by the evaluation task, it is obligatory that researchers develop clinically-meaningful assays. Given this, one important outcome of the Stoner et al. (1994) study was that it demonstrated the utility of CBM for assessing the effects of methylphenidate on academic performance. A second important outcome was that the study showed that there are individual differences in the pattern of responding to methylphenidate, with results for a given person influenced by both dose and response measure.

In some cases, the apparent effects of a psychotropic drug depend not only on the domain of behavior that is sampled, but also upon the specific procedure that is used. To emphasize this point, Figure 9-5 (Poling, 1986) was constructed to show how a hypothetical response would be scored during baseline (no drug) and treatment (drug administered) conditions under a variety of measurement systems, all involving direct observation of behavior. Rate and duration data are reported, as are data obtained with time sampling and intermittent time sampling procedures. In time sampling, an observational period is divided into discrete intervals and the observer records whether or not the behavior appeared in each interval, whereas in intermittent time sampling observation occurs in only a few intervals, typically selected at random. With either observational system, partial interval or whole interval recording may be used. In partial interval recording, an observer scores (indicates that the target behavior occurred in) any interval in which the response definition was met, regardless of the duration of occurrence of the behavior. In whole interval recording, an interval is scored only if the response definition was met throughout the interval.

For the data in Figure 9-5, depending on how behavior was quantified, one could reasonably conclude that the drug decreased, increased, or had no effect on the behavior being measured. Although the data in Figure 9-5 obviously were contrived to support a point, that point is valid: Persons interested in meaningful clinical drug evaluations cannot afford to be cavalier with respect to either general or specific aspects of behavioral assessment. They do make a difference.

The cardinal rule in selecting an observation system is to be sure that the system adopted maximally reflects the aspects of behavior that the drug is prescribed to change. Beyond this,

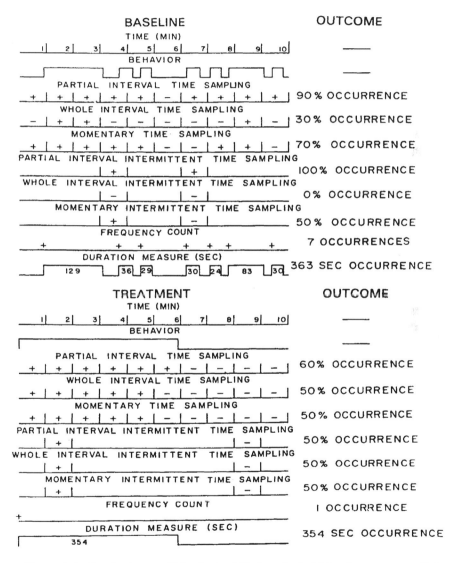

Figure 9-5. *Results that would be obtained if a hypothetical behavior were quantified using various strategies of direct observation.*

systems that arrange frequent observation are to be preferred to those that fail to do so, for the more frequently behavior is sampled, the greater the likelihood that obtained data will actually reflect the level of occurrence of the behavior. Finally, because all drugs can deleteriously affect behavior, an acceptable observational system must make provision for the detection of countertherapeutic effects.

Self-reports, direct observation, and a variety of rating scales can be used to index adverse physiological and behavioral effects of psychotropic medications (see Brown & Sawyer, 1998; Kalachnik et al., 1998; Wilson, Lott, & Tsai, 1998). Unfortunately, because the range of potential adverse effects of many psychotropic drugs is wide and the range of behaviors that an investigator can monitor limited, it is practically impossible ever to be sure that a drug is not producing some undesirable side effect. Perhaps the best that a clinical investigator can do is to become familiar with the known physiological and behavioral actions of the drug being investigated and to search systematically for undesirable manifestations of these actions. Phenothiazine antipsychotics (e.g., chlorpromazine), for example, are known to be associated with weight gain, corneal edema, Parkinsonian reactions, akathisia, and tardive dyskinesia (Poling, Gadow, & Cleary, 1991). Anyone evaluating such drugs, whether in the context of research or everyday clinical practice, should look for these side effects throughout the period of drug administration. A conscientious investigator should also take steps to ascertain whether the drug was interfering with the acquisition or performance of appropriate behavior. Such side effects can best be detected through the direct observation of a range of important behaviors, but self-reports and nonsystematic clinical observations are often useful in their initial detection. Analogue measures, including performances on laboratory tasks, also can provide valuable indications of behavioral side effects, and of therapeutic effects as well. The primary limitation of such measures is that their ecological validity, that is, the extent to which results obtained with them generalize to the situation of clinical concern, cannot be assumed, but must be demonstrated empirically.

One easily overlooked potential side effect of pharmacotherapies involves their ability to influence the outcome of nonpharmacological interventions. Assessing the interaction of medications and other treatments is in principle simple enough – the effects of each intervention alone on the behavior(s) of interest are determined and compared to the effects of the two together – but poses practical problems. This is evident when one considers that each of the treatments should be evaluated at a number of parametric values (e.g., several drug doses should be assessed), and their interactions at all combinations of values studied. Doing so would entail considerable time and effort and probably could not be accomplished in many clinical settings. In such cases, it might appear possible to diminish effort by considering only the most effective value of each treatment. Yet this cannot be accomplished without parametric evaluation, for how else can the most effective treatment values be determined?

Given that drugs can affect may aspects of a client's behavior, it is obvious that no single study can adequately profile a drug's clinically significant effects. Characteristically, a series of studies, each building on prior findings, are required before a drug's effects can be specified with anything approaching confidence. For example, in considering the study by Stoner et al. (1994) and other prior studies of methylphenidate, Gulley and Northrup (1997) pointed out that:

> [This literature] suggests a number of limitations to previous evaluations of the effects of MPH [methylphenidate]. First, an overwhelming majority of studies have evaluated treatment effects based on subjective parent report, teacher report, and behavior rating scales. Unfortunately, these procedures are subject to informant bias and are often technically inadequate (Stoner, Carey, Ikeda, & Shinn, 1994). Second, most studies of children's response to MPH have reported results based on between-group statistical analyses. The use of single-case designs combined with standard drug evaluation procedures (i.e., double-blind placebo controls) has been rare. Third, only a few studies have included an adequate range of doses to evaluate individual dose-response relations. Finally, previous research has frequently included assessments of only one area of functioning (typically disruptive behavior). Thus, simultaneous effects (positive or negative) across other important areas of functioning (e.g., academics) often remain unknown. (pp. 627-628).

Gulley and Northrup attempted to avoid these limitations in their study, which used a multielement design to evaluate comprehensively the effects of methylphenidate in two boys diagnosed with ADHD. In a multielement (or alternating-treatments) design, behavior is measured repeatedly under rapidly alternating values of the independent variable, and in this study the boys received 0.0 (placebo), 0.1, 0.2, and 0.3 mg/kg doses of methylphenidate on different days. Dependent measures included observations of disruptive and social behavior, academic measures (curriculum based measurement of math and reading), a global behavior rating scale (the ADHD Rating Scale), and a measure of stimulant medication side effects (Side Effects Rating Scale). The two subjects were observed in their classroom setting on a daily basis by trained observers.

Results, which were analyzed by visual inspection, showed that for both subjects one or more doses of methylphenidate were associated with improvement in behavioral, academic, and social measures relative to placebo. As in the study by Stoner et al. (1994), the effects of a given dose differed across the two students and across the three domains. For one subject, disruptive behavior, socially inappropriate behavior, and teacher ratings of problem behavior was lowest (best) at 0.3 mg/kg, but academic measures were highest (best) at 0 mg/kg (placebo). For the second subject, global behavior ratings were lowest (indicating the best performance) at 0.0 mg/kg (placebo), but disruptive and socially inappropriate behaviors were lowest (best) at 0.2 or 0.3 mg/kg.

Perhaps the biggest strength of this study is that it describes highly specific and individualized dose-dependent patterns of responding in different domains of functioning. Although its findings support the general conclusion that methylphenidate is useful in treating the problem behaviors characteristic of children with an ADHD diagnosis, those findings also indicate that the degree of improvement obtained differs as a function of the kind of behavior measured, the dose in question, and the individual.

Neither the Stoner et al. (1994) nor the Gulley and Northrup (1997) study support strong actuarial predictions concerning the likelihood that methylphenidate will produce a positive outcome. Only two subjects were used in each study, and it is tenuous to generalize in a statistical sense from such a small, nonrandom sample to a population at large. Traditional drug studies, where many subjects are studied, although often in relatively little detail, have long played a valuable role in generating data that allow for actuarial predictions concerning the likelihood that an untreated individual with a particular diagnosis will respond favorably to a particular medication. An example of the traditional approach follows.

Traditional Drug Evaluations: An Example with Clozapine

In the last 15 years, a number of "atypical" antipsychotic medications have come to the market. These drugs are labeled "atypical" because they do not belong to the same chemical classes as the traditional medications used to manage schizophrenia and other psychotic disorders, and because they produce fewer extrapyramidal side effects. One such drug that has received considerable attention, particularly for its efficacy in clients previously resistant to other forms of pharmacotherapy, is clozapine (Clozaril). Pharmacologically, clozapine is nonselective in that it has antagonistic actions at serotonergic, adrenergic, histaminergic, cholinergic, and dopaminergic sites (Baldessarini, 1996). Clozapine has high affinity for D-1 dopamine receptors, and it is theorized that blockade of these receptors underlies its clinical effectiveness (e.g., Coward, Imperato, Urwyler, & White, 1989).

Clozapine has been investigated as a treatment for individuals experiencing chronic schizophrenic behaviors who have previously not responded to other types of antipsychotic drug treatment. We will consider one such clinical trial as an example of the traditional approach to clinical drug evaluation.

The study of interest was conducted by Kane et al. (1988) and is fairly representative of many large scale clinical trials. Kane et al. investigated clozapine and chlorpromazine in a sample of 268 individuals diagnosed predominantly with undifferentiated type schizophrenia. All subjects were psychiatric inpatients at one of 16 facilities. Prior to the Kane et al. study, all of the subjects had participated in a trial of haloperidol (Haldol) and had showed no improvement as indexed by two separate rating scales (the Brief Psychiatric Rating Scale, BPRS, and the Clinical Global Impression Scale, CGI).

In the Kane et al. (1988) study, subjects were randomly assigned to either a chlorpromazine (plus benztropine mesylate to reduce extrapyramidal side effects) group or a clozapine group. Over the course of the study, doses for individual participants were titrated and BPRS and CGI scores were collected on a weekly basis. Motoric side effects were also assessed throughout the study using two movement disorder rating scales. All of the rating scales were completed by staff who were working with the individuals in their respective inpatient settings.

Data for the clozapine and chlorpromazine groups were expressed as mean changes from baseline scores on the BPRS and CGI. Post-treatment change scores were significantly higher (more positive) for the clozapine group than for the chlorpromazine group from the first week of the study to its end. Therefore, the behavior of the average client was significantly better when the treatment drug was clozapine than when it was chlorpromazine. Figure 9-6 shows the BPRS data.

Of course, average improvement is not necessarily indicative of the performance of any one individual, and in fact most clients in the clozapine group did not show clinical improvement. With clinical improvement defined as either a 20% reduction (improvement) in BPRS scores plus CGI scores of mild, or BPRS total scores of less than 35, 30% of the clozapine group showed improvement compared to only 4% for the chlorpromazine group. Interestingly, in this multi-site study, 14 out of 16 centers demonstrated the pattern of clozapine superiority. Two of the 16 centers either showed no difference or showed chlorpromazine superiority.

This study provides clinically useful actuarial information, insofar as its results suggest that a) clozapine is more effective that chlorpromazine in treating clients diagnosed with undifferentiated type schizophrenia when improvement is indexed in terms of BPRS and CGI scores, and b) clozapine will produce benefit in about one in three clients with this diagnosis who have been unresponsive to other forms of pharmacotherapy. Unfortunately, the study revealed nothing about the characteristics that differentiate drug responders and nonresponders. It also failed to provide a fine-grained analysis of drug effects in individual subjects, or an analysis of dose-response relations.

The single traditional drug study summarized thus far (Kane et al., 1988), and all three of the behavior-analytic studies (Gulley & Northrup, 1997; Marholin et al, 1979; Stoner et al., 1994), evaluated drug effects over relatively brief periods (weeks

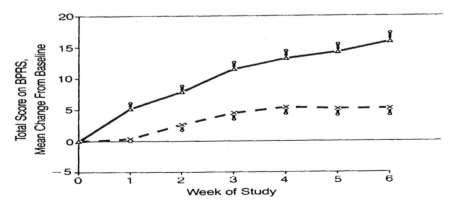

Figure 9-6. *Mean change from baseline in total score on the Brief Psychiatric Rating Scale for people treated with clozapine (solid line, n = 126) or chlorpromazine and benztropine mesylate (broken line, n = 139) during each week of the study. Taken from Kane et al. (1988) and reproduced by permission.*

or months). In fact, it appears that most behavior-analytic drug evaluations fail to provide long-term follow-up data. This is understandable in view of the practical problems associated with conducting clinical drug evaluations and the pressures on researchers to publish. Moreover, brief studies can provide potentially important information about drug effects. Nonetheless, people frequently take psychotropic medications for many years, and short-term and long-term drug effects are not necessarily equivalent. Therefore, longitudinal studies are important.

Most longitudinal research that has been published involves comparing people treated with a particular medication to people with the same diagnosis who receive another medication, or no pharmacotherapy at all. Such methods do not support strong conclusions and there is a surprisingly large gap in our understanding of the long-term effects of many psychotropic medications in populations that commonly receive those drugs. This point is cogently made by Brown and Sawyer (1998) in a review of the long-term cognitive and behavioral effects of psychotropic medications in children:

> Compared to the numerous well-controlled studies on the short-term effects of psychotropic medications for pediatric populations, surprisingly few investigations examined the long-term efficacy and safety of these medications for children and adolescents. Possible exceptions are investigations that examined the outcomes for children, adolescents, and young adults who received stimulant medication. Because of methodological limitations and problems with research design, these studies provide only limited information about the long-term effects of stimulant medication. In contrast to the efficacy of stimulant medication on measures of cognitive functioning in the short term, results from longitudinal follow-up studies are disappointing. Conclusions from these studies generally provide little support that long-term stimulant drug administration influences achievement. Similarly, research data provide limited support that stimulant medication improves peer relationships, aggression, and delinquency in the long run. These results are rather discouraging. However, the limitations in research design in these studies preclude definitive conclusions about the long-term effects of these agents. (p. 84)

Given the conclusions of Brown and Sawyer (1998), which are justified, it is apparent that further, better-controlled research concerning long-term drug effects is needed. This point was highlighted at a recent consensus development conference sponsored by the National Institutes of Health. The results of the meeting indicated that a priority for future research with individuals diagnosed with ADHD was to investigate long-term benefits and risks associated with the use of stimulant medications.

Predicting Drug Effects in Untreated Individuals

As each of the studies summarized in this chapter indicates, individuals often differ in how they respond to psychotropic drugs. This occurs even for people who have received the same psychiatric diagnosis. Large group studies, like the one conducted by Kane et al. (1988), are invaluable for making predictions about the probable proportion of individuals with a particular diagnosis who will respond favorably to a given medication. As noted above, the findings of Kane and his colleagues suggest that about one in three persons with a diagnosis of schizophrenia who are unresponsive to traditional antipsychotic medications will show clinically significant improvement when treated with clozapine. Studies of small numbers of individuals, no matter how intensive and well designed, do not support such actuarial predictions.

In a general way, traditional clinical evaluations have clearly established that people with similar symptoms - and resultant psychiatric diagnoses - are apt to respond similarly to particular drugs. For example, as discussed in the example of paroxetine, serotonin-specific reuptake inhibitors are likely to reduce troublesome behaviors in people with a diagnosis of depression. Such drugs are not, however, usually effective in people diagnosed with ADHD or schizophrenia. For those individuals, more frequent successes would occur with stimulants (e.g., methylphenidate) and antipsychotics (e.g., chlorpromazine, clozapine), respectively. Psychiatric diagnosis provides a general strategy for matching clients to drug treatments.

As discussed previously, however, individuals with the same diagnostic label frequently differ substantially in their response to a particular medication. In principle, at least, it should be possible to delineate the variables that modulate the behavioral effects of psychotropic medications across individuals, and some advances have been made in so doing. For instance, as Kollins, Shapiro, Newland, and Abramowitz (1998) pointed out,

> [Research has shown that the likelihood of individuals with a diagnosis of ADHD responding favorably to methylphenidate] is enhanced if they exhibit low levels of internalizing symptoms (DuPaul, Barkley, & McMurray, 1994), high levels of aggression (Hinshaw, 1991), and high levels of behavioral problems in general (Handen, Janosky, McAuliffe, Breaux, & Feldman, 1994). A multivariate model that included high IQ, high levels of inattentiveness, young age, low severity of the disorder, and low rates of anxiety predicted a favorable response most effectively (Buitelaar, Van der Gaag, Swaab-Barneveld, & Kuiper, 1995). Whether or not these factors can be used clinically to match treatment to problem behavior remains to be empirically determined, however. (p. 1)

These findings, which indicate that fine-grained differences in the behaviors of children diagnoses with ADHD may predict their response to medication, suggest that ADHD is not a homogeneous condition. Rather, it appears that there may be subtypes of ADHD that can be defined in terms of specific behaviors and that these subtypes differ in their sensitivity to stimulant medication. Further research is required, however, to determine if this is the case and to develop diagnostic procedures that allow clients to be matched with effective interventions.

Attempts to determine the behavioral variables that influence clients' responsiveness to psychotropic medications are not limited to children with ADHD and stimulants. For example, several studies (reviewed by Sandman et al., 1998) suggest that naltrexone, as opiate antagonist, is useful in treating self-injurious behavior (SIB) in people with mental retardation. But beneficial effects are not observed in all such individuals: "The symptom of self-injury appears to be selectively influenced by naltrexone, although the effect may occur only for some people and only for certain types of SIB" (Sandman et al., 1998, p. 297). The characteristics that differentiate people whose SIB is adequately managed by naltrexone from those in whom this does not occur cannot presently be specified with confidence, but it does appear that the specific form and location of the SIB may be an important variable. This effect is evident in a recent study by Thompson, Hackenberg, Cerutti, Baker, and Axtell (1994).

Thompson et al. (1994) used time sampling procedures to quantify the frequency of SIB and a rating scale to quantify its intensity in eight adults with severe or profound mental retardation and long histories of pernicious SIB. Side effects were quantified with a checklist and sleep and vital sign measurements also were recorded. The study comprised four phases: baseline, placebo, 50 mg/day naltrexone, and 100 mg/day naltrexone. Conditions were double blind (neither the subjects nor the observers were aware of experimental conditions) and each subject was exposed to all conditions. The first condition for all participants was a 2- to 3-week baseline period. After baseline, each of the other three conditions was arranged for a 2-week period, with conditions arranged in a different order across subjects. Some subjects also received clonidine, a drug that reduces opiate withdrawal effects.

During baseline, all subjects occasionally engaged in high levels of SIB. These episodes were separated by periods in which relatively little SIB occurred. Naltrexone at both doses (50 and 100 mg/day) generally reduced SIB in subjects who struck their head with their hands or against objects or who engaged in self-biting. In contrast, skin-scratching, pinching, and poking fingers into the mouth, nose, and ears were not reduced by naltrexone. Serious side effects were not observed in any subjects, nor were drug-induced changes in sleeping or vital signs.

These data suggest that the form and/or location of SIB may influence whether or not such behavior is reduced by naltrexone. If additional studies confirm that this is the case, clinicians may be able to predict accurately whether or not a person with SIB who has not received naltrexone will respond favorably to the drug by determining the form and location of the behavior. If, for instance, face-slapping or head-banging is the response of concern, the data reported by Thompson et al. (1994) predict a favorable response. But, if the response is scratching the skin with the fingernails, those data suggest that naltrexone would not be effective.

Behavioral Mechanisms of Clinical Drug Effects

As discussed in previous chapters, making sense of drug effects requires understanding of the processes whereby a drug produces those effects. In most areas of pharmacology and medicine, these processes - which are referred to as mechanisms of drug action - involve events at the biochemical level. For example, as described earlier in this chapter, amoxicillin disrupts cell wall synthesis in gram-negative bacteria and is therefore bactericidal with respect to *Streptococcus pyogenes*. Neurochemical mechanisms of actions are commonly invoked in attempting to explain the effects of psychotropic medications. For instance, it is plausible that some forms of SIB lead to the release of endogenous morphine-like substances (endorphins) in the brain (Thompson et al., 1994; Sandman et al., 1998). These substances serve as positive reinforcers, thereby increasing the likelihood of subsequent self-injury. Naltrexone blocks the reinforcing effects of endorphins and, through the behavioral process of extinction, reduces SIB. But this occurs only if SIB is maintained by endorphin release. SIB maintained in other ways (e.g., because it produces attention from caregivers) is not reduced by naltrexone. If this analysis is correct, it may be the case that in the Thompson et al. (1994) study described above, SIB that involved damage to the face, but not self-injury that involved scratching the skin, was maintained by endorphin release. Undoubtedly due to ethical and practical considerations, this possibility was not evaluated by Thompson et al. (1994). For those same reasons, it would be difficult to evaluate in other studies. At the present time, clients' overt behaviors provide a better means of predicting drug effects than do the neurochemical events that accompany those behaviors.

In fact, as explained in the example of using paroxetine to treat depression, the relation between neurochemical events and behavioral events, and how psychotropic drugs affect that relation, characteristically cannot be described in detail. Behavior and serotonin reuptake are events that occur at different levels of analysis and are described in different dimensions and terms (see Marr, 1990 for an interesting discussion of this general topic). It is not presently possible to reduce behavior to neuropharmacology.

Nonetheless, relatively few attempts have been made to explain the mechanisms of action of psychotropic drugs at other levels of analysis. As discussed in Chapter 1, behavioral pharmacologists have proposed that the concept of behavioral mechanisms of drug action is generally useful in explaining the behavioral effects of drugs, and it is possible that the concept may be profitably applied to psychotropic medications. A case in point is a recent study by Northup, Fusilier, Swanson, Roane, and Borrero (1997), described below, who examined the possibility that methylphenidate functions as an establishing operation (EO) when administered to children diagnosed with ADHD.

Methylphenidate as an Establishing Operation in Children Diagnosed with ADHD

An EO is a stimulus or event that alters the reinforcing efficacy of another stimulus (Michael, 1982). For example, deprivation is a commonly used establishing operation in nonhuman research since it "establishes" food or water as an effective reinforcer. Northup and his colleagues hypothesized that one of the potential functions of methylphenidate in changing behavior is to alter the reinforcing efficacy of other stimuli and events in a person's environment. This hypothesis has empirical support. For example, it has been shown in nonhuman species that methylphenidate alters the reinforcing efficacy of a sucrose solution in reliable ways that can be described mathematically by the matching law (e.g., Heyman, 1992).

Northup and his colleagues studied the behavior of three children diagnosed with ADHD who were receiving methylphenidate daily. In the context of a summer day treatment program, the children worked in 5-minute segments completing math problems. They were able to earn token coupons for completing a set number of problems (determined individually for each child during baseline). A variety of different colored coupons were used; they represented six different kinds of available reinforcers. The reinforcer classes that were selected included edible items, other tangible items, activities, teacher attention, peer attention, and escape from academic programs. The relative efficacy or reinforcing value of each class was determined based on the number of coupons a child selected for each class. For example, one subject (Scott) was able to select a coupon for every four completed math problems. Once Scott had finished four problems, he was able to select any one of the different coupons representing the different reinforcer classes.

The distribution of choices across reinforcer classes was examined for each child both on and off medication (under placebo conditions) to identify possible differences in reinforcer efficacy. Results showed that for all three children methylphenidate functioned to change the reinforcing efficacy of at least one reinforcer class. For example, under placebo conditions, Tim's most preferred reinforcer class was edible items. At 20 mg methyphenidate, however, both activities and tangible nonfood items were preferred over edible items. Similar results were obtained across the other two subjects as well. In all three, activities functioned as a more potent reinforcer following methylphenidate administration compared to placebo. In contrast, edible items were more effective as reinforcers when drug was absent than when it was present.

The capacity of methylphenidate to act as an EO is important with respect to one of the potential side effects of the drug, that is, its capacity to alter the effectiveness of behavioral interventions. That is, the effectiveness of behavior-change programs that utilize reinforcement - and most behavioral interventions used to treat children diagnosed with ADHD do so (e.g., Barkley, 1991) - will differ in the presence and absence of methylphenidate if the drug alters the reinforcing capacity of the objects and events arranged to strengthen behavior. In addition, reinforcer assessments conducted in the absence of drug may yield information that is inaccurate in the presence of drug, and vice versa. Clearly, the demonstration that methylphenidate has EO effects in applied situations helps to understand how the drug may influence behavior in children diagnosed with ADHD.

Methylphenidate as a Discriminative Stimulus in Children Diagnosed with ADHD

Of course, the behavioral mechanisms of action of methylphenidate relevant to its clinical effects are not limited to its EO properties. As Kollins et al. (1998) pointed out:

Conceptualizing methylphenidate as a stimulus embedded in a pattern of ongoing behavior may offer new insights into the behavioral mechanisms of action underlying the improvements noted with this drug. For example, methylphenidate may function as a discriminative stimulus for differential reinforcement in children for whom it is administered for behavior problems; it may exert direct motoric or cognitive effects that, in turn, could be discriminated; it may somehow alter the reinforcing efficacy of other stimuli, thus altering the probability of future behavior; or it may function in more than one of these capacities to produce behavioral change. (p. 1)

To examine the possibility that methylphenidate might serve as a discriminative stimulus in clinical settings, Kollins et al. (1998) attempted to train children to discriminate between their typical dose of methylphenidate (10-20 mg) and placebo capsules. Twelve children with a diagnosis of ADHD who were being treated with methylphenidate were studied in a series of three experiments. The general procedure involved administering methylphenidate or placebo, then, several hours later, having the child report whether he or she had taken "medicine" or "no medicine" that day. During training, correct responses were reinforced with money. During testing, with the training dose and other doses, differential reinforcement was not arranged. The general deportment of all children was indexed with a rating scale, and participant-rated effects of the drug also were recorded.

In general, results revealed that the subjects could learn to discriminate methylphenidate from placebo. For this to occur, however, it frequently was necessary to instruct the children to pay attention to the drug effects, to provide immediate feedback following their discrimination responses, and to have those responses occur at the time of peak drug effects. Results revealed no clear relation between accurate discrimination and behavioral change as indexed by the rating scale. The rating scale did not appear to be sensitive to behavioral change, however, insofar as most subjects' scores did not change when they were on and off medication.

It is noteworthy that participant-rated effects were absent in many children under conditions where methylphenidate served as a discriminative stimulus. Although some researchers have emphasized that the discriminative and participant-rated effects of drugs are overlapping, but not isomorphic (e.g., Preston & Bigelow, 1991), it is all too easy to reason that drug-discrimination assays reveal "how a drug makes people feel," which is information revealed more easily by simply asking them. This clearly is not the case, at least when the effects of methylphenidate in children with a diagnosis of ADHD are considered.

Although the data reported by Kollins et al. (1998) demonstrate that methylphenidate *could* improve the behavior of children diagnosed with ADHD by acting as a discriminative stimulus, they do not demonstrate such an effect. Further research is needed to determine whether the conditions of differential reinforcement required to establish methylphenidate as discriminative for appropriate behavior actually occur in clinical settings and, if so, whether they establish the drug as a discriminative stimulus.

The clinical significance of identifying methylphenidate as an establishing operation or as a discriminative stimulus in children to whom it is administered for behavioral problems is currently unknown, but it is the case that examining behavioral mechanisms of drug action may help to account for the variability in clients' responses to psychotropic drugs that are commonly observed. Although both of the studies discussed here involve the stimulant, methylphenidate, similar work in clinical settings with other behaviorally active drugs may provide useful information. For example, it has been clearly shown that a number of clinically prescribed anxiolytic drugs (e.g., diazepam: Rush, Critchfield, Troisi, & Griffiths, 1995; triazolam: Rush, Madakisira, Goldman, Woolverton, & Rowlett, 1997) can function as discriminative stimuli. However, the discriminative stimulus effects of these drugs have not been systematically examined in the clinical population to whom the drugs are prescribed (i.e., individuals experiencing anxiety disorders). The reinforcing effects, however, of one anxiolytic, diazepam, have been studied in anxious individuals. Chutuape and deWit (1995) showed that following sessions in which 20 mg diazepam (administered in five 4 mg divided doses) was administered under double-blind conditions, individuals with a history of clinical anxiety problems were more likely to choose diazepam in subsequent blind choice sessions. Similar research that further investigates the stimulus properties of clinically used drugs may help to elucidate the manner in which these compounds interact with other environmental events to influence clinical efficacy.

Concluding Comments

Many different drugs are used clinically to alter behavior, and new psychotropic medications are constantly under development. The effects of such drugs can be evaluated using a wide range of specific methods, which can be generally categorized as involving either single-case or group approaches to research. Despite common arguments to the contrary, neither approach is intrinsically good or evil. Instead, they are based upon different assumptions and provide fundamentally different kinds of information. Large scale clinical trials provide important information regarding which compounds are likely to be effective for the largest number of individuals with a particular behavior disorder, and a great deal has been written concerning this approach to drug evaluation.

Single-case approaches, in contrast, are less useful for fostering actuarial predictions. But they do allow for a careful evaluation of interactions between drugs and other environmental stimuli that may be unique to each individual participant. Such studies are invaluable for providing a detailed description of a drug's behavioral effects and how those effects differ across individuals, for isolating behavioral mechanisms of drug action, and for determining the variables that modulate a drug's clinical effectiveness.

The single-case approach to applied research is best developed in applied behavior analysis, and the tactics and strategies commonly used in applied behavior analysis can be readily adapted to clinical drug assessment (Poling & Ehrhardt, 1999). Two important characteristics of this approach are given short shrift in many clinical drug evaluations. One is carefully defining target behaviors and ensuring that those behaviors are accurately assessed. In drug evaluations, this means specifying exactly how a person's behavior should change if the drug produces a therapeutic effect and determining how such a change can be detected. The second is assessing the social validity of an intervention, that is, whether people with a legitimate interest in a given drug treatment are satisfied with its goals, procedures, and results (Wolf, 1978). Poling and LeSage (1995) point out that social validity data are not commonly reported in drug studies involving people with mental retardation, a group that merits special protections, and suggest that collecting and reporting such data would be valuable in many areas of clinical psychopharmacology.

Be that as it may, basic research reviewed throughout this book has made it clear that the strategies and tactics characteristic of behavior analysis are useful in assessing behavioral loci of drug action, behavioral mechanisms of drug action, and the variables that modulate drug effects. Research in all of the areas are directly relevant to clinical drug evaluation.

References

American Psychiatric Association. (1994). *Diagnostic and statistical manual of mental disorders, fourth edition.* Washington, DC: Author.

Baldessarini, R. J. (1996). Drugs and the treatment of psychiatric disorders: Psychosis and anxiety. In J. G. Hardmann, L. E. Limbird, P. B. Molinoff, R. W. Ruddon, & A. G. Gilman (Eds.), *The pharmacological basis of therapeutics* (pp. 399-430). New York. McGraw-Hill.

Barkley, R. A. (1991). *The hyperactive child: A handbook for diagnosis and treatment.* New York: Guilford Press.

Barlow, D. H., Hayes, S. C., & Nelson, R. O. (1984). *The scientist-practitioner: Research and accountability in clinical and educational settings.* New York: Pergamon Press.

Baumeister, A. A., Sevin, J. A., & King, B. H. (1998). Neuroleptics. In S. Reiss & M. G. Aman (Eds.), *Psychotropic medications and developmental disabilities: The international consensus handbook* (pp. 133-150). Columbus, OH: The Ohio State University Nisonger Center.

Buitelaar, J. K., Van der Gaag, R. J., Swaab-Barneveld, H., & Kuiper, M. (1995). Prediction of clinical response to methylphenidate in children with attention deficit hyperactivity disorder. *Journal of the American Academy of Child and Adolescent Psychiatry, 34,* 1025-1032.

Brown, R. T., & Sawyer, M. G. (1998). *Medications for school-age children.* New York: Guilford Press.

Coward, D. M., Imperato, A., Urwyler, S., & White, T. G. Biochemical and behavioral properties of clozapine. *Psychopharmacology, 99,* Supplement: s6-s12.

Chutuape, M.A. & de Wit, H. (1995). Preference for ethanol and diazepam in anxious volunteers: A test of the self-medication hypothesis. *Psychopharmacology, 121,* 91-103.

DeMers, S. T. (1994). Legal and ethical issues in school psychologists' participation in psychopharmacological interventions with children. *School Psychology Quarterly, 9,* 41-52.

DuPaul, G. J., & Barkley, R. A. (1993). Behavioral contributions to pharmacotherapy: The utility of behavioral methodology in medication treatment of children with attention deficit hyperactivity disorder. *Behavior Therapy, 24,* 47-65.

DuPaul, G. J., Barkley, R. A., & McMurray, M. B. (1991). Therapeutic effects of medication on ADHD: Implications for school psychologists. *School Psychology Review, 20,* 203-221.

DuPaul, G. J., Barkley, R. A., & McMurray, M. B. (1994). Response of children with ADHD to methylphenidate: Interaction with internalizing symptoms. *Journal of the American Academy of Child and Adolescent Psychiatry, 33,* 894-903.

Gadow, K. D., & Poling, A. (1986). *Methodological issues in human psychopharmacology: Advances in learning and behavioral disabilities.* Greenwich, CT: JAI Press.

Gadow, K. D., & Poling, A. (1988). *Pharmacotherapy and mental retardation.* Boston: College-Hill.

Greiner, T. (1958). Problems of methodology in research with drugs. *American Journal on Mental Deficiency, 64,* 346-352.

Guiltieri, C. T., Schroeder, S. R., Hicks, R. E., & Quade, D. (1986). Tardive dyskinesia in young mentally retarded individuals. *Archives of General Psychiatry, 43,* 335-340.

Gulley, V. & Northup, J. (1997). Comprehensive school based assessment of the effects of methylphenidate. *Journal of Applied Behavior Analysis, 30,* 627-638.

Handen, B. L., Janosky, J., McAuliffe, S., Breaux, A. M., & Feldman, H. (1994). Prediction of response among children with ADHD and mental retardation. *Journal of the American Academy of Child and Adolescent Psychiatry, 33,* 1185-1193.

Heyman, G. M. (1992). Effects of methylphenidate on response rate and measures of motor performance and reinforcement efficacy. *Psychopharmacology, 109,* 145-152.

Hinshaw, S. P. (1991). Stimulant mediation and the treatment of aggression in children with attentional deficits. *Journal of Clinical Child Psychology, 20,* 301-312.

Kalachnik, J. E. (1988). Medication monitoring procedures. In K. D. Gadow & A. Poling, *Pharmacology and mental retardation* (pp. 231-268). Boston: College-Hill Press.

Kalachnik, J. E., Leventhal, B. L., James, D. H., Sovner, R., Kastner, T. A., Walsh, K., Weisblatt, S. A., & Klitzke, M. G. (1998). Guidelines for the use of psychotropic medication. In S. Reiss & M. G. Aman (Eds.), *Psychotropic medications and developmental disabilities: The international consensus handbook* (pp.45-72). Columbus, OH: The Ohio State University Nisonger Center.

Kane, J., Honigfeld, G., Singer, J., Meltzer, H., & the Clozaril Collaborative Stud Group. (1988). Clozapine for the treatment-resistant schizophrenic. *Archives of General Psychiatry, 45,* 789-796.

Kennedy, C. H., & Meyer, K. A. (1998). The use of psychotropic medication for people with severe disabilities and challenging behavior: Current status and future directions. *Journal of the Association for Persons with Severe Handicaps, 23,* 83-97.

Kollins, S. H., Shapiro, S. K., Newland, M. C, & Abramowitz, A. (1998). Discriminative and subject-rated effects of methylphenidate in children diagnosed with Attention Deficit Hyperactivity Disorder. *Experimental and Clinical Psychopharmacology, 6,* 1-15.

Marholin, D., Touchette, P. E., & Stewart, R. M. (1979). Withdrawal of chronic chlorpromazine medication: An experimental analysis. *Journal of Applied Behavior Analysis, 12,* 150-171.

Marr, M. J. (1990). Behavioral pharmacology: Issues of reductionism and causality. In J. E. Barrett, T. Thompson, & P. B. Dews (Eds.) *Advances in Behavioral Pharmacology* (Volume 7, pp. 1-12). Hillsdale, NJ. Lawrence Erlbaum.

Michael, J. (1982). Distinguishing between discriminative and motivational functions of stimuli. *Journal of the Experimental Analysis of Behavior, 37,* 149-155.

Northup, J., Fusilier, I., Swanson, V., Roane, H., & Borrero, J. (1997). An evaluation of methylphenidate as a potential establishing operation for some common classroom reinforcers. *Journal of Applied Behavior Analysis, 30,* 615-625.

Poling, A. (1986). *A primer of human behavioral pharmacology.* New York: Plenum Press.

Poling, A. (1994). Pharmacological treatment of behavioral problems in people with mental retardation: Some ethical considerations. In L. J. Hayes, G. J. Hayes, S. C. Moore, & P. M. Ghezzi (Eds.), *Ethical issues in developmental disabilities* (pp. 149-177). Reno, NV: Context Press.

Poling, A., & Cleary, J. (1986a). The role of applied behavior analysis in evaluating medication effects. In A. Poling & R. W. Fuqua (Eds.), *Research methods in applied behavior analysis: Issues and advances* (pp. 299-312). New York: Plenum Press.

Poling, A., & Cleary, J. (1986b). Within-subject designs. In K. D. Gadow & A. Poling (Eds.), *Methodological issues in human psychopharmacology: Advances in learning and behavioral disabilities* (Suppl. 1, pp. 115-136). Greenwich, CT: JAI Press.

Poling, A., & LeSage, M. (1995). Evaluating psychotropic drugs in people with mental retardation: Where are the social validity data? *American Journal on Mental Retardation, 100,* 193-200.

Poling, A., Gadow, K. D., & Cleary, J. (1991). *Drug therapy for behavior disorders.* New York: Pergamon Press.

Poling, A., & Ehrhardt, K. (1999). Applied behavior analysis, social validation, and the psychopharmacology of mental retardation. *Mental Retardation and Developmental Disabilities Research Reviews, 5,* 342-347.

Preston, K. L., & Bigelow, G. E. (1991). Subjective and discriminative effects of drugs. *Behavioural Pharmacology, 2,* 293-313.

Rapport, M. D. (1987). Attention deficit disorder with hyperactivity. In M. Hersen & V. B. Van Hasselt (Eds.), *Behavior therapy with children and adolescents: A clinical approach* (pp. 325-361). New York: Wiley.

Rush, C. R., Critchfield, T. S., Troisi II, J. R. & Griffiths, R. R. (1995). Discriminative stimulus effects of diazepam and buspirone in normal volunteers. *Journal of the Experimental Analysis of Behavior, 63,* 277-294.

Rush, C. R., Madakisira, S., Goldman, N. H., Woolverton, W. L. & Rowlett, J. K. (1997). Discriminative stimulus effects of zolpidem in pentobarbital trained subjects: II. Comparison with triazolam and caffeine in humans. *Journal of Pharmacology and Experimental Therapeutics, 280,* 174-188.

Sandman, C. A., Thompson, T., Barrett, R. P., Verhoeven, W. M. A., McCubbin, J. A., Schroeder, S. R., & Hetrick, W. P. (1998). Opiate blockers. In S. Reiss & M. G. Aman (Eds.), *Psychotropic medications and developmental disabilities: The international consensus handbook* (pp. 291-302). Columbus, OH: The Ohio State University Nisonger Center.

Shapiro, E. S., & Kratochwill, T. R. (1988). *Behavioral assessment in schools: Conceptual foundations and practical applications.* New York: Guilford.

Singh, N. N., & Beale, I. L. (1986). Behavioral assessment of pharmacotherapy. *Behavior Change, 3,* 34-40.

Sprague, R. L., & Werry, J. L. (1971). Methodology of psychopharmacological studies with the retarded. In N. R. Ellis (Ed.), *International review of research in mental retardation* (Vol. 5, pp. 147-219). New York: Academic Press.

Stoner, G., Carey, S. P., Ikeda, M. J., & Shinn, M. R. (1994). The utility of curriculum-based measurement for evaluating the effects of methylphenidate on academic performance. *Journal of Applied Behavior Analysis, 27,* 101-113.

Thompson, T., Hackenberg, T., Cerutti, D., Baker, D., & Axtell, S. (1994). Opioid antagonist effects on self-injury in adults with mental retardation: Response form and location as determinants of medication effects. *American Journal on Mental Deficiency, 99,* 85-102.

Wilson, J. G., Lott, R. S., & Tsai, L. (1998). Side effects: Recognition and management. In S. Reiss & M. G. Aman (Eds.), *Psychotropic medications and developmental disabilities: The international consensus handbook* (pp. 95-114). Columbus, OH: The Ohio State University Nisonger Center.

Wolf, M. M. (1978). Social validity: The case for subjective measurement or how applied behavior analysis is finding its heart. *Journal of Applied Behavior Analysis, 11,* 203-215.

Wysocki, T., & Fuqua, R. W. (1982). Methodological issues in the evaluation of drug effects. In S. E. Breuning & A. Poling (Eds.), *Drugs and mental retardation* (pp. 138-167). Springfield, IL: Charles C Thomas.

Chapter 10

Drug Abuse

Sean Laraway[1], Susan Snycerski[1],
Tom Byrne[2], and Alan Poling[1]

*[1]Western Michigan University and
[2]Massachusetts College of Liberal Arts*

Some patterns of drug-self administration harm the user or other individuals without producing offsetting therapeutic or other benefit. The harm may involve direct physical damage, as when chronic high-dose alcohol intake eventually leads to cirrhosis, or indirect physical damage, as when an intoxicated driver maims innocents in an automobile accident. The unwise use of drugs is a major cause of suffering and death. For example, in summarizing data reported in monographs published by the National Institute on Drug Abuse (NIDA), Hollinger (1997) reports that each year tobacco, alcohol, cocaine, and heroin cause 390,000, 80,000, 2,200, and 2,000 deaths in the United States, respectively.

Of course, drug-related behaviors can be damaging even if they cause no physical harm. A person forced to engage in prostitution or breaking and entering to support a $200-a-day heroin habit certainly has a drug-related problem. So, too, does a college undergraduate who rarely drinks but who has just been arrested for driving under the influence of alcohol, or a middle-school student whose learning is impaired by lunch-time marijuana use. The misuse of drugs can cause medical, interpersonal, financial, vocational, educational, and legal problems.

Drug Abuse and Related Terms

Several terms, among them drug abuse, drug addiction, and drug dependence, have been used to refer to harmful patterns of drug self-administration. Unfortunately, each of these terms has multiple and overlapping definitions. As we use the term, **drug abuse** occurs when nonmedicinal use of a drug creates a problem for the individual who self-administers the drug or for those who have a legitimate interest in that person's activities. A problem in this sense is a current state of affairs that is described as needing change in a particular direction. Such change, if affected, constitutes solution of the problem. Those with a legitimate interest in a person exhibiting drug-related problems include all individuals who are, or might be, harmed by the irresponsible drug use or who have a legal and generally recognized right to work toward controlling it. Parents, for instance, have a legitimate interest in their children's drug-related problems, as do spouses in their mates' drug abuse.

Society at large has an accepted interest in many drug-related problems; laws exist and are enforced to ensure that interest is realized.

In the United States (and much of the rest of the world), the use of certain drugs is illegal. Such "illicit" or "unsanctioned" drugs are sometimes viewed as having properties that are fundamentally different from those of legal ("licit") substances, which are often not even termed "drugs" in the vernacular (as in the common verbal construction "alcohol and drug abuse"). Consider the following statement from the White House Conference for a Drug Free America (1988; quoted in Abadinsky, 1993): "The use of *illicit* drugs affects moods and emotions; chemically alters the brain; and causes loss of control, paranoia, reduction of inhibition, and unprovoked anger" (pp. 1-2; emphasis added). Two aspects of this statement are misleading. One is that it suggests that *only* illicit drugs produce the listed effects; the other is that it suggests that *all* illicit drugs produce these effects. In truth, licit as well as illicit drugs can affect brain chemistry and behavior and, as evidenced throughout this book, effects differ widely across drugs and settings.

Principles of drug action are not affected by the legal system; it is foolish to think of legal drugs as "good" and illegal drugs as "bad." It is possible to use an unsanctioned drug without abusing it, at least in the sense that we use the term, and it is also possible to abuse a sanctioned drug. In fact, whether or not the use of a particular drug is condoned by a society is often unrelated to the harmful consequences associated with use of that drug. Consider the lethality of alcohol (ethanol). Although most people who consume the drug do not abuse it, alcohol causes at least 25 times the number of deaths that can be attributed to all illegal drugs combined (Julien, 1996). Of course, the harm caused by alcohol is not limited to fatalities. For instance, the drug is linked to child and spouse abuse, and the National Institute on Alcohol Abuse and Alcoholism (1990) concluded that: "In both animal and human studies, alcohol, more than other drug, has been linked with a high incidence of violence and aggression" (p. 92). Precedent, not pharmacology, dictates alcohol's status as a widely used and accepted recreational drug. The same it true of tobacco.

None of the foregoing should be taken as evidence that alcohol or tobacco are "bad" or that illegal drugs are "better." The point is that all drugs with the potential for recreational use pose risks for users. Even substances that are used purely as medications can be harmful. In fact, one study estimated that adverse reactions from legally prescribed medicines are responsible for approximately 106,000 deaths each year, making adverse drug reactions between the fourth and sixth leading cause of death (Lazarou, Pomranz, & Corey, 1998). Drugs can be dangerous, but they also can be valuable. We humans derive great benefit from our medications, and we *use* as well as *abuse* recreational drugs. As the next section illustrates, we have done so for millennia.

Historical Overview

Humans have used drugs from at least the Neolithic period for religious, medicinal, and recreational purposes (Devereux, 1997; Grinspoon & Bakalar, 1997; Leakey, 1994; Schultes & Hofmann, 1992). As Jaffe (1990) notes:

As far back as recorded history, every society has used drugs that produce effects on mood, thought, and feeling. Moreover, there were always a few individuals who digressed from custom with respect to the time, the amount, and the situation in which these drugs were to be used. Thus, both the nonmedical use of drugs and the problem of drug abuse are as old as civilization itself. (p. 522)

Even a cursory examination of human history reveals the importance of drugs in the evolution of human cultures. For example, in a number of ancient religions, a shaman used hallucinatory drugs to induce ecstatic, visionary experiences; such experiences were seen as a means to commune with spirits, foretell the future, and diagnose and cure diseases (Devereux, 1997; Furst, 1976; Grinspoon & Bakalar, 1997; McKenna, 1992; Schultes & Hofmann, 1992). The shaman functioned as a healer, forecaster, and religious figure in the community, and drug-induced ecstatic experiences were an integral part of the religious and medicinal practices of many ancient cultures. The drugs used by the ancients to produce those experiences, and for other purposes, include many substances used recreationally and medicinally today. Among them are coca (cocaine), tobacco, datura, peyote, cannabis, opium, the *Psilocybe* mushroom, and the *Aminita muscaria* mushroom (Grinspoon & Bakalar, 1997; McKenna, 1992; Ray & Ksir, 1993; Schultes & Hofmann, 1992). Cannabis, for example, has been used for centuries by Indian saddhus (holy men) in their devotions, and the Indian vedas describe this plant as one of the divine nectars, given to humans by the gods (Schultes & Hofmann, 1992).

Psychoactive plants often were considered sacraments in the cultures in which they were used, much like the Eucharist is held a sacrament in Catholicism. In fact, the Aztecs called the *Psilocybe* mushroom, *teonanacatl*, meaning "God's flesh" (Devereux, 1997; Grinspoon & Bakalar, 1997). The belief that the sacred plant is actually the flesh of a god is held by many other indigenous peoples. For instance, the Huichol people of Mexico worship the peyote cactus as "The Elder Brother Deer." The peyote cactus is ritually "hunted" during an annual pilgrimage and its "flesh" allows those religious seekers who participate in the sacred communion to "see their lives" (Furst, 1976). Reverence for sacred plants continues to this day in many cultures throughout the world (Schultes & Hofmann, 1992).

Apart from religious and medicinal uses, ancient humans also used drugs for purely recreational purposes (although the distinctions between these different types of uses are to some extent arbitrary; Schultes & Hofmann, 1992). For example, alcohol, in the form of beer, wine, or mead, has been used as an intoxicant since at least 6000 BC, and probably before, and there were very few ancient cultures that did not utilize the fermentation process to produce alcoholic beverages (McKim, 1997). The importance of alcohol in the ancient world is confirmed by references to alcoholic preparations in the Egyptian Book of the Dead (3000 BC), the Code of Hammurabi (2225 BC), and *The Law*, by Plato (360 BC) (McKim, 1997). The Bible makes several references to alcoholic beverages; most are admonitions to refrain from drinking to excess (Poling, Schlinger, Starin, & Blakely, 1990).

Drug use did not wane with the passing centuries, and it came to North America from Asia with the earliest inhabitants. The Europeans who came later brought with them their favored substances and, by the end of the Nineteenth Century, recreational use of alcohol and caffeine was widespread in the United States (Segal, 1988). Other drugs were also gaining in popularity, including those found in patent medicines, which often contained morphine or cocaine, as well as alcohol (Segal, 1988).

By the early Twentieth Century, Americans were consuming more drugs than ever before, including some, such as heroin, that were unavailable to previous generations (Inciardi, 1992; Segal, 1988). Widespread and troublesome patterns of drug use lead some Americans to join the temperance movement, which blamed all of society's ills on the use of drugs. This movement attributed crime, violence, sexual impropriety, insanity, and general moral decay directly to alcohol, coffee, tobacco, cannabis, cocaine, and opium (Segal, 1988).

The Prohibitionist Model of Drug Abuse

Not content with using moral persuasion to convince people to remain sober, the prohibition movement began exerting political influence, which eventually resulted in legislative action. The prohibition movement's efforts culminated in the ratification in 1917 of the **Eighteenth Amendment to the U.S. Constitution**, which made the production, sale, and use of alcohol illegal. Rather than make America alcohol-free, as was intended, Prohibition instead created a black market in which organized crime thrived by meeting the American public's unabated demand for alcohol. Americans eventually realized that Prohibition caused more harm than legal alcohol. In 1931, the Eighteenth Amendment to the Constitution was nullified with the ratification of the Twenty-First Amendment (Segal, 1988).

Despite the fact that Prohibition was a failure, the prohibitionist model upon which the Eighteenth Amendment was based remained intact and relatively untarnished after Prohibition ended. The emphasis merely shifted from alcohol to other "sinful" drugs, particularly cannabis (Segal, 1988), which was frequently associated in the popular press with "degenerate Spanish-speaking residents" (i.e., Mexican immigrants) (Musto, 1973). Thus, even though Prohibition was a failure, its underlying philosophy was not discredited, but rather was strengthened and incorporated into subsequent federal drug control efforts. Today, the prohibitionist model, sometimes referred to as "zero-tolerance" (Inciardi, 1992), remains the official federal approach to drug use and abuse in the United States.

The prohibitionist model is, in part, a product of the Judeo-Christian cultural heritage, which sees behavior as the result of an individual's free choice and physical pleasure as "sinful" (Inciardi, 1992). Consequently, those who engage in pleasurable activities are considered "sinners" in need of punishment. According to the prohibitionist model, it is the state's duty to mete out the punishment to those who use (certain) drugs. Former President Ronald Reagan (1982) stated it thus: ". . . individuals are responsible for their actions . . . evil is frequently a conscious choice, and . . . retribution must be swift and sure" (p. 1313). As White (1979) points out, a key element in the prohibitionist model "is the arbitrary designation of 'good' and 'evil' drugs with evil drugs possessing powers that can overwhelm all efforts at human control. 'The Devil made him do it' is changed to 'the drug made him do it'" (p. 174). As discussed previously, legal drugs commonly are construed as "good," whereas illegal drugs are construed as "bad." There is absolutely no empirical basis for such a distinction.

Although drug users are no longer referred to as "sinners" by most people who advocate zero tolerance, the view that drug use results from something inherently wrong or evil in the person is still very much a part of the prohibitionist model. For example, in his discussion of the War on Drugs, Inciardi (1992) identifies the premises upon which zero tolerance is based; these premises include: a) if there were no drug abusers there would be no drug problem; b) drug abuse starts with a willful act; c) drug users are powerless to act against outside influences such as peer pressure is erroneous; and d) most illegal drug users can choose to stop their drug-taking behaviors and must be held accountable if they do not. It follows from this view that drug users do not deserve sympathy or compassion because they "choose" to abuse drugs. In other words, drug users are "free" to stop at any time, but they do not stop because they are simply bad people who deserve nothing but punishment. If one conceptualizes drug abuse as the result of some inherent badness within the individual, there is little that can be done to treat such an individual; thus, punishment remains the only alternative. Given these basic premises, one should not be surprised that the prohibitionists place the majority of their emphasis on law enforcement and imprisonment.

The prohibitionist model may have some intuitive appeal because it directly follows from the common Western view that human behavior is freely chosen, but there is little empirical evidence to demonstrate that policies based on the model actually decreases drug use and abuse. For example, in 1988, federal spending on the War on Drugs was slightly under $5 billion (Office of National Drug Control Policy, 1998), while the number of persons reporting past month use of any illegal drug was slightly over 13 million (Substance Abuse and Mental Health Services Administration, 1998). By 1997, the total federal drug control budget grew to almost $15 billion (Office of National Drug Control Policy, 1998), while the number of persons reporting past month use of any illegal drug was slightly under 14 million (NIDA, 1998). Despite the threefold increase in spending on drug control efforts, the number of illegal drug users has increased slightly. As it did in the 1920s, prohibition once again has failed to control drug abuse.

The Disease Model of Drug Abuse

Another old and popular conception of drug abuse is the disease model, which suggests less draconian strategies for dealing with drug abusers than does the prohibitionist model. In this model, which is most often applied to alcoholism, drug abuse is viewed as a chronic and progressive disease that merits medical treatment.

One of the earliest suggestions that alcoholism was a disease was made by Benjamin Rush, a signer of the Declaration of Independence and Surgeon General of the United States (Rivers, 1994). The modern version of the disease model came to prominence in the middle of the twentieth century with the rise of the Alcoholics Anonymous movement (McKim, 1997), and was given some degree of scientific legitimacy with the publication of Jellinek's *The Disease Concept of Alcoholism* in 1960. The disease model of alcoholism was once strongly rejected by the American Medical Association, but is now strongly endorsed by that agency. Some have argued that the medical profession embraced the disease concept of drug abuse after it came to realize the financial and political gains associated with labeling drug-related problems a disease (e.g., Peele, 1989).

Perhaps for similar reasons, the American Psychiatric Association (APA) also embraces a disease model, although it uses the term "disorder" rather than "disease" when referring to drug abuse (McKim, 1997). Because of its approval by the APA, this model is likely to be employed by clinicians in their diagnosis and treatment of substance abuse. For example, in diagnosing substance abuse, clinicians are likely to use criteria from the *Diagnostic and Statistical Manual of Mental Disorders - Fourth Edition (DSM-IV)* (APA, 1994). According to *DSM-IV*, a substance (drug) abuse disorder involves:

A maladaptive pattern of substance use leading to clinically significant impairment or distress, as manifested by one or more of the following: (1) recurrent substance use resulting in a failure to fulfill major role obligations . . . (2) recurrent substance use in situations in which it is physically hazardous (e.g., driving an automobile or operating a machine when impaired by substance use) . . . (3) recurrent substance-related legal problems . . . [and] (4) continued substance use despite having persistent or recurrent social or interpersonal problems caused or exacerbated by the effects of the substance. (pp. 182-183)

One major problem with the disease model is that there is sufficient variability in patterns of drug abuse to render questionable the value of subsuming all of those "symptoms" under the rubric of a single disease. A second problem is that the physical cause of the drug-related problems is unspecified. The lack of a causal mechanism makes it virtually impossible to identify suitable treatments.

Aside from conceptual difficulties, the disease model also fails as a basis for treating drug abuse. The 12-step program, as exemplified by Alcoholics Anonymous (AA), is perhaps the most well-known method of treating drug abuse. It is based, in part, on a disease model, and has the virtue of viewing alcohol abusers as "sick people who need help," not as "sinners who deserve punishment." Nonetheless, the effectiveness of AA in treating alcohol abuse is questionable (Akers, 1992). In fact, when compared to behavioral treatments, 12-step treatment programs based on the disease model are not as effective in retaining clients in treatment or in engendering abstinence (Higgins et al., 1991; Higgins et al., 1994). The disease model has many supporters (see Maltzman, 1994), but few virtues.

Contemporary Drug Use in America

Today in America, drug use is widespread. Consider that approximately 80% to 90% of Americans over the age of 11 years (about 180 million people) consume caffeine, primarily in the form of coffee, weekly (Strain, Mumford, Silverman, & Griffiths, 1994). Their average per capita consumption is 200 mg per day (about the amount in two cups of coffee) (Barone & Roberts, 1984; Clementz & Dailey, 1988). This is enough caffeine to produce withdrawal symptoms upon abstention in some regular users (Griffiths & Mumford, 1995).

According to the most recent National Household Survey on Drug Abuse (NIDA, 1998), alcohol is second only to caffeine as Americans' drug of choice, and approximately 50% of U.S. citizens over 12 years of age (111 million) consumed alcohol at least once in the month before they completed the survey. Tobacco, in the form of both smoked and smokeless products, is the third most popular drug in America. It is used by approximately 30% of Americans over the age of 12 years (71 million) (NIDA, 1998). Figure 10-1 depicts the number of individuals in the United States reporting use of various drugs in the month before they completed the NIDA survey.

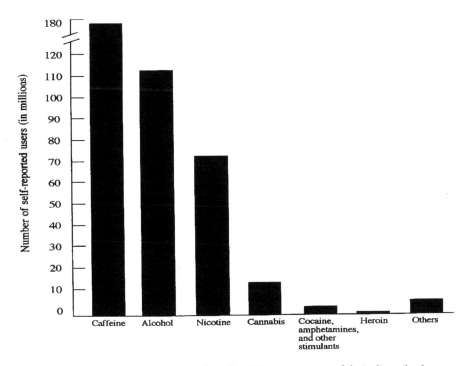

Figure 10-1. *Number of individuals in the U.S. reporting use of the indicated substance in the month prior to completing the most recent NIDA survey.*

As Figure 10-1 shows, most Americans consume one drug or another on at least a monthly basis. It should be noted that these data are based on self-reports and thus may not accurately reflect actual level of drug use. In addition, these data do not include certain segments of the population, such as the homeless and school truants and dropouts, who are believed to have higher than average rates of drug use. It is probable, but by no means certain, that the actual prevalence of drug use is slightly higher than is reflected in the National Household Survey.

In considering the data presented in Figure 10-1, it is important to recognize that these are data for drug *use*, not drug *abuse*. Unless one adopts a moralistic position, in which any use of a particular substance is tantamount to abuse, it is possible to self-administer a drug and not abuse it. For instance, far more people drink alcohol than abuse it. Determining why this is so requires an understanding of the variables that contribute to drug abuse.

Although the specific problems that result from inappropriate drug use can vary greatly in form and severity, there is one element common to all cases of drug abuse: Drug-related behaviors create a problem that can be solved only if these behaviors are changed. Drug abuse inevitably involves, and is in fact defined by, inappropriate drug-seeking and drug-taking. Behavioral pharmacologists emphasize that drug-seeking and drug-taking are operant responses that should be conceptualized no differently from other undesirable behaviors controlled by other response-produced events. The variables that influence operant behavior in general, and drug self-administration in particular, have been studied at considerable length, and a behavior-analytic model of drug abuse has gained acceptance in many quarters. Its primary features are outlined below.

The Behavior-Analytic Model of Drug Abuse

As discussed in Chapter 5, behavioral pharmacologists have demonstrated convincingly that a variety of opiates, sedatives, stimulants, and other drugs will maintain the drug taking of nonhumans in environments devoid of obvious predisposing factors (e.g., Griffiths, Bigelow, & Henningfield, 1980). That is, laboratory animals need not be stressed, food-deprived, provided with nondrug reinforcers, or treated in any unusual manner to establish drug self-administration. This finding called into question the long-held belief that drug abuse in humans was a symptom of an underlying psychopathology, and suggested that people took recreational drugs simply because the short-term sensory consequences of the drugs were pleasurable.

In addition, the availability of animal self-administration assays provided a basis for examining the kinds of variables that influence drug intake. The relevance of data collected with nonhumans to understanding human drug self-administration depends upon the extent to which (1) drugs that serve as positive reinforcers for nonhumans serve a similar function for humans; (2) humans and nonhumans are similarly sensitive to the effects of self-administered drugs, and (3) similar variables control humans' and nonhumans' drug intake. After reviewing the self-administration literature, Johanson (1978) and Griffiths et al. (1980) contended that these assumptions are generally well supported. Results of animal studies, combined with controlled human research in laboratory settings (Chapter 6), naturalistic observations, and treatment outcome studies (see below), provide ample support for conceptualizing abused drugs as positive reinforcers and drug self-administration as operant behavior. As Kelleher and Goldberg (1976) note: "The advantage of considering drug-seeking behaviors in terms of reinforcement is not that this explains why drugs can act as reinforcers but rather that drug-seeking behavior can be analyzed functionally in the same way as other operant behavior" (p. 294). From this perspective, drug reinforcers are not fundamentally different from other reinforcers and abusive patterns of drug self-administration are not fundamentally different from other unhealthy behavior patterns.

It is, for instance, not surprising that it is very difficult for most people to stop smoking cigarettes. Cigarettes are easy to obtain and relatively cheap. Each inhalation of cigarette smoke, a response that requires minimal effort, is followed almost immediately by the arrival of nicotine molecules in the brain, an event that serves as a powerful positive reinforcer. Moreover, it is a reinforcer that is effective hundreds of times a day. There are no short-term aversive consequences of smoking, but a smoker who fails to smoke feels poorly. Given these features, cigarette smoking is difficult to give up, even though it dramatically increases the risk of lung cancer, emphysema, and other health problems.

Cigarette smoking is not fundamentally different from another huge public-health problem, overeating. High-calorie food is a powerful positive reinforcer readily available and relatively cheap in the U.S. Eating such food is easy and can be repeated several times a day, with no short-term aversive consequences. Not surprisingly, many people in the U.S. overeat and experience serious health problems (e.g., heart disease) as a consequence. Nonetheless, they have difficulty dieting.

Not all people with ready access to cigarettes become "addicted" to them, however, and some who do are able to quit. Similarly, many people follow healthy diets, despite the widespread availability of sweetened fats. Even when stimuli that potentially are powerful positive reinforcers are available, patterns of intake are not fixed, but vary as a function of a wide range of historical and current variables. Several of these variables are discussed below.

Imitation and Rules

Obviously, no one abuses a drug without having been exposed to it. If a drug is available, initial exposure to it characteristically involves imitative or rule-governed behavior. In Western cultures children receive extensive imitation training, therefore, a young person who observes the behavior of someone who is important to him or her is likely to imitate that individual (Guerin, 1994). The imitating individual may receive social reinforcers, such as praise, for imitation, or the correspondence between the imitator's behavior and the behavior of the model may function as a form of generalized reinforcement. The last mechanism seems to be involved when children buy and "smoke" candy cigarettes and cigars in an attempt to be more like adults who smoke. It is unlikely that children would purchase and consume such items if they had no models to imitate.

It is also possible that the imitating individual observes the consequences of the model's behavior and is affected by them. A common tactic used by the tobacco and alcohol industries is the production of advertisements implying that the use of their products is associated with success, sex, or status. For example, a common cigarette advertisement shows a man holding a pack of brand-name cigarettes as an attractive woman looks at him with obvious interest, even though she is with another man. This advertisement implies that smoking this particular brand of cigarettes will make the smoker more appealing to beautiful women, to the point where they will leave their significant others for the smoker. For many men, this is a powerful outcome, even if it is merely implied. Viewing the ad may directly increase the likelihood that such people will smoke the "sexy" brand, as a form of imitative behavior. Doing so may also cause them to formulate verbal rules that lead to smoking.

As discussed in Chapter 8, verbal stimuli in the form of **rules** can influence many important human behaviors, including drug use (see Poling & LeSage, 1992). As we use the term, rules are stimuli that specify relations among responses and stimuli and alter behavior by changing the function of other stimuli (Blakely & Schlinger, 1987; Schlinger & Blakely, 1987). Rules may, for instance, cause previously neutral stimuli to act as powerful positive reinforcers. Consider a young woman who is told by her friends that "smoking cigarettes make you look more mature." If looking more mature is important to her, then this rule may increase the likelihood that the young woman will try her first cigarette and that smoking cigarettes will be a reinforcing event.

Several studies have demonstrated the ability of rules to alter the behavioral function of drugs (see Poling & LeSage, 1992). For example, a series of studies by Hughes and his associates (Hughes, Pickens, Spring, & Keenan, 1985; Hughes et al., 1989b; Hughes, Gulliver, Amori, Mireault, & Fenwick, 1989a) that are described in some detail in Chapter 8 demonstrate that whether or not nicotine in chewing gum serves as a positive reinforcer in cigarette smokers trying to quit depends on what they are told regarding the availability of nicotine and its subjective effects.

Self-generated as well as other-generated rules can influence the effects of drugs, including whether they are self-administered. Differences in rule-governed behavior may well contribute to differences in drug effects across people. One of the beneficial effects of rules is to bring behavior under the control of long-delayed consequences; another is to bring behavior under the control of consequences that would be harmful if directly experienced. Although this possibility is difficult to test empirically, it may be that drug self-administration in drug abusers is controlled primarily by the drug's immediate pharmacological consequences; that is, for such individuals, drug-taking is not rule-governed. Or it may be that drug abusers follow rules that generate harmful patterns of self-administration (e.g., "I can have one more beer and drive home O.K.; I've done it before"). In contrast, people who use drugs responsibly appear to generate and follow gainful rules (e.g., "I'd better switch to soda; I have to drive home").

Behavior analysts have only recently begun to explore the variables that control rule generation and rule following (e.g., Hayes & Chase, 1991). Like contingency-governed behavior, rule-governed behavior is operant behavior. All operant behavior is plastic, in that it varies within and across people as a function of historical and current variables. Those variables reside in the environment, and are potentially capable of being measured and manipulated.

Social Contingencies

Another possible reason for using a drug is that social reinforcers may become available as a result of drug use. For example, a teenager may receive praise or attention from friends for trying beer for the first time, or for "chugging" (rapidly drinking) several beers. In this situation, the behavior of drinking is reinforced by the resulting praise, and the taste and smell of the beer may become conditioned reinforcers due to their proximity to social reinforcers (Higgins, Hughes, & Bickel, 1989; Johanson, Mattox, & Schuster, 1995). It is also the case that in some social circles young people can escape from teasing, disapproval, name-calling, or ostracism if they use a particular drug. Here, drug use would be strengthened by negative social reinforcement. In both scenarios, the social variables that contribute to drug use could be subsumed under the term "peer pressure."

Social interactions form the basis of drug-using subcultures. In general, a **drug-using subculture** consists of an interrelated network of persons who maintain behavioral practices involving the use of a certain drug as a main focus of activity. These behaviors typically involve searching for, obtaining, and self-administering the chosen drug, as well as talking about the drug-related behaviors. Participating in a drug subculture increases the likelihood that a person will come under the control of the social contingencies maintained by the group, hence increasing the likelihood that the person will self-administer the chosen drug. Furthermore, the drug subculture may come to act as social support network for the individual, who may not have access to alternative support networks. It is also possible that as the person becomes more involved in the drug subculture, people outside the drug-using subculture may lose their influence and disappear from the drug user's life, further increasing the likelihood of self-administration.

For example, as drug self-administration increases and progresses toward abuse, drug-related behaviors can weaken contingencies that otherwise would discourage abusive intake. Envision a happily married couple, one of whom has recently secured employment as a construction laborer. Neither has a drug abuse problem, but the newly hired spouse begins to stop regularly after work to have a few drinks with fellow laborers. At first, the drinking involves little time and less alcohol, for the reinforcers associated with home and spouse are preferred to those associated with bar and coworkers. As days pass, however, the homebound mate wearies of waiting, and begins to behave differently upon the companion's return from work. No longer is dinner kept waiting and plans laid for a happy evening. Arguments, beginning with "Where the hell have you been?" become commonplace as the evening hour grows less pleasant - and less reinforcing - for both partners. As the home environment becomes less reinforcing, the bar grows relatively more so. Hence more time is spent in the bar and more alcohol is drunk. This in its turn further increases marital discord in an ever worsening spiral that may well end in both divorce and a drug abuse problem.

The scenario just described is overly simple, but it does emphasize an important point: Drug-related behaviors may reduce an individual's access to other reinforcers and thereby increase the relative time and effort directed to drug seeking and drug taking. Moreover, some individuals who experience drug-related problems have never acquired a behavioral repertoire adequate for attaining any of a range of significant positive reinforcers, such as a good job, a reasonable place of residence, rewarding friends, and satisfying lovers. In the absence of strong competing reinforcers, the relative power of drugs and drug-related activities to control behavior is magnified immensely. This has significant treatment implications, for, as Ray (1983) notes, "In fact, treatment for many drug abusers is habilitation, not rehabilitation" (p. 28).

In considering the relative reinforcing value of environments that are and are not associated with drug use, it is interesting that many drugs used recreationally, including alcohol and d-amphetamine, increase human social interaction and the reinforcing value of such interaction. For example, Higgins et al. (1989) gave volunteers the opportunity to engage in one of two mutually-exclusive concurrent options, either speaking with a volunteer or providing a speech monologue for money. Subjects chose the social reinforcement option significantly more often when they received d-amphetamine than when they received placebo. They reported that the drug made them feel more friendly, elated, and energetic, measures that are associated with increased sociability. These results indicate that d-amphetamine acted as a establishing operation that increased the reinforcing effectiveness of social reinforcement relative to monetary reinforcement. Note that choosing the social option necessarily resulted in loss of the opportunity to earn money, a powerful reinforcer under most conditions. Drugs that increase social contact, such as d-amphetamine, increase the likelihood that the interoceptive stimuli produced by the drug will be paired with social reinforcers, thereby changing these stimuli into conditioned reinforcers. Such pairings could give a drug an added degree of reinforcing effectiveness, hence increasing the frequency of self-administration.

As we have seen, many of the variables involved in drug use could result in changing formerly neutral or aversive stimuli into reinforcing stimuli. This could occur through direct pairing with potent reinforcers, such as when drug use is followed by social reinforcement as in the Higgins et al. (1989) study just described, or through the statement of a rule, such as "This pill will make you feel really good." Such acquired reinforcing properties could well function to increase the frequency of subsequent drug use. The taste of a cigarette, for instance, might become a conditioned reinforcer as a result of being paired with attention, thus contributing to the maintenance of smoking (Jaffe, 1990). A similar process has been demonstrated in a study by Johanson et al. (1995), in which placebo pills that were paired with monetary reinforcers became potent reinforcers in their own right. These placebo pills subsequently maintained significantly more self-administration than placebo pills that were paired with lower monetary values (see Chapter 6 for a more detailed discussion of this study).

Stressful Environments

"Stress" generally refers to behavioral and physiological responses to aversive stimuli, termed stressors, and stressful environments contain a high density of aversive stimuli. Studies with nonhumans reveal that self-administration of cocaine and other drugs often increases when subjects are exposed to electric shocks and other stressors (Piazza & Le Moal, 1998). For example, Shaham and Stewart (1995) demonstrated that exposure to intermittent electric shock reinstated heroin self-administration in rats even though up to six weeks had passed, and many sessions of extinction had been arranged, since the last drug injection. Similar results were obtained by Erb, Shaham, and Stewart (1996), who used cocaine as the reinforcer.

In sum, results with nonhumans suggest that humans exposed to stressful environments may be more likely to self-administer drugs. Consistent with this analysis are the results of retrospective studies which indicate that stress contributes to the acquisition and maintenance of drug self-administration in humans (e.g., Gawin, 1991; Johanson & Fischman, 1989). For example, a large number of American soldiers used heroin and other drugs in Vietnam, which undoubtedly qualified as a "stressful" environment (Segal, 1988). Most of them did not, however, continue to use the same drugs upon returning to the States (Robins, Davis, & Goodwin, 1974). There were, of course, many variables in addition to stress that contributed to drug use and abuse among these soldiers. Neither stress nor any of the other variables we are considering cause drug abuse in a simple, linear fashion. Instead, each of them potentially contributes to its occurrence.

Impoverished Environments

Environments with a high density of aversive stimuli may also provide a low density of positive non-drug reinforcers. As suggested in the example of the married couple presented earlier in this chapter, the lack of alternative reinforcers can function to increase drug use (Schuster, 1986). Behavior analysts have developed **matching theory** to provide a quantitative description of the allocation of behavior when two or more reinforcers are concurrently available. This theory states that behavior is distributed across concurrently available alternative behaviors in the same proportion that reinforcers are distributed across these alternatives (McDowell, 1988). That is, the rate of behavior on, or time allocated to, one response alternative is directly related to the rate of reinforcement for that response alternative. Thus, richer sources of reinforcement will control proportionally more behavior than leaner sources. Furthermore, response rates on a single response alternative are a function of the availability of reinforcers for that behavior relative to all other sources of reinforcement in the environment. In general, as the overall environment becomes richer in terms of reinforcement density, the number of responses on the single response alternative decreases (McDowell, 1988).

It is evident from matching theory that, if a person lives in an impoverished environment, he or she likely will spend much time and effort engaging in those behaviors that result in what few reinforcers are available, including drugs. Evidence for this interpretation is provided by Kirby, Marlowe, Lamb, and Platt (1997), who identified the social characteristics of urban crack cocaine-dependent individuals: " . . . [They] are typically poorly educated, unemployed, lacking in both communication and vocational skills, estranged from family and friends, and homeless" (p. 420). Such persons may well have very few available sources of reinforcement apart from drugs, including crack cocaine.

Economic Conditions

In recent years, the field of behavioral economics has applied economic principles to the analysis of operant behavior, including drug self-administration. In essence, behavioral economics involves determining the importance of a commodity to an individual by ascertaining how consumption of that commodity changes as a function of its price. Price refers to the amount of resources (time, behavior, money) required to produce a commodity, and is often operationally defined in laboratory studies as the number of responses required to produce a reinforcer, such as delivery of a drug. In such studies, consumption characteristically is defined as the number of drug deliveries obtained in a specified period.

The log-log plot of consumption against price increases is termed the **demand function**. Inelastic demand, indicating that the commodity is very important to the individual - that is, a "need" - is shown by a function with a slope less steep than - 1 (work increases as price increases), where the slope is a measure of the elasticity. Elastic demand, suggesting that the commodity is a "luxury," is shown by a function with a slope steeper than -1 (work decreases as price increases). Many demand functions are curvilinear and equations have been developed for describing such functions (e.g., Hursh & Winger, 1995). The interpretation of curvilinear demand functions is not fundamentally different from the interpretation of linear functions. If demand for a particular drug is relatively inelastic, strategies that increase the unit (i.e., per reinforcer) price of that drug, in terms of the amount of time, money, or behavior required to produce it, should be minimally effective. On the other hand, if demand is highly elastic, slight increases in price should significantly reduce consumption. As an example of applying demand analyses to reducing drug abuse, McKim (1997) relates that the overall elasticity of demand for cigarettes is about -0.7. Elasticity of demand varies, however, for different segments of the population. In one study (Lewitt, 1989), demand in smokers less than 20 years of age was found to be elastic; the slope of the demand curve was -1.40. In older smokers, however, demand was relatively inelastic. For them, the slope of the demand curve was -0.4. As McKim (1997) relates, these figures indicate that:

> [I]ncreasing the price of cigarettes will have a considerable impact on the initiation rate of young smokers - but it may not have a large effect on the smoking behavior of older, established smokers. Since most people become smokers before the age of 20, price increases will have a considerable effect

not only at the time they are put into effect, but will decrease cigarette consumption far into the future (Lewitt, 1989). (p. 180)

Consistent with this analysis are data indicating that the relative price of cigarettes has increased over the past 30 years, while the relative number of cigarette smokers has decreased. However, despite substantial price increases, experienced smokers - for whom demand is inelastic - have trouble quitting.

Older people differ from younger people in several regards that might influence demand for cigarettes. One obvious difference is that older people, on whole, have more money. There is no doubt that income, defined as the resources available to obtain reinforcers within a given period of time, combines with price to determine consumption (DeGrandpre, Bickel, Rizvi, & Hughes, 1993). In fact, changing income has been demonstrated to affect, and sometimes even reverse, choice for a variety of reinforcers, including drugs (e.g., Carroll, Rodefer, & Rawleigh, 1995; DeGrandpre et al., 1993).

A study by DeGrandpre et al. (1993) provides a clear example of the effects of income manipulations on human drug intake. In this study, nicotine-dependent smokers had concurrent access to two brands of cigarettes, their preferred brand and a nonpreferred brand. The nonpreferred brand always was one-fifth the price of the preferred brand and income was varied across sessions. In general, as income increased, self-administration of the preferred brand increased while self-administration of the less expensive nonpreferred brand decreased. Subjects were exposed to an additional condition in which income was held constant and the price of the nonpreferred brand was increased. In most subjects, increasing the price of the nonpreferred brand decreased their consumption of that brand. Thus, when an individual's income is sufficient he or she will tend to consume more of a preferred drug reinforcer. Similarly, when the price of a preferred drug reinforcer is relatively low compared to alternative reinforcers, the person will consume more of the preferred drug reinforcer.

In the DeGrandpre et al. (1993) study, two alternative drug reinforcers were available. In this case, the nonpreferred brand substituted for the preferred brand when income was low, but not when income was high. Laboratory studies indicate that under some conditions non-drug reinforcers also can substitute for drug reinforcers (e.g., Carroll, 1993).

In sum, research and theorizing in behavioral economics provides evidence that patterns of drug use are influenced by a person's income and by the price and availability of drug and alternative reinforcers. Although these are by no means the only variables that contribute to drug use and abuse, they certainly are important ones, and demand curve analyses provide a powerful, quantitative method for assessing their effects. Matching theory analyses serve a similar function.

Respondent Conditioning Variables

When an individual consistently uses a drug in the same environment, features of the environment can control certain drug-related responses. This occurs via respondent conditioning, in which a neutral stimulus (environmental feature) is predictably followed by an unconditional stimulus (US), the drug. Eventually, as a result of repeated pairings, the formerly neutral stimulus becomes a conditional stimulus (CS) and elicits conditional responses (CRs) that may be similar to the unconditional responses (URs) produced by the drug. In this case, if the effects of the drug are positively reinforcing, then drug-related stimuli may come to serve as conditioned positive reinforcers. This occurs, for instance, in the "needle freak" phenomenon. Individuals who earn this sobriquet report that the act of preparing and injecting their drug of choice is most pleasant. In the words of an occasional heroin user, "Sometimes I think that if I just shot water I'd enjoy it as much" (unnamed, quoted in Powell, 1973, p. 591). Perhaps, but only so long as injections were at least occasionally paired with heroin injections.

> "Needle freaks" are not commonly encountered. However: There is widespread clinical speculation that rituals and other stimuli associated with drug use become potent conditioned reinforcers which maintain involvement in the drug-using lifestyle and contribute significantly to relapse. For instance, the taste of cigarettes or strong alcoholic drinks are generally considered unpleasant by the inexperienced user; however, after a history involving repeated pairing with the associated drug effects, these tastes apparently become quite powerful conditioned reinforcers in experienced users. (Griffiths et al., 1980, p. 53).

In the "needle freak" phenomenon, conditional responses controlled by pre-drug stimuli are similar to the unconditional responses produced by the drug, insofar as both are perceived as pleasant. It is often the case, however, that with respondent drug conditioning the CS elicit CRs *opposite* to those produced by the drug (see Chapter 3). Such responses, termed "compensatory responses," attenuate the URs produced by the drug, hence diminishing the experienced drug effects (Cunningham, 1993). In a sense, environmental stimuli that regularly precede drug administration physiologically "prepare" the organism for the upcoming drug administration by producing responses to compensate for the unconditioned drug effects. Because pre-drug stimuli often produce compensatory responses that are the opposite of the drug effect, in the absence of drug such compensatory responses would be expected to resemble withdrawal symptoms. Experiencing those withdrawal symptoms may increase the reinforcing effectiveness of the drug. In other words, the environmental stimuli (i.e., CSs) that have been paired with drug administration (i.e., US) may become establishing operations for the drug by producing compensatory responses. If this is the case, an increase in the value of a drug reinforcer will be accompanied by an increase in drug-seeking behaviors, eventually resulting in drug self-administration.

There is a second plausible mechanism whereby environmental stimuli could, through respondent conditioning, increase the reinforcing effectiveness of a drug. This mechanism involves the pairing of environmental stimuli with drug abstinence and its attendant withdrawal syndrome. If a drug-dependent individual is unable to procure drug in time to prevent withdrawal syndrome, he or she may begin to experience the unpleasant effects of a withdrawal syndrome in the presence of certain environmental stimuli. Such stimuli could be the person's home, neighborhood, or friends with whom the person uses or seeks drugs. Probably the stimulus most likely to be reliably paired with withdrawal syndrome is the person from which the drug-dependent individual purchases the drug. Because of this pairing, stimuli related to the dealer would precipitate withdrawal syndrome, although other environmental stimuli likely would have similar effects.

Evidence for this phenomenon is provided in a study by Goldberg, Woods, and Schuster (1969), who found that stimuli paired with nalorphine, an opiate antagonist that produces an immediate withdrawal syndrome in opiate-dependent organisms, also induced withdrawal syndrome in morphine-dependent monkeys and increased morphine self-administration. Subsequent presentation of these conditioned stimuli produced an increase in the reinforcing efficacy of morphine and evoked self-administration behavior. In this study, the stimuli paired with the nalorphine-induced withdrawal syndrome were analogous to stimuli in the natural environment that are paired with a withdrawal syndrome brought on by continued abstinence from the drug.

Clinical observations of drug-dependent humans lend further support to the notion that stimuli paired with drug administration can elicit withdrawal symptoms and thereby a) increase the reinforcing capacity of the drug in question, and b) evoke drug-seeking behavior (Cunningham, 1993; Hinson & Siegel, 1980; O'Brien, Ehrman, & Ternes, 1986). Put differently, such stimuli can serve as establishing operations. Wikler (1965), for instance, noted that former drug-dependent individuals receiving treatment sometimes showed signs of withdrawal syndrome months after their last drug administration, a phenomenon Wikler termed **conditioned abstinence** (sometimes referred to as **conditioned withdrawal**) Some of the individuals that Wikler observed exhibited these symptoms in group therapy during explicit descriptions of drug use. Apparently, the verbal stimuli themselves were able to precipitate the onset of withdrawal syndrome. Wikler's (1965) findings fit nicely with the experimental findings of Goldberg et al. (1969), confirming the important role of respondent conditioning factors in human drug use and abuse.

Other Variables

As discussed in Chapter 1, behavioral pharmacologists recognize that genotype influences behavior, including drug self-administration. It is, for example, widely known that children with one or both parents diagnosed as alcoholic are at increased risk for receiving the same diagnosis, even if they are raised by adoptive parents (e.g., Petrakis, 1985; Schuckit, 1992). Such individuals may differ with respect to brain chemistry, a proposition discussed in Chapter 4, and may therefore be more sensitive to alcohol as a reinforcer. Some support for this proposition comes from animal studies (e.g., George & Goldberg, 1989; George, Ritz, & Elmer, 1991), which show that the effectiveness of ethanol as a positive reinforcer a) differs across some existing rodent strains, and b) can be readily varied through selective breeding.

It is unlikely, however, that a simple difference in reinforcing effectiveness is responsible for the role of inheritance in alcohol abuse. Other effects, such as an individual's initial sensitivity to the drug, probably play a role as well. The effects of such variables were recently demonstrated by Kurtz, Stewart, Zweifel, Li, and Froehlich (1996), who studied the influence of genetic differences in responses to the behaviorally-disruptive effects of alcohol in alcohol-preferring (P) and alcohol-nonpreferring (NP) lines of rats. These lines of rats were selectively bred to drink high (P) and low (NP) amounts of an alcohol solution when given free access to the drug, food, and water. Each group of rats was given two injections of alcohol separated by either 1 or 2 days. As the dependent variable, Kurtz et al. measured alcohol's effects on the latency to lose the righting reflex and the time to recover the righting reflex. The loss of the righting reflex was determined by placing each rat on its back every 30 s after the injection until the rat was unable to right itself. The time between the injection and the rat's inability to right itself was defined as the latency of loss of righting reflex.

When given an initial behaviorally-disruptive dose of alcohol, P rats exhibited a significantly longer latency to lose the righting reflex and a significantly shorter time to recover the righting reflex than did NP rats. These results indicate that, with respect to behavioral impairment, the P rats were less sensitive to alcohol than were the NP rats. Furthermore, when one day separated the two alcohol injections, the P rats recovered the righting reflex more rapidly following the second injection compared to the first injection, indicating that the P rats developed tolerance to the disruptive effects of alcohol. The NP rats recovered the righting reflex more slowly following the second alcohol injection than they did after the first injection, indicating that these rats developed sensitization to the disruptive effects of alcohol. These differences between the two lines of rats disappeared when the alcohol injections were separated by two days.

In this study, a genetic difference in preference for alcohol was associated with decreased initial sensitivity to alcohol and with the rapid development of tolerance to alcohol. The findings of Kurtz et al. suggest that genetic differences among individuals in initial sensitivity to alcohol and/or the rapid development of tolerance to alcohol may contribute to differences in susceptibility to alcohol abuse and dependence. Support for this interpretation is provided by a study by Schuckit (1994), who found that sons of alcoholics generally were less affected by alcohol than were other young men of the same age. In Schuckit's study, those men who were least affected by alcohol when tested at the age of 22 years were most likely to be alcohol dependent 10 years later. However, as Kurtz et al. caution:

> It is unlikely that any single trait, such as alcohol sensitivity or the rapid development of alcohol tolerance is sufficient for the expression of the alcohol drinking phenotype. Instead, the presence of certain environmental variables and alcohol-related traits may serve to increase the probability of high alcohol drinking behavior, and a combination of these variables and traits may act additively or interact synergistically to produce high alcohol drinking behavior. (p. 590)

Schuckit (1994) did not assess the reinforcing effectiveness of alcohol, and it is not clear whether it is related to intrinsic tolerance. In any case, most people who abuse alcohol do not have an alcohol-abusing parent, and the mechanism through which genotype contributes to drug abuse remains speculative.

As an aside, there is a recognized genetic mutation that does appear to reduce the likelihood of alcohol abuse (O'Brien, 1996). Alcohol is inactivated (oxidized) primarily by two enzymes, alcohol dehydrogenase, which acts to produce acetaldehyde, and acetaldehyde dehydrogenase, which acts to convert acetaldehyde to acetyl CoA. Acetyl CoA is oxidized through the citric acid cycle or used in a variety of anabolic reactions (Hobbs, Ral, & Verdoorn, 1996). By virtue of inheritance, a substantial number of people of Asian descent produce a form of acetaldehyde dehydrogenase that is less effective than the more common version. They rapidly convert alcohol to acetaldehyde, but not acetaldehyde to acetyl CoA. Thus, acetaldehyde - which is toxic - rapidly accumulates. As a result, "The drinker . . . experiences a very unpleasant facial flushing reaction that may attenuate the probability of becoming an alcoholic" (O'Brien, 1996, p. 559).

In passing, it is worth noting that **disulfiram** (Antabuse) which sometimes is used to treat alcohol abuse, works by interfering with the action of acetaldehyde dehydrogenase. (Actually, to be precise, metabolites of disulfiram, not the drug itself, appear to do so). The result is that, when a person who has taken disulfiram consumes alcohol, acetaldehyde rapidly accumulates.

[Consequently], within about 5 to 10 minutes, the face feels hot, and soon afterwards it is flushed and scarlet in appearance. As the vasodilation spreads over the whole body, intense throbbing is felt in the head and neck, and a pulsating headache may develop. Respiratory difficulties, nausea, copious vomiting, sweating, thirst, chest pain, considerable hypotension, orthostatic syncope, marked uneasiness, weakness, vertigo, blurred vision, and confusion are observed. . . . As little as 7 ml of alcohol will cause mild symptoms in sensitive persons, and the effect, once elicited, lasts between 30 minutes and several hours. (Hobbs et al., 1996, p. 391)

Given these effects, it is obvious that alcohol will not serve as a positive reinforcer for a person who has taken disulfiram. In fact, the behavioral action of the latter drug is in this case an EO effect - it alters (reduces) the reinforcing effectiveness of another stimulus (alcohol). The allele (form of a gene) associated with an ineffective form of acetaldehyde dehydrogenase does likewise, through a very similar mechanism. Clearly, genotype can play an important role in determining a person's likelihood of abusing alcohol and, perhaps, of abusing drugs in general.

Another variable that is correlated with drug abuse is the presence of psychiatric problems. For example, studies have found that 70-80% of opiate-dependent persons have a psychiatric diagnosis other than opiate dependence (Rounsaville, Weissman, Kleber, & Wilber, 1982; Woody, Luborsky, McLellan, O'Brien, & Beck, 1983). Moreover, drug abuse is prevalent in persons with schizophrenia (Smith & Hucker, 1994). The link between psychiatric conditions and drug abuse is by no means simple. One possibility is that drugs are used to self-medicate the negative effects resulting from the psychiatric condition (O'Brien et al., 1986). It may also be that people with psychiatric conditions are especially likely to live in stressful environments, to have limited access to nondrug reinforcers, and to receive social reinforcers contingent upon drug use. Another possibility is that persons with psychiatric disorders may be especially prone to lack sufficient self-regulatory repertoires to control their own drug use. A final possibility, of course, is that excessive drug use causes, or exacerbates existing, psychiatric conditions. It is, for example, known that stimulants such as amphetamine and cocaine worsen the symptoms of schizophrenia, and that prolonged exposure to such drugs can induce behavior changes closely resembling those indicative of schizophrenia. In addition, terminating exposure to stimulants characteristically induces depression.

Regardless of whether they are causal, a wide range of variables are correlated with an individual's risk of developing an abusive pattern of drug use. Behavior analysts are aware of those variables, and are endeavoring to determine how they are related to substance abuse. Understanding the variables that contribute to a behavioral problem provides a good start for its treatment. As discussed in the next section, treating drug abuse is very difficult, but some interventions based upon the behavior-analytic model of drug abuse are promising.

Treating Drug Abuse

A substantial number of people with drug-related problems eventually are able to solve those problems on their own, but many end up receiving treatment from professionals. The drug treatment literature is gargantuan. Given that there are several alternative theoretical models of drug abuse, it should come as no surprise that there are several different approaches to treatment. This section provides an overview of selected treatments based on the behavior-analytic model of drug abuse. For a behavior analyst, the first step in treating drug abuse is to identify and target those behaviors that produce outcomes that cause significant harm to the individual or to other people. Characteristically, the target behavior to be changed is the self-administration of the abused drug and the desired outcome is abstinence. This outcome has been reliably obtained through the community reinforcement approach (CRA) (Hunt & Azrin, 1973; Sisson & Azrin, 1989) and contingency-management procedures (Stitzer & Bigelow, 1983; Shaner et al., 997).

In the **community reinforcement approach**, an attempt is made to develop community-based sources of reinforcement that can compete with drug reinforcers. Competing reinforcers arranged in CRA procedures include employment, improved interpersonal (e.g., marital) relationships, and new recreational activities. As part of the CRA program, clients attend behavioral therapy sessions that involve employment and career counseling, assertiveness training, relaxation training, and counseling that targets participation in non-drug-related recreational and social activities (Budney, Higgins, Delaney, Kent, & Bickel, 1991). These therapy sessions are intended to increase drug users' participation in non-drug activities, so that they can contact the naturally-occurring reinforcement contingencies related to these activities. As pointed out earlier in our discussion of the matching law, increasing the number of alternative reinforcers should decrease the amount of behavior allocated to obtaining the drug reinforcer and reduce the number of drug reinforcers obtained (e.g., Carroll, 1985; McDowell, 1988). Moreover, successful behavioral therapy enables the client to gain the social skills and rule-governed behavior needed to remain abstinent, thus increasing her or his self-control and independence from the therapist and therapeutic situation.

Contingency management is another example of a therapeutic approach that involves the reinforcement of alternatives to drug-related activities. Under **contingency management procedures,** clients receive tangible reinforcers, such as money or privileges, for providing evidence of drug abstinence, usually in the form of drug-free urine samples (Silverman et al., 1996). A promising variation of contingency management procedures is **voucher-based reinforcement therapy.** Voucher-based reinforcement procedures were developed by Stephen Higgins and his colleagues at the University of Vermont to initiate and maintain cocaine abstinence (e.g., Budney & Higgins, 1998; Higgins et al., 1991; Higgins et al., 1993; Higgins et al., 1994).

Under this procedure, clients receive vouchers for providing drug-free urine samples. Vouchers have monetary values and are exchangeable for goods and services that are consistent with treatment goals, and voucher exchanges are monitored by treatment staff to insure this outcome. An important feature of the voucher system is that the value of the vouchers starts low and is systematically increased as the number of consecutive drug-free urine samples provided by the client is increased. Thus, clients can earn more valuable vouchers by continuing to remain drug-free. If the client produces a drug-positive urine, the value of the vouchers is reset to the initial low value. The purpose of the voucher system is to produce prolonged periods of drug abstinence.

Controlled clinical trials evaluating the voucher system have demonstrated that it is more effective than traditional forms of therapy, such as standard drug abuse counseling (Budney & Higgins, 1998). For instance, Higgins et al. (1991) compared a procedure that combined CRA and contingency-management procedures (i.e., vouchers for drug-free urine) with a standard 12-step drug counseling program for the treatment of cocaine abuse. Abstinence from cocaine was determined by collecting urine samples and analyzing them for benzoylecgonine, a metabolite of cocaine. In this study, 13 cocaine-dependent clients participated in the outpatient behavioral treatment procedures and 12 cocaine-dependent clients participated in the 12-step counseling procedures. In general, characteristics of subjects in the two groups were similar, although the group given the behavioral treatment did report significantly more cocaine use per week before entering treatment and had significantly more intravenous (IV) users than the group given 12-step counseling. Given these two significant differences between groups, one might expect that the group exposed to the behavioral treatment would more resistant to treatment than the other group.

In actuality, 11 out of 13 clients in the behavioral-treatment group completed 12 weeks of behavioral treatment, but only 5 out of 12 clients completed 12 weeks of the 12-step program; this difference was statistically significant. As one might surmise, keeping clients in treatment is an important, and difficult, accomplishment which increases the likelihood that clients will obtain the skills needed to remain abstinent and contact non-drug reinforcers. In fact, clients given the behavioral treatment achieved significantly longer periods of continuous abstinence than clients given the 12-step counseling. For example, 6 out of 13 clients exposed to the behavioral treatment achieved 8 weeks of continuous cocaine abstinence. None of the 12 clients exposed to the 12-step treatment did so. 12 clients exposed to the 12-step treatment did so.

Similar results were obtained by Higgins et al. (1993), who randomly assigned 38 clients to either a CRA and voucher condition or a 12-step program. As in the Higgins et al. (1991) study, subjects in the behavioral treatment group stayed in treatment significantly longer than subjects in the 12-step treatment group. Specifically, 58% of the clients in the former group completed 24 weeks of treatment, whereas only 11% of those in the 12-step treatment group did so. Moreover, 42% of the clients in the behavioral treatment group achieved 16 weeks of continuous cocaine abstinence, whereas only 5% of the clients in the 12-step treatment group achieved this level of abstinence. Figure 10-2 depicts these results.

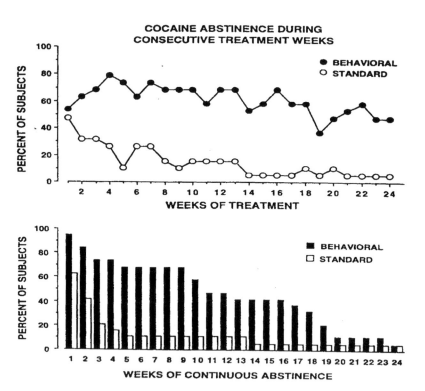

Figure 10-2. *Percent of subjects treated for cocaine abuse who remained abstinent for the indicated number of weeks while receiving behavioral or standard (12-step) treatment. Data are from Higgins et al. (1993) and reproduced by permission.*

Contingency management procedures have been demonstrated to be effective in increasing abstinence from cocaine (e.g., Shaner et al., 1997), nicotine (e.g., Stitzer, Rand, Bigelow, & Mead, 1986), benzodiazepines (e.g., Stitzer, Bigelow, & Liebson, 1979), and opioids (e.g., Silverman et al., 1996). Furthermore, contingency management has been shown to be successful with diverse populations, such as small-city cocaine users (e.g., Higgins et al., 1994), inner-city cocaine users (e.g., Kirby et al., 1997), schizophrenic nicotine users (e.g., Roll, Higgins, Steingard, & McGinley, 1998), homeless and schizophrenic cocaine users (e.g., Shaner et al., 1997), and inner-city opiate users (e.g., Silverman et al., 1997), among others.

Perhaps the most obvious criticism that could be leveled at behavioral treatments such as those used by Higgins and his colleagues is that they require the use of monetary incentives to produce their effects. Objections that have been raised to use of monetary reinforcers include: 1) monetary reinforcers are contrived, 2) the use of monetary reinforcers will result in "symptom substitution" because the underlying problem (i.e., the substance abuse disorder or disease) has not been solved, 3) providing monetary reinforcers for drug abstinence is immoral because people should not be paid to abstain from illegal and dangerous activities, and 4) monetary reinforcers are costly (Higgins et al., 1991). A fifth objection is that procedures based on monetary reinforcers fail to provide effective treatment for a substantial number of drug abusers.

The first criticism is based on an arbitrary distinction. Monetary reinforcers are environmental events that can alter drug-taking behavior, just as drug reinforcers are environmental events that can alter drug-taking behavior. The studies discussed above demonstrated that monetary reinforcers can compete effectively with drug reinforcers. Because these events (i.e., money and drugs) can serve similar behavioral functions, there seems to be no scientific basis by which to distinguish one event as "contrived" and another as "natural." Neither cocaine nor money would be available to serve as positive reinforcers were it not for the efforts of humans.

The second criticism is based on the disease model of drug abuse which, as discussed previously, is at best of questionable validity. In addition, the criticism appears to have no empirical basis - people who refrain from using one drug characteristically do not begin using another drug or develop other troublesome behaviors. For example, in the Higgins et al. (1991) study, there was relatively little use of drugs other than cocaine (the targeted drug) and cannabis. Although the group that received the behavioral treatment used significantly more cannabis than the group that received 12-step treatment, cannabis use and cocaine abstinence were not significantly related, as would be expected if cannabis was substituting for cocaine.

The third criticism is moralistic and is based on the prohibitionist model of drug abuse. From this perspective, people can and should refrain from using drugs because using drugs is immoral; a society should not have to pay people to behave "morally" and should, in fact, punish them if they fail to do so. For those hold this view, treatment effectiveness is irrelevant and all treatments that "reward" drug abusers for abstention are unacceptable. Although this view is held by a surprising number of people, it is inconsistent with a scientific analysis of human behavior in general, and of drug use in particular. This view is also immoral, insofar as it would deprive drug abusers of interventions that reduce suffering and save lives.

The fourth criticism is more legitimate than the first three. Providing monetary incentives can be costly. For example, in the study by Higgins et al. (1994), subjects in the behavioral treatment group could have earned a maximum of $1,022 in incentives, or $6.08 per treatment day, if they were continuously abstinent for the entire 24 weeks of treatment. The actual average total cost per client for this group was $601, or $3.58 per treatment day. Although this may appear to be a substantial amount of money, consider the alternatives. Other interventions, such as 12-step programs, can be quite costly, as well as ineffective. Ineffective interventions have "hidden costs" because of their failure to retain clients in treatment. Among these hidden costs are those associated with inpatient hospitalizations due to drug overdose, medical care for HIV/AIDS and other diseases that are related to certain forms of drug abuse, and medical care for drug-exposed neonates (Budney et al., 1991; Higgins et al., 1991; Higgins et al., 1994). There are also additional costs to society that result from continued drug abuse, including those associated with lost job productivity, industrial accidents, traffic accidents, crimes committed by drug-dependent persons, and child neglect and abuse. In short, the money spent on drug abuse treatment is a good investment for society. For example, Lewis (1994) reported that for every dollar spent on treating abuse of alcohol and other drugs in California, seven dollars were saved. Good treatment programs are a blessing as well as a bargain: They save lives and tears, as well as dollars.

The fifth criticism is legitimate. There is as yet no treatment that produces long-term amelioration of drug-related problems in all clients, or anything approaching that number. While a number of studies have shown that behavioral interventions are more effective than traditional approaches to treating drug abuse, there is a clear need to increase further the effectiveness of interventions. Behavioral-analytic approaches to treating drug abuse are not panaceas, but they are nonetheless extremely useful tools for dealing with one of society's most vexing, and enduring, problems.

Concluding Comments

Drug use and abuse are complex phenomena that can be viewed meaningfully from biological, sociocultural, and behavior-analytic perspectives. In the interest of brevity, many important topics, including pharmacological strategies for treating drug abuse and approaches to preventing drug abuse, have been ignored totally in the present chapter. Others that were introduced, such as the role of genetics, verbal behavior, and cultural practices in drug abuse, were not given adequate attention. Nonetheless, it is our hope that sufficient information was provided to convince the reader of the viability of the behavior-analytic model of drug use and abuse. That model considers drug self-administration to be learned behavior that is, in general, determined by the same classes of variables that affect other kinds of learned behavior.

One advantage of this conception is that it suggests strategies for treating (and preventing, although we did not cover this topic) drug abuse. In general, behavioral approaches to treating drug abuse often involve arranging the client's environment so that a) drug use and abstinence are easily detected, b) drug abstinence is rewarded as quickly as possible, c) drug use results in loss of reinforcers, and d) the density of non-drug reinforcers is increased so as to compete with the reinforcing effects of drugs (Higgins et al., 1991). As evidenced in the studies summarized in this chapter, behavioral treatments such as contingency management have been empirically demonstrated to be more effective than traditional treatment interventions, such as 12-step approaches. Because behavioral programs seek to identify the functional relations that exist between the client's environment and his or her drug-using behaviors, such programs can more effectively alter the environmental conditions that maintain these behaviors than those programs that view drug abuse as the result of an underlying disorder or the fault of the individual user. Equally important, because the behavioral model conceptualizes drug use and abuse as operant behavior that is controlled by the person's environment, clinicians committed to this model focus their energy on finding pragmatic and humane solutions to solving behavioral problems. There is no room in the behavioral model for blaming the user for her or his excessive drug use, just as their is no room for blaming the child who engages in self-injurious behavior for such behavior. Operant behaviors - including drug self-administration - are primarily a result of a person's history of interactions with the environment and current environmental variables. Therefore, laying blame is pointless and a waste of valuable resources that could be better used to help those who are literally trapped in unsafe behavior patterns.

References

Abadinsky, H. (1993). *Drug abuse: An introduction.* Chicago: Nelson-Hall.

Akers, R. L. (1992). *Drugs, alcohol, and society: Social structure, process, and policy.* Belmont, CA: Wadsworth.

American Psychiatric Association. (1994). *Diagnostic and statistical manual of mental disorders* (4th ed.). Washington, DC: Author.

Barone, J. J., & Roberts, H. (1984). Human consumption of caffeine. In P. B. Dews (Ed.), *Caffeine: Perspectives from recent research* (pp. 59-73). Berlin: Springer-Verlag.

Blakely, E., & Schlinger, H. (1987). Rules: Function-altering contingency-specifying stimuli. *The Behavior Analyst, 10,* 183-187.

Budney, A. J., & Higgins, S. T. (1998). *A community reinforcement approach: Treating cocaine addiction* (Manual 2). NIDA Therapy Manuals for Drug Addiction. (NIH Publication No. 98-4309). Rockville, MD: National Institute on Drug Abuse.

Budney, A. J., Higgins, S. T., Delaney, D. D., Kent, L., & Bickel, W. K. (1991). Contingent reinforcement of abstinence with individuals abusing cocaine and marijuana. *Journal of Applied Behavior Analysis, 24,* 657-665.

Carroll, M. E. (1985). Concurrent phencyclidine and saccharin access: Presentation of an alternative reinforcer reduces drug intake. *Journal of the Experimental Analysis of Behavior, 43,* 131-144.

Carroll, M. E. (1993). The economic context of drug and nondrug reinforcers affects acquisition and maintenance of drug reinforced behavior and withdrawal effects. *Alcohol and Drug Dependence, 33,* 201-210.

Carroll, M. E., Rodefer, J. S., & Rawleigh, J. M. (1995). Concurrent self-administration of ethanol and an alternative nondrug reinforcer in monkeys: effects of income (session length) on demand for drug. *Psychopharmacology, 120,* 1-9.

Clementz, G. L., & Dailey, J. W. (1988). Psychotropic effects of caffeine. *American Family Physician, 37,* 167-172.

Cunningham, C. L. (1993). Pavlovian drug conditioning. In F. van Haaren (Ed.). *Methods in behavioral pharmacology* (pp. 349-377). Amsterdam: Elsevier.

DeGrandpre, R. J., Bickel, W. K., Rizvi, S. A. T., & Hughes, J. R. (1993). Effects of income on drug choice in humans. *Journal of the Experimental Analysis of Behavior, 59,* 483-500.

Devereux, P. (1997). *The long trip: A prehistory of psychedelia.* New York: Arkana Books.

Erb, S., Shaham, Y., & Stewart, J. (1996). Stress reinstates cocaine-seeking behavior after prolonged extinction and a drug-free period. *Psychopharmacology, 128,* 408-412.

Furst, P. T. (1976). *Hallucinogens and culture.* San Francisco, CA: Chandler & Sharp.

Gawin, F. H. (1991). Cocaine addiction: Psychology and neurophysiology. *Science, 251,* 293-296.

George, F. R., & Goldberg, S. R. (1989). Genetic approaches to the analysis of addiction processes. *Trends in Pharmacological Science, 10,* 78-83.

George, F. R., Ritz, M. C., & Elmer, G. I. (1991). The role of genetics in vulnerability to drug dependence. In J. Pratt (Ed.), *The biological basis of drug tolerance and dependence* (pp. 265-295). London: Academic Press.

Goldberg, S. R., Woods, J. H., & Schuster, C. R. (1969). Morphine: Conditioned increases in self-administration in rhesus monkeys. *Science, 166,* 1306-1307.

Griffiths, R. R., Bigelow, G. E., & Henningfield, J. E. (1980). Similarities in animal and human drug taking behavior. In N. K. Mello (Ed.), *Advances in substance abuse* (vol. 1, pp. 1-90). Greenwich, CT: JAI Press.

Griffiths, R. R., & Mumford, G. K. (1995). Caffeine—A drug of abuse? In F. E. Bloom & D. J. Kupfer (Eds.), *Psychopharmacology: The fourth generation of progress* (pp. 104-137). New York: Raven Press.

Grinspoon, L., & Bakalar, J. B. (1997). *Psychedelic drugs reconsidered.* New York: The Lindesmith Center.

Guerin, B. (1994). *Analyzing social behavior: Behavior analysis and the social sciences.* Reno, NV: Context Press.

Hayes, L J., & Chase, P. N. (1991). *Dialogues on verbal behavior.* Reno, NV: Context Press.

Drug Abuse   245

Higgins, S. T., Budney, A. J., Bickel, W. K., Feorg, F. E., Donham, R., & Badger, G. J. (1994). Incentives improve outcome in outpatient behavioral treatment of cocaine dependence. *Archives of General Psychiatry, 51,* 568-576.

Higgins, S. T., Budney, A. J., Bickel, W. K., Hughes, J. R., Feorg, F. E., & Badger, G. J. (1993). Achieving cocaine abstinence with a behavioral approach. *American Journal of Psychiatry, 150,* 763-769.

Higgins, S. T., Delaney, D. D., Budney, A. J., Bickel, W. K., Hughes, J. R., Feorg, F., & Fenwick, J. W. (1991). A behavioral approach to achieving initial cocaine abstinence. *American Journal of Psychiatry, 148,* 1218-1224.

Higgins, S. T., Hughes, J. R., & Bickel, W. K. (1989). Effects of *d*-amphetamine on choice of social versus monetary reinforcement: a discrete-trial test. *Pharmacology Biochemistry and Behavior, 34,* 297-301.

Hinson, R. E., & Siegel, S. (1980). The contribution of Pavlovian conditioning to ethanol tolerance and dependence. In H. Rigter & J. C. Crabbe (Eds.), *Alcohol tolerance and dependence* (pp. 181-199). Amsterdam: Elsevier/North-Holland.

Hobbs, W. R., Rall, T. W., & Verdoorn, T. A. (1996). Hypnotics and sedatives: Ethanol. In J. G. Hardman, L. E. Limbird, P. B. Molinoff, R. W. Ruddon, & A. G. Gilman (Eds.), *The pharmacological basis of therapeutics* (pp. 361-396). New York: McGraw-Hill.

Hollinger, M. A. (1997). *Introduction to pharmacology.* Washington, DC: Taylor & Francis.

Hughes, J. R., Gulliver, S. B., Amori, G., Mireault, G., & Fenwick, J. E. (1989a). Effects of instructions and nicotine on smoking cessation, withdrawal symptoms and self-administration of nicotine gum. *Psychopharmacology, 99,* 486-491.

Hughes, J. R., Pickens, R. W., Spring, W., & Keenan, R. M. (1985). Instructions control whether nicotine will serve as a reinforcer. *Journal of Pharmacology and Experimental Therapeutics, 235,* 106-112.

Hughes, J. R., Strickler, G., King, D., Higgins, S. T., Fenwick, J. W., Gulliver, S. B., & Mireault, G. (1989b). Smoking history, instructions and the effects of nicotine: Two pilot studies. *Pharmacology Biochemistry and Behavior, 34,* 149-155.

Hunt, G. M., & Azrin, N. H. (1973). A community-reinforcement approach to alcoholism. *Behavior Research and Therapy, 14,* 339-348.

Hursh, S. R., & Winger, G. (1995). Normalized demand for drugs and other reinforcers. *Journal of the Experimental Analysis of Behavior, 64,* 373-384.

Inciardi, J. A. (1992). *The War on Drugs II.* Mountain View, CA: Mayfield.

Jaffe, J. H. (1990). Drug addiction and drug abuse. In A. G. Gilman, T. W. Rall, A. S. Nies, & P. Taylor (Eds.), *The pharmacological basis of therapeutics* (pp. 522-573). New York: Pergamon Press.

Jellinek, E. M. (1960). *The disease concept of alcoholism.* New Brunswick, NJ: Hillhouse.

Johanson, C. E. (1978). Drugs as reinforcers. In D. E. Blackman & D. J. Sanger (Eds.), *Contemporary research in behavioral pharmacology* (pp. 325-448). New York: Plenum Press.

Johanson, C. E., & Fischman, M. W. (1989). The pharmacology of cocaine related to its abuse. *Pharmacological Reviews, 41*, 3-52.

Johanson, C. E., Mattox, A., & Schuster, C. R. (1995). Conditioned reinforcing effects of capsules associated with high versus low monetary payoff. *Psychopharmacology, 120*, 42-48.

Julian, R. M. (1996). *A primer of drug action.* New York: W. H. Freeman.

Kelleher, R. T., & Goldberg, S. R. (1976). General introduction: Control of drug-taking behavior by schedules of reinforcement. *Pharmacological Reviews, 27*, 291-299.

Kirby, K. C., Marlowe, D. B., Lamb, R. J., & Platt, J. C. (1997). Behavioral treatments of cocaine addiction: Assessing patient needs and improving treatment entry and outcome. *Journal of Drug Issues, 27*, 417-429.

Kurtz, D. L., Stewart, R. B., Zweifel, M., Li, T.-K., & Froehlich, J. C. (1996). Genetic differences in tolerance and sensitization to the sedative/hypnotic effects of alcohol. *Pharmacology Biochemistry and Behavior, 53*, 585-591.

Lazarou, J., Pomeranz B. H. , & Corey, P. N. (1998). Incidence of adverse drug reactions in hospitalized patients: A meta-analysis of prospective studies. *Journal of the American Medical Association, 279*, 1200-1205.

Leaky, L. (1994). *The origins of humankind.* New York: Basic Books.

Lewis, D. C. (1994). More evidence that treatment works. *The Brown University Digest of Addiction Theory and Application, 13*, 12-43.

Lewitt, E. M. (1989). US tobacco taxes: Behavioral effects and policy implications. *British Journal of Addiction, 84*, 1217-1235.

Maltzman, I. (1994). Why alcoholism is a disease. *Journal of Psychoactive Drugs, 26*, 13-31.

McDowell, J. J. (1988). Matching theory in natural human environments. *The Behavior Analyst, 11*, 95-109.

McKenna, T. (1992). *Food of the gods: A radical history of plants, drugs, and human evolution.* New York: Bantam Books.

McKim, W. (1997). *Drugs and behavior.* Upper Saddle River, NJ: Prentice-Hall.

Musto, D. (1973). *The American disease: Origins of narcotic control.* New Haven, CT: Yale University Press.

National Institute on Alcohol Abuse and Alcoholism. (1990). *Alcohol and health: Neuroscience.* Rockville, MD: Author.

National Institute on Drug Abuse (July, 1998). *National household survey on drug abuse: Preliminary findings.* Rockville, MD: Author.

O'Brien, C. P. (1996). Drug addiction and drug abuse. In J. G. Hardman, L. E. Limbard, P. B. Molinoff, R. W. Ruddon, & A. G. Gilman (Eds.), *The pharmacological basis of therapeutics* (pp. 557-577). New York: McGraw-Hill.

O'Brien, C. P., Ehrman, R. N., & Ternes, J. W. (1986). Classical conditioning in human opioid dependence. In S. R. Goldberg & J. P. Stolerman (Eds.), *Behavioral analysis of drug dependence* (pp. 329-356). Orlando, FL: Academic Press.

Office of National Drug Control Policy. (1998). *FY 1999 drug budget program highlights* [on line]. Available:http://www.whitehousedrugscontrolpolicy.gov/policy/budge

Petrakis, P. L. (1985). *Alcoholism: An inherited disease.* Washington, DC: US Government Printing Office.

Peele, S. (1989). *Diseasing of America: Addiction treatment out of control.* Lexington, MA: Lexington Books.

Piazza, P. V., & Le Moal, M. (1998). The role of stress in drug self-administration. *Trends in Pharmacological Sciences, 19,* 67-74.

Poling, A., & LeSage, M. (1992). Rule-governed behavior and human behavioral pharmacology: A brief commentary on an important topic. *The Analysis of Verbal Behavior, 10,* 37-44.

Poling, A., Schlinger, H., Starin, S., & Blakely, E. (1990). *Psychology: A behavioral overview.* New York: Plenum Press.

Powell, D. H. (1973). A pilot study of occasional heroin users. *Archives of General Psychiatry, 28,* 586-594.

Ray, O. (1983). *Drugs, society, and human behavior.* St. Louis: Mosby.

Ray, O., & Ksir, C. (1993). *Drugs, society, and human behavior.* St. Louis, MO: Mosby-Year Book.

Reagan, R. (October, 14, 1982). Remarks announcing federal initiatives against drug trafficking and organized crime. *Public papers of the Presidents of the United States, Ronald Reagan, August 1 to December 31, 1982.*

Rivers, P. C. (1994). *Alcohol and human behavior: Theory, research, and practice.* Englewood Cliffs, NJ: Prentice Hall.

Robbins, L. N., Davis, D. H., & Goodwin, D. W. (1974). Drug use by U.S. Army enlisted men in Vietnam: A followup on their return home. *American Journal of Epidemiology, 99,* 235-249.

Roll, J. M., Higgins, S. T., Steingard, S., & McGinley, M. (1998). Use of monetary reinforcement to reduce the cigarette smoking of persons with schizophrenia: A feasibility study. *Experimental and Clinical Psychopharmacology, 6,* 157-161.

Rounsaville, B. J., Weissman, M. M., Kleber, H., & Wilber, C. (1982). Heterogeneity of psychiatric diagnosis in treated opiate addicts. *Archives of General Psychiatry, 39,* 161-166.

Schlinger, H, & Blakely, E. (1987). Function-altering effects of contingency-specifying stimuli. *The Behavior Analyst, 10,* 41-45.

Schuckit, M. A. (1992). Advances in understanding the vulnerability to alcoholism. In C. E. O'Brien & J. H. Jaffe (Eds.), *Addictive states* (pp. 93-108). New York: Raven Press.

Schuckit, M. A. (1994). Low level of response to alcohol as a predictor of future alcoholism. *American Journal of Psychiatry, 151,* 184-189.

Schultes, R. E., & Hofmann, A. (1992). *Plants of the gods: Their sacred, healing, and hallucinogenic powers.* Rochester, VT: Healing Arts Press.

Schuster, C. R. (1986). Implications of laboratory research for the treatment of drug dependence. In S. R. Goldberg & I. P. Stolerman (Eds.), *Behavioral analysis of drug dependence* (pp. 357-385). Orlando, FL: Academic Press.

Segal, B. (1988). *Drugs and behavior: Cause, effects, and treatment.* New York: Gardner Press.

Shaham, Y., & Stewart, J. (1995). Stress reinstates heroin-seeking in drug-free animals: An effect mimicking heroin, not withdrawal. *Psychopharmacology, 119,* 334-341.

Shaner, A., Roberts, L. J., Eckman, T. A., Tucker, D. E., Tsuang, J. W., Wilkins, J. N., & Mintz, J. (1997). Monetary reinforcement of abstinence from cocaine among mentally ill patients. *Psychiatric Services, 48,* 807-810.

Silverman, K., Wong, C. J., Higgins, S. T., Brooner, R. K., Montoya, I. D., Contereggi, C., Umbricht-Schneiter, A., Schuster, C. R., & Preston, K. L. (1996). Increasing opiate abstinence through voucher-based reinforcement therapy. *Drug and Alcohol Dependence, 41,* 157-165.

Sisson, R., & Azrin, N. H. (1989). The community reinforcement approach. In R. K. Hester & W. R. Miller (Eds.), *Handbook of alcoholism treatment approaches: Effective alternatives* (pp. 242-257). New York: Pergamon Press.

Smith, J., & Hucker, S. (1994). Schizophrenia and substance abuse. *British Journal of Psychiatry, 165,* 13-21.

Stitzer, M. L., & Bigelow, G. E. (1983). Contingent payment for carbon monoxide reduction: Effect of pay amount. *Behavior Therapy, 14,* 647-656.

Stitzer, M. L., Bigelow, G. E., & Liebson, I. (1979). Reducing benzodiazepine self-administration with contingent reinforcement. *Addictive Behaviors, 4,* 245-252.

Stitzer, M. L., Rand, C. S., Bigelow, G. E., & Mead, A. M. (1986). Contingent payment procedures for smoking reduction and cessation. *Journal of Applied Behavior Analysis, 19,* 197-202.

Strain, E. C., Mumford, G. K., Silverman, K., & Griffiths, R. R. (1994). Caffeine dependence syndrome. *Journal of the American Medical Association, 272,* 1043-1048.

Substance Abuse and Mental Health Services Administration. (August, 1998). *Preliminary estimates from the 1997 National Household Survey on Drug Abuse* [on line]. Available: http://www.samhsa.gov/oas/nhsda/nhsda97/

White, W. (1979). Themes in chemical prohibition. In W. P. Link, L. P. Miller, & B. Fisher (Eds.), *Drugs in perspective* (participant's manual) (pp. 171-181). Rockville, MD: National Institute on Drug Abuse.

Wikler, A. (1965). Conditioning factors in opiate addiction and relapse. In D. I. Wiher & G. G. Kassenbaum (Eds.), *Narcotics* (pp. 85-100). New York: McGraw-Hill.

Woody, G. E., Luborsky, L., McLellan, A. T., O'Brien, C. P., & Beck, A. T. (1983). Psychotherapy for opiate addicts. *Archives of General Psychiatry, 40,* 639-648.

Subject Index

Absorption, 44-45
Accumulation, 55
Action potential, 70-71
Acute drug administration, 55
Amotivational syndrome, 131-134
Animals as subjects, see *nonhumans as subjects*
Animal models, 19-20
Antecedent stimuli and drug effects, 169-172
Assays of drug effects, 96-108; 111-137; 191-215
Behavior analysis, 9-22, 25-41
Behavior analysis and clinical drug assessment, 195-206
Behavior analytic model of drug abuse, 226-238
Behavioral loci of drug action, 21
Behavioral mechanisms of drug action, 21, 211-214
Behavioral tolerance, 172-175
Behavioral toxicology, 20
Behavioral economics, 232-233
Biological models of mental illness, 80-81
Biotransformation, 45, 51-52
Blood-brain barrier, 50-51
Central nervous system, 67
Chronic drug administration, 55
Classical conditioning, see *respondent conditioning*
Classification of drugs, 43-46
Clinical drug assessment, 191-215
Collateral responses, 116
Community reinforcement approach to treatment, 238-239
Conditional discrimination, 34
Conditional response, 26
Conditional stimulus, 26, 141-146
Conditioned abstinence, 235
Conditioned reinforcement, 30, 128-130
Conditioned withdrawal, 143, 235
Consequence-dependent drug effects, 177-179; see also *Establishing operation*
Contingency management approach to treatment, 239
Cross tolerance, 52
Deactivation of neurotransmitters, 80
Delayed-matching-to-sample procedure, 99-100, 120-122
Depot binding, 50
Dimensions of behavior, 89-90
Discriminative stimulus, 32-34, 134-137